Obesity and Pregnancy

Obesity and Pregnancy

Edited by Marshalla Ortega

AMERICAN
MEDICAL PUBLISHERS
www.americanmedicalpublishers.com

American Medical Publishers,
41 Flatbush Avenue,
1st Floor, New York,
NY 11217, USA

Visit us on the World Wide Web at:
www.americanmedicalpublishers.com

ISBN: 978-1-63927-157-3

Cataloging-in-Publication Data

Obesity and pregnancy / edited by Marshalla Ortega.
p. cm.
Includes bibliographical references and index.
ISBN 978-1-63927-157-3
1. Obesity in women. 2. Pregnancy. 3. Pregnancy--Complications. I. Ortega, Marshalla.
RG580.O24 O24 2022
618.242--dc23

Table of Contents

Preface

Maternal obesity is associated with neonatal death, elective preterm delivery or delivery of a baby with an extremely low birth weight. Babies surviving such odds are often seen to have severe neurodevelopmental impairments. Maternal obesity has severe impacts on offspring development such as congenital anomalies, diabetes, etc. There are various ways to regulate obesity during pregnancy, such as by altering diet and exercising regularly. A healthy and well-balanced diet during pregnancy is necessary for a healthy pregnancy. Gastric bypass surgery is a common intervention to curb appetite and control body weight. The aim of this book is to present researches that have transformed our understanding of obesity and its impact on pregnancy. Some of the diverse topics covered herein address the varied management strategies of obesity during gestation. For all readers who are interested in obstetrics, the case studies included in this book will serve as an excellent guide to develop a comprehensive understanding.

This book unites the global concepts and researches in an organized manner for a comprehensive understanding of the subject. It is a ripe text for all researchers, students, scientists or anyone else who is interested in acquiring a better knowledge of this dynamic field.

I extend my sincere thanks to the contributors for such eloquent research chapters. Finally, I thank my family for being a source of support and help.

Editor

1

Knowledge translation tool to improve pregnant women's awareness of gestational weight gain goals and risks of gaining outside recommendations

Sarah D McDonald[1,2,3*], Christina K Park[3], Eleanor Pullenayegum[4], Keyna Bracken[5], Wendy Sword[3,6], Helen McDonald[7], Binod Neupane[3], Valerie H Taylor[8], Joseph Beyene[3], Valerie Mueller[1] and Melissa Brouwers[3,9]

Abstract

Background: There is an urgent need to prevent excessive pregnancy weight gain, a contributor to both maternal and child obesity. However, the majority of women had reported not being counseled to gain an appropriate amount of gestational weight by their health care providers. We developed a knowledge translation (KT) tool designed to facilitate the clinical interaction between pregnant women and their health care providers (HCPs). We piloted the tool on the impact on women's knowledge of gestational weight gain (GWG) goals, and evaluated its potential in promoting appropriate knowledge about GWG within the 2009 Institute of Medicine guidelines.

Methods: We conducted a prospective cohort study, comparing women's knowledge about GWG after the KT tool to women from the same clinics and care providers the year prior. Our primary outcome was the proportion of women who reported receiving an appropriate GWG recommendation from their care provider. We evaluated knowledge on a survey conducted at enrollment in the cohort at ≤ 20 weeks gestation and evaluated participant satisfaction with the KT tool in the third trimester. We performed univariate and multivariable logistic regression analyses for differences in outcomes with historical controls from the same clinics. Our *a priori* sample size calculation required 130 participants to demonstrate a 15% increase in reported counseling about gestational weight gain.

Results: One hundred and forty-six women were recruited and 131 (90%) completed the enrollment survey. Women who received the KT tool were more likely to report receiving a specific GWG recommendation from their HCP (adjusted odds ratio [AOR] 3.45, 95% confidence interval [CI] 2.22-5.37) and discussing GWG topics with their HCP (AOR 7.96, 95% CI 4.41-14.37), and believing that there were risks to their infants with inadequate GWG (AOR 2.48, 95% CI 1.14-5.37). Half of women (49.5%) indicated that they would recommend the tool to a friend.

Conclusions: Women who received the KT tool reported receiving more counseling on GWG from their HCPs and were more aware of the risks of gaining outside appropriate GWG recommendations. The association between GWG education and GWG requires further research.

Keywords: Knowledge translation, Intervention studies, Surveys, Gestational weight gain, Lifestyle factors, Counseling

* Correspondence: mcdonals@mcmaster.ca
[1]Department of Obstetrics & Gynecology, McMaster University, 1280 Main St. West, Hamilton, ON L8S 4L8, Canada
[2]Department of Radiology, McMaster University, 1280 Main St. West, Hamilton, ON L8S 4L8, Canada
Full list of author information is available at the end of the article

Background

High weight gain during pregnancy has serious implications, including increased risk of later obesity for both mothers [1] and their infants [2]. Other risks of high gestational weight gain (GWG) include being large for gestational age [3] and preterm birth [4] for infants, and postpartum weight retention [5] and cesarean delivery [6] for mothers, which were some of the outcomes considered in the development of the 2009 Institute of Medicine (IOM) gestational weight gain guidelines, along with childhood obesity and small for gestational age [7]. Approximately 10.9% (95% CI 10.7-11.1) of cesarean sections overall were attributable to above recommended GWG and this proportion was even more striking in multiparous women with no prior cesarean at 23.6% (95% CI 23.0-24.2%) [8].

Previous work has shown that up to 88% of women reported not being counseled to gain the appropriate amount of weight by their antenatal care providers [9]. Furthermore, 70% of women indicated that either a chart or a website showing how much weight should be gained each week and in total would be helpful [9]. Over three quarters of practitioners reported that a tool that would calculate GWG would be helpful [10].

Computer- and web-based platforms are effective at influencing patient and practitioner decision behavior [11-14]. For instance, a systematic review found that computerized clinical decision support systems improved practitioner performance, leading to improved diagnosis, preventive care, disease management, drug dosing, or drug prescribing [14]. A systematic review of interactive health communication applications reported a significant positive effect on patients' knowledge, social support, self-efficacy, and behavioral outcomes over time [13]. Another systematic review demonstrated that most patients welcomed a patient-held record [12]. As these aspects were relatively easy to implement and were sustainable, we developed a knowledge translation (KT) tool for GWG. Our tool was designed to present information in "clear, concise, and user friendly formats and ideally to provide explicit recommendations" to meet participants' knowledge needs and influence their behavior [15].

The primary objective of this study was to pilot a KT tool designed to improve women's knowledge of GWG, thereby assessing suitability for further study. We additionally sought to assess participants' evaluations of the tool.

Methods

Study design

We conducted a prospective cohort study, comparing women receiving the KT tool ("KT group") to historical controls ("control group") in a non-randomized comparison. Historical controls were used as data from the same clinics from only one year prior to the present study were available to determine if the KT tool improved outcomes in women in the same geographical setting. In addition, the use of historical controls reduced the additional burden on the participating clinics and avoided contamination of the KT group into the control group.

The intervention

A website ("Me and My Baby") was developed with advice from prenatal care providers, which required the input of a woman's prepregnancy height and weight. The KT tool then presented a graph showing the upper and lower limits for recommended weight gain specific for each woman's prepregnancy body mass index (BMI) according to the 2009 IOM guidelines [7] also adopted by Health Canada [16], the federal department responsible for helping Canadians maintain and improve their health, plotted on a graph against the number of weeks gestation. This graph was unique for each woman as the weekly and final optimal weight gain range was specific to her prepregnancy weight. For instance, for a woman who was 165 cm and 150 lbs, the points plotted would show two diverging lines, one from 150 lbs to 185 lbs (the upper GWG limit for a woman of her weight and BMI) and the other from 150 lbs to 175 lbs (the lower GWG limit). The tool also presented risks of excess and inadequate weight gain (care providers were encouraged to personalize them further based on the individual woman), and nutritional suggestions on how to achieve the recommended intake of 300 additional calories per day during pregnancy [17]. The website provided a print-out that could be could be folded to carry in a wallet for the participant's own reference, while one remained in the clinical chart throughout pregnancy. This print-out was designed to facilitate prenatal discussions regarding GWG between women and their health care providers. A sample of the KT tool is shown in Figure 1.

Practitioners were encouraged to use the KT tool print-out as a starting point for GWG discussion with participants, and to write in participant-specific risks with excess or inadequate GWG that would be particularly motivating. We assessed knowledge immediately after the visit in which the tool would have been introduced to the women.

Study population

Four local clinics in Hamilton, Ontario, a city of 520,000 [18], took part in this study: one obstetric clinic with a yearly roster of 300 pregnant patients, two midwifery practices with a combined 730 clients per year, and one family medicine practice with 50–75 pregnant patients per year. Eligibility criteria for women included being ≤ 20 weeks gestation with a live singleton pregnancy, and the ability to read English well enough to complete the surveys. Women were excluded from the study if they

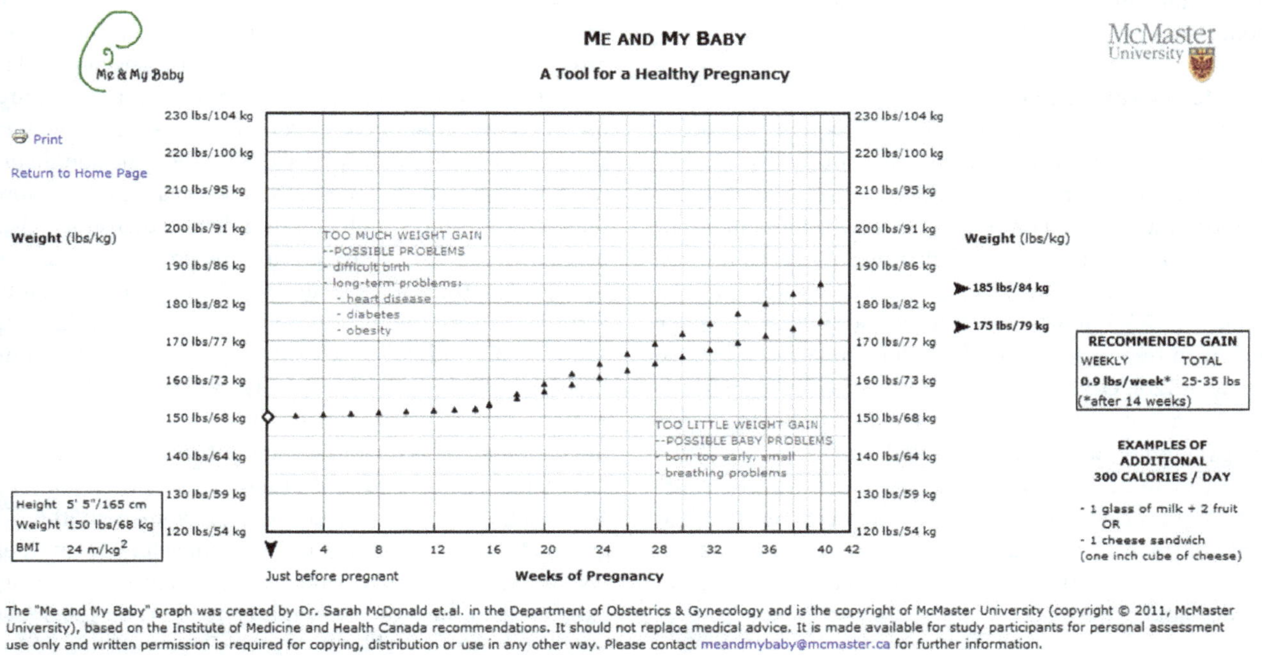

Figure 1 Sample of Me And My Baby knowledge translation tool. Legend: A sample Me and My Baby knowledge translation tool for a woman in the normal body mass index (BMI) range (18.5-24.9 m/kg^2).

experienced fetal demise during their pregnancy or were pregnant with twins, triplets, or higher order multiples.

Recruitment and study conduct

Approval from Hamilton Health Sciences/McMaster University Faculty of Health Sciences/St. Joseph's Hospital Research Ethics Boards was obtained before the study commenced (Project #11-285). The study was explained to eligible women by the clinic staff and all participants provided written informed consent prior to study inclusion. Participants reported their prepregnancy weight and height to clinic staff who inserted this information into the KT tool website and printed two copies of the participant's individualized tool, one for the women to bring to each appointment and one for their medical charts. Women did not log into the website themselves. Pregnant women typically had appointments with their health care providers according to the usual antenatal schedule: every month until 24 weeks gestation, every two weeks until 36 weeks gestation, and weekly thereafter until giving birth. Health care providers were instructed to plot women's weights on the print-out of the tool at each visit and to discuss their GWG progress.

Data collection

Self-administered surveys were conducted by participants either on paper or electronically at enrolment (≤20 weeks gestation) to evaluate knowledge outcomes and in the third trimester (approximately 36 weeks gestation) to evaluate the tool. Up to three reminders were sent for each survey, using a modified Dillman approach [19] to maximize response rates.

Outcomes

Our primary knowledge outcome was the proportion of women who reported receiving a GWG recommendation within guidelines from their health care provider, which was assessed at the enrolment survey at ≤ 20 weeks gestation. Other GWG knowledge aspects, such as plans for weight gain and beliefs about risks with inadequate or excess GWG, were also measured at the enrolment survey ≤ 20 weeks gestation. The survey was based on a previous questionnaire conducted in the same four clinics the year before this current study [9]. Women from the previous questionnaire served as the historical control group for our analysis. We assessed participants' evaluations of the tool, such as satisfaction with it, at approximately 36 weeks gestation.

Historical control group

Women in the historical control group was had at least one prenatal visit, could read English sufficiently well to complete the survey, and had a live singleton gestation to be eligible to participant. Similar to the present study, the women were invited to participate in the study by clinic staff and prenatal care providers. The objectives of the study that provided the controls were to determine the proportion of women who reported being counseled at all by their health care providers and the proportion of women who were counseled appropriately according to the guidelines. The study methods and findings were published elsewhere [9].

Sample size calculation

As our objective was to pilot the KT tool, we calculated a sample size of 130 participants as sufficient to demonstrate feasibility, based on a 15% increase in participants reporting a correct GWG recommendation from health care providers (above 12% of historical controls, n = 310) and allowing for 15% dropout as well as 15% missing data, with 85% power. KT interventions vary considerably with respect to reported absolute impact on physician behavior [20]. Grimshaw et al. [20] reported median behavior change ranging between 1% (passive educational workshops) and 21% (patient-directed interventions), thus an estimate of 15% for this intervention was appropriate as the health care providers who were involved have demonstrated above average willingness to improve knowledge and participate in shared decision-making with participants.

Statistical analysis

Demographic variables and knowledge outcomes were compared between the KT group and the control group, including age, parity, and prepregnancy BMI using student's *t*-test for continuous variables and chi-squared tests for categorical variables. Variables that were statistically significant in univariate logistic regression at $p \leq 0.10$ were included in the multivariable logistic regression model using the enter method. In the event of high correlation (correlation coefficient ≥ 0.70) between variables, the most biologically relevant variable was selected. We maintained a relaxed rule of at least five events per variable in the initial multivariable model for each outcome [21]. The multivariable model for each outcome was based on the complete case scenario, where data from subjects with missing outcome or exposure variables were discarded. Data were analyzed using SAS 9.2 (SAS Inc, Cary, NC).

Results

Women were recruited into the study from July to October 2011. The clinic staff kept an accurate tally of all eligible women and the number enrolled, declined and not approached for the first ten days of screening. Of the eligible women, 81% were enrolled, 17.4% declined and 1.6% were not approached. A total of 146 women were initially enrolled in the intervention study; 90% (n = 131) completed the enrolment survey and 72% (n = 105) of women completed the subsequent third trimester survey.

The women in the KT group were similar to those in the control group on most demographic factors (Table 1). The mean gestational age was 17.2 weeks (SD 5.5) at enrolment for the KT group and 30.9 weeks (SD 7.5) for the control group ($P < 0.001$). The mean gestational age in the present survey is much less than in the control group as it was part of our eligibility criteria for the KT group to be ≤20 completed weeks of gestation. The women in the control group did not have this requirement, as we attempted to sample consecutive women, and the visit frequency increases in later gestation, hence women were farther along in their pregnancies. Therefore, there was greater sampling of women further along their pregnancies in the control group. The groups also differed in education (secondary or less was 14.7% in the KT group and 23.5% in the control group; any post-secondary was 85.3% in KT and 76.5% in control; $p = 0.039$) and chronic health conditions (29.8% KT, 19.1% control; $p = 0.015$).

Univariate analysis on knowledge outcomes between knowledge tool and control groups

More than twice the proportion of women in the KT group reported receiving GWG counseling from their health care provider to gain a specific amount or range compared to the women in the control group (60.5% vs. 29.2%, $p < 0.001$) (Table 2). Eighty-six percent (85.7%) of women in the KT group compared to 47.2% in the control group reported that their health care provider discussed GWG-related topics, such as nutrition/healthy eating, appropriate weight gain, risks of gaining too much weight, and/or exercise ($p < 0.001$).

More women in the KT group than in the control group believed that there were risks to themselves with excess GWG (79.2% vs. 63.3%, $p = 0.014$), and risks to themselves (34.4% versus 21.3%, $p = 0.044$) and their infants (62.4% vs. 37.8%, $p = 0.001$) with inadequate GWG.

About one fourth (24.0%) of women reported being counseled to consume a specific amount or range of additional calories each day by their health care providers in the KT group, compared to 17.9% in the control group ($p = 0.139$).

The proportion of women who planned to gain below, within, and above the IOM guidelines in the KT group were 33.9%, 33.9%, and 32.3%, respectively, compared to the control group, 24.3%, 36.8%, and 39.0%, respectively ($p = 0.124$). The proportion of women who reported being recommended to gain within the IOM guidelines was 51.6% in the KT group and 48.4% in the control group ($p = 0.772$).

Univariate and multivariable logistic regression on knowledge outcomes

The knowledge outcomes that were considered for the univariate and multivariable logistic regression analyses were: 1) reported receiving health care provider counseling to gain a specific amount or range of gestational weight, 2) reported discussing GWG topics with the health care provider, 3) believed that there were risks to themselves with excess GWG, 4) believed that there were risks to

Table 1 Demographic characteristics of knowledge tool group and control group

Variables	Subcategories (If applicable)	Knowledge tool group (n = 131) N (%)*, unless otherwise indicated	Control group (n = 310) [9]† N (%)*, unless otherwise indicated	p-value
Maternal age	Mean (±SD), years	30.1 (5.5)	29.5 (5.7)	0.365
Gestational age at enrolment	Mean (±SD), years	17.2 (5.5)	30.9 (7.5)	<0.001‡
Ethnicity	Caucasian	96 (75.6)	229 (74.1)	0.747
Marital status	Married	95 (74.8)	203 (65.5)	0.156
	Common-law	17 (13.4)	53 (17.1)	
	Other	15 (11.8)	54 (17.4)	
Education	Secondary or less	19 (14.7)	72 (23.5)	0.039‡
	Any post-secondary	110 (85.3)	234 (76.5)	
Income	Low (< $20,000)	19 (15.7)	52 (19.8)	0.115
	Middle ($20,000 to $80,000)	40 (33.1)	106 (40.3)	
	High (> $80 000)	62 (51.2)	105 (39.9)	
Current smoker		14 (10.8)	32 (10.4)	0.897
Chronic health conditions§		39 (29.8)	56 (19.1)	0.015‡
Pregnancy history	First time giving birth	62 (47.7)	132 (44.7)	0.437
	One previous birth	50 (38.5)	107 (36.3)	
	Two or more previous births	18 (13.9)	56 (19.0)	
Prepregnancy BMI	Mean (±SD), kg/m^2	24.7 (5.7)	25.1 (6.7)	0.492
	Underweight (BMI <18.5 kg/m^2)	11 (8.5)	20 (6.8)	0.789
	Normal weight (BMI 18.5-24.9 kg/m^2)	67 (51.4)	164 (56.2)	
	Overweight (BMI 25.0-29.9 kg/m^2)	33 (25.4)	65 (22.3)	
	Obese (BMI >30 kg/m^2)	19 (14.6)	43 (14.7)	

Abbreviations: *BMI* Body Mass Index, *IQR* interquartile range, *N/A* not applicable, *n* sample size, *SD* standard deviation.
*Participants with missing values were discarded from percentage calculations. There may be discrepancies in percentage calculations in previously published data if missing values were not discarded.
†Reprinted from The American Journal of Obstetrics and Gynecology, Vol 205, Sarah D. McDonald, Eleanor Pullenayegum, Valerie H. Taylor, Olha Lutsiv, Keyna Bracken, Catherine Good, Eileen Hutton, Wendy Sword, Despite 2009 guidelines, few women report being counseled correctly about weight gain during pregnancy, Pages No. 333.e1-333.e6, Copyright (2011), with permission from Elsevier.
‡Statistically significant difference ($p < 0.05$).
§Included depression, anxiety, obsessive compulsive disorder, eating disorders, digestive disorders, high blood pressure, diabetes, hypoglycemia, thyroid disorders, asthma, Reynaud's phenomenon, arthritis, pituitary microadenoma, polycystic ovary syndrome, and eczema.

themselves with inadequate GWG, and 5) believed that there were risks to their infants with inadequate GWG (Tables 3, 4, 5, 6 and 7).

Biologically plausible variables selected for both univariate and multivariable analyses for each knowledge outcome included: study group (intervention vs. control group), maternal age (continuous variable, per year), ethnicity (Caucasian vs. non-Caucasian), education (any post-secondary education vs. secondary education or less), income (middle income as reference group), chronic health condition (yes vs. no), pregnancy history (first birth vs. one or more previous births) and prepregnancy BMI (normal weight as reference group).

In multivariable analyses for knowledge outcomes, women who reported receiving health care provider counseling to gain a specific amount or range were more likely to be in the KT group (adjusted odds ratio [AOR] 3.45, 95% confidence interval [CI] 2.22-5.37), to be giving birth for the first time (AOR 1.75, 95% CI 1.15-2.67), and to be overweight (AOR 1.80, 95% CI 1.08-3.01). Women who reported discussing GWG topics with their health care providers were more likely to be in the KT group (AOR 7.96, 95% CI 4.41-14.37) and to be giving birth for the first time (AOR 2.60, 95% CI 1.66-4.07), and were less likely to be Caucasian (AOR 0.52, 95% CI 0.31-0.89). However, women who believed that there were risks to themselves

Table 2 Univariate analysis of participant report of knowledge outcomes associated with knowledge tool group and control group

Variables	Subcategories (If applicable)	Knowledge tool group (n = 131) N (%)*, unless otherwise indicated	Control group (n = 310) [9]† N (%)*, unless otherwise indicated	p-value
Reported receiving GWG counseling from HCP	To gain a specific amount or range‡	78 (60.5)	90 (29.2)	<0.001§
	To gain within IOM guidelines	32 (51.6)	31 (48.4)	0.722
	Discussed GWG topics with HCP**	108 (85.7)	142 (47.2)	<0.001§
Believed that there were risks in gaining excess GWG	To themselves	95 (79.2)	50 (63.3)	0.014§
	To their infants	75 (63.6)	42 (56.0)	0.295
Believed that there were risks in gaining inadequate GWG	To themselves	42 (34.4)	17 (21.3)	0.044§
	To their infants	73 (62.4)	28 (37.8)	0.001§
Reported receiving counsel to consume an amount or range of additional calories each day by HCP		31 (24.0)	55 (17.9)	0.139
Amount or range of additional calories recommended each day for those counseled to do so by HCP	0-100 calories	0 (0.0)	2 (3.7)	0.007§
	100-300 calories	23 (76.7)	23 (42.6)	
	300-500 calories	5 (16.7)	6 (11.1)	
	>500 calories	0 (0.0)	2 (3.7)	
	Could not recall how many calories	2 (6.7)	21 (38.9)	
Reported receiving counsel to take vitamins by HCP		12 (98.4)	301 (97.7)	0.628
Reported discussing nutrition/healthy eating with HCP††		77 (61.1)	210 (69.1)	0.110
Reported discussing appropriate weight gain with HCP††		82 (65.1)	142 (47.2)	0.001§
Reported discussing risks of gaining too much weight with HCP††		38 (30.4)	79 (26.5)	0.415
Reported discussing exercise with HCP††	Discussed	70 (55.6)	162 (53.8)	0.743
Planned GWG	Below IOM guidelines	43 (33.9)	66 (24.3)	0.124
	Within IOM guidelines	43 (33.9)	100 (36.8)	
	Above IOM guidelines	41 (32.3)	106 (39.0)	
Difference between planned GWG and reported weight gain recommendation by HCP, kg‡‡	Mean of differences (SD)	0.5 (4.5)	0.9 (3.0)	0.536

Abbreviations: *BMI* Body Mass Index, *GWG* gestational weight gain, *HCP* health care provider, *IOM* Institute of Medicine, *IQR* interquartile range, *PDA* personal digital assistant, *SD* standard deviation.

*Participants with missing values were discarded from percentage calculations. There may be discrepancies in percentage calculations in previously published data if missing values were not discarded.

†Reprinted from The American Journal of Obstetrics and Gynecology, Vol 205, Sarah D. McDonald, Eleanor Pullenayegum, Valerie H. Taylor, Olha Lutsiv, Keyna Bracken, Catherine Good, Eileen Hutton, Wendy Sword, Despite 2009 guidelines, few women report being counseled correctly about weight gain during pregnancy, Pages No. 333.e1-333.e6, Copyright (2011), with permission from Elsevier.

‡The numerator was calculated by determining how many patients answered the question "Has your doctor, midwife, nurse practitioner or nurse made a recommendation about how much weight you should gain during pregnancy (total amount of weight)?" with either "Yes" or "I can't remember".

§Statistically significant difference ($p < 0.05$).

**The numerator value was calculated by counting the number of participants who responded that their health care provider discussed the following topics: nutrition/healthy eating, appropriate weight gain, risks of gaining too much weight, and exercise (the denominator is equivalent to the total number of participants who provided an answer to any of the topics mentioned).

††The responses to these questions are taken from the Enrolment Survey only. The questions were asked in the subsequent third trimester survey.

‡‡Calculated by woman's planned gestational weight gain subtracted by weight gain recommended by health care provider.

with excess GWG differed in education (AOR 13.47, 95% CI 4.03-44.97 for any post-secondary education) and income (AOR 3.63, 95% CI 1.38-9.52 for high income), but not by study group. Additionally, women who believed that there were risks to themselves with inadequate GWG only differed in BMI with normal weight women as the

Table 3 Univariate and multivariable analysis of variables associated with participant report of receiving health care provider counseling to gain a specific amount or range

Variable	Comparison groups	Crude odds ratio (95% CI)	P-value	Adjusted odds ratio (95% CI)	P-value
Study group	KT group vs. control group [9] (reference)	3.70 (2.38-5.56)	<0.001*	3.45 (2.22-5.37)	<0.001†
Maternal age	Age as a continuous variable (per year)	1.00 (0.96-1.03)	0.865	-	-
Ethnicity	Caucasian vs. non-Caucasian (reference)	1.16 (0.74-1.82)	0.526	-	-
Education	Any post-secondary education vs. secondary education or less (reference)	1.21 (0.74-1.97)	0.440	-	-
Income	Low vs. middle income (reference)	1.06 (0.59-1.92)	0.845	-	-
	High vs. middle income (reference)	1.24 (0.78-1.95)	0.364	-	-
Smoking	Current smoker vs. non-smoker (reference)	1.19 (0.63-2.22)	0.592	-	-
Chronic health condition	Has chronic health condition vs. does not have chronic health condition (reference)	1.00 (0.62-1.59)	0.988	-	-
Pregnancy history	First birth vs. one or more previous birth (reference)	1.73 (1.17-2.57)	O0.006*	1.75 (1.15-2.67)	0.010†
Prepregnancy BMI	Underweight vs. normal weight (reference)	1.42 (0.66-3.08)	0.369	1.42 (0.64-3.17)	0.392
	Overweight vs. normal weight (reference)	1.72 (1.06-2.78)	0.028*	1.80 (1.08-3.01)	0.024†
	Obese vs. normal weight (reference)	1.26 (0.71-2.24)	0.434	1.32 (0.71-2.46)	0.378

Abbreviations: *BMI* body mass index, *CI* confidence interval, *KT* knowledge translation.
*Variable was included in multivariable logistic regression model ($p \leq 0.10$).
†Variable was statistically significant in multivariable logistic regression model ($p < 0.05$).

reference group (AOR 0.44, 95% CI 0.19-0.98 for overweight; and AOR 0.05, 95% CI 0.01-0.36 for obese women). Women who believed that there were risks to their infants with inadequate GWG were more likely to: be in the KT group (AOR 2.48, 95% CI 1.14-5.37), have any post-secondary education (AOR 5.36, 95% CI 1.50-19.17), have a chronic health condition (AOR 3.39, 95% CI 1.32-8.69), and be normal weight than obese (AOR 0.09, 95% CI 0.03-0.31).

With regard to the missing data, of the outcomes considered for multivariable analysis, there were no significant differences in percent missing between the KT group and control group for "reported receiving health care provider counseling to gain a specific amount or

Table 4 Univariate and multivariable analysis of variables associated with participant report of discussing gestation weight gain topics with health care provider

Variable	Comparison groups	Crude odds ratio (95% CI)	P-value	Adjusted odds ratio (95% CI)	P-value
Study group	KT group vs. control group [9] (reference)	6.67 (3.85-11.11)	<0.001*	7.96 (4.41-14.37)	<0.001†
Maternal age	Age as a continuous variable (per year)	0.99 (0.95-1.02)	0.467	-	-
Ethnicity	Caucasian vs. non-Caucasian (reference)	0.67 (0.42-1.06)	0.091*	0.52 (0.31-0.89)	0.018†
Education	Any post-secondary education vs. secondary education or less (reference)	1.52 (0.95-2.43)	0.083*	1.43 (0.83-2.47)	0.196
Income	Low vs. middle income (reference)	0.81 (0.45-1.43)	0.462	-	-
	High vs. middle income (reference)	1.32 (0.83-2.08)	0.239	-	-
Smoking	Current smoker vs. non-smoker (reference)	0.74 (0.40-1.37)	0.344	-	-
Chronic health condition	Has chronic health condition vs. does not have chronic health condition (reference)	1.00 (0.63-1.61)	0.987	-	-
Pregnancy history	First birth vs. one or more previous birth (reference)	2.24 (1.49-3.35)	0.001*	2.60 (1.66-4.07)	<0.001†
Prepregnancy BMI	Underweight vs. normal weight (reference)	1.76 (0.77-4.02)	0.178	-	-
	Overweight vs. normal weight (reference)	1.40 (0.85-2.30)	0.182	-	-
	Obese vs. normal weight (reference)	0.86 (0.49-1.53)	0.616	-	-

Abbreviations: *BMI* body mass index, *CI* confidence interval, *KT* knowledge translation.
*Variable was included in multivariable logistic regression model ($p \leq 0.10$).
†Variable was statistically significant in multivariable logistic regression model ($p < 0.05$).

Table 5 Univariate and multivariable analysis of variables associated with the belief that there are risks to themselves in gaining excess gestational weight

Variable	Comparison groups	Crude odds ratio (95% CI)	P-value	Adjusted odds ratio (95% CI)	P-value
Study group	KT group vs. control group [9] (reference)	2.22 (1.16-4.17)	0.015*	1.53 (0.66-3.53)	0.323
Maternal age	Age as a continuous variable (per year)	1.09 (1.02-1.16)	0.008*	0.95 (0.87-1.04)	0.285
Ethnicity	Caucasian vs. non-Caucasian (reference)	1.15 (0.54-2.44)	0.718	-	-
Education	Any post-secondary education vs. secondary education or less (reference)	12.32 (5.19-29.25)	<0.001*	13.47 (4.03-44.97)	<0.001†
Income	Low vs. middle income (reference)	0.50 (0.20-1.26)	0.141	0.76 (0.25-2.30)	0.632
	High vs. middle income (reference)	4.25 (1.83-9.90)	0.001*	3.63 (1.38-9.52)	0.009†
Smoking	Current smoker vs. non-smoker (reference)	0.18 (0.07-0.47)	0.001*	0.95 (0.23-3.91)	0.947
Chronic health condition	Has chronic health condition vs. does not have chronic health condition (reference)	2.43 (1.01-1.16)	0.009*	2.34 (0.78-7.04)	0.132
Pregnancy history	First birth vs. one or more previous birth (reference)	1.65 (0.88-3.11)	0.122	-	-
Prepregnancy BMI	Underweight vs. normal weight (reference)	0.48 (0.17-1.39)	0.175	-	-
	Overweight vs. normal weight (reference)	0.92 (0.42-1.98)	0.825	-	-
	Obese vs. normal weight (reference)	0.58 (0.24-1.43)	0.238	-	-

Abbreviations: *BMI* body mass index, *CI* confidence interval, *KT* knowledge translation.
*Variable was included in multivariable logistic regression model ($p \leq 0.10$).
†Variable was statistically significant in multivariable logistic regression model ($p < 0.05$).

range" (1.5% KT and 0.7% control), reported discussing gestational weight gain topics with health care provider" (3.8% KT and 2.9% control), and "believed that there are risks to themselves in gaining excess gestational weight gain" (8.4% KT and 15.6% control). There were differences between the outcomes of "believed that there are risks to themselves in gaining inadequate gestational weight" (6.9% KT and 15.6% control) and "believed that there are risks to their infants in gaining gestational weight" (10.7% and 21.1%). The respondents in both groups were more likely to live in high-income than middle- or low-income households than those who did not respond for these outcomes (respectively: for "risks to themselves", 94.2% vs. 82.7%, $p = 0.01$; and for "risks to their infants", 90.8% vs. 77.3%, $p = 0.008$).

Table 6 Univariate and multivariable analysis of variables associated with the belief that there are risks to themselves in gaining inadequate gestational weight

Variable	Comparison groups	Crude odds ratio (95% CI)	P-value	Adjusted odds ratio (95% CI)	P-value
Study group	KT group vs. control group [9] (reference)	1.96 (1.01-3.70)	0.046*	1.99 (0.92-4.30)	0.080
Maternal age	Age as a continuous variable (per year)	1.00 (0.94-1.06)	0.991	-	-
Ethnicity	Caucasian vs. non-Caucasian (reference)	0.78 (0.38-1.64)	0.522	-	-
Education	Any post-secondary education vs. secondary education or less (reference)	2.11 (0.82-5.42)	0.121	-	-
Income	Low vs. middle income (reference)	1.07 (0.36-3.19)	0.910	1.06 (0.33-3.40)	0.916
	High vs. middle income (reference)	2.18 (1.01-4.70)	0.046*	2.18 (0.97-4.93)	0.061
Smoking	Current smoker vs. non-smoker (reference)	0.54 (0.17-1.68)	0.286	-	-
Chronic health condition	Has chronic health condition vs. does not have chronic health condition (reference)	1.06 (0.52-2.17)	0.874	-	-
Pregnancy history	First birth vs. one or more previous birth (reference)	1.46 (0.79-2.70)	0.229	-	-
Prepregnancy BMI	Underweight vs. normal weight (reference)	0.27 (0.07-0.99)	0.048*	0.34 (0.09-1.30)	0.115
	Overweight vs. normal weight (reference)	0.44 (0.21-0.90)	0.025*	0.44 (0.19-0.98)	0.044†
	Obese vs. normal weight (reference)	0.05 (0.01-0.37)	0.003*	0.05 (0.01-0.36)	0.003†

Abbreviations: *BMI* body mass index, *CI* confidence interval, *KT* knowledge translation.
*Variable was included in multivariable logistic regression model ($p \leq 0.10$).
†Variable was statistically significant in multivariable logistic regression model ($p < 0.05$).

Table 7 Univariate and multivariable analysis of variables associated with the belief that there are risks to their infants in gaining inadequate gestational weight

Variable	Comparison groups	Crude odds ratio (95% CI)	P-value	Adjusted odds ratio (95% CI)	P-value
Study group	KT group vs. control group [9] (reference)	2.70 (1.49-5.00)	0.001*	2.48 (1.14-5.37)	0.021†
Maternal age	Age as a continuous variable (per year)	0.98 (0.93-1.04)	0.565	-	-
Ethnicity	Caucasian vs. non-Caucasian (reference)	1.82 (0.89-3.70)	0.105	-	-
Education	Any post-secondary education vs. secondary education or less (reference)	4.43 (1.79-10.97)	0.001*	5.36 (1.50-19.17)	0.010†
Income	Low vs. middle income (reference)	0.53 (0.20-1.40)	0.199	0.56 (0.17-1.88)	0.350
	High vs. middle income (reference)	1.96 (1.00-3.85)	0.050*	1.52 (0.67-3.45)	0.315
Smoking	Current smoker vs. non-smoker (reference)	0.34 (0.11-1.00)	0.051*	0.87 (0.18-4.15)	0.866
Chronic health condition	Has chronic health condition vs. does not have chronic health condition (reference)	3.02 (1.44-6.32)	0.003*	3.39 (1.32-8.69)	0.011†
Pregnancy history	First birth vs. one or more previous birth (reference)	2.43 (1.36-4.36)	0.003*	2.10 (1.00-4.42)	0.051
Prepregnancy BMI group	Underweight vs. normal weight (reference)	0.50 (0.17-1.46)	0.206*	0.82 (0.21-3.14)	0.775
	Overweight vs. normal weight (reference)	0.45 (0.23-0.89)	0.022*	0.45 (0.20-1.05)	0.064
	Obese vs. normal weight (reference)	0.14 (0.05-0.37)	<0.001*	0.09 (0.03-0.31)	<0.001†

Abbreviations: *BMI* body mass index, *CI* confidence interval, *KT* knowledge translation.
*Variable was included in multivariable logistic regression model ($p \leq 0.10$).
†Variable was statistically significant in multivariable logistic regression model ($p < 0.05$).

Knowledge translation tool evaluation

Women's evaluation of the KT tool is shown in Table 8. About half of women reported "definitely yes" or "probably yes" to recommending the tool to a friend (49.5%). Most women felt the tool could be improved by one or more changes, including having a bigger graph (54.3%), more information on food servings (43.8%), or more information on exercise (30.5%), while 14.3% of women felt the tool should remain unchanged.

When asked if their health care provider showed them the tool at each visit, 24.2% of women reported "always", 13.1% "usually", 9.1% "about half the time", 18.2% "occasionally" and 35.4% "never".

Sixty percent (59.6%) of women reported that their health care providers marked their weights on the tool, and 40.4% of women reported that they marked their own weights. If using the tool in the future, most women (60.6%) preferred to have both their health care provider mark their weights in their chart and also mark their weight themselves on their own copy. The majority of women would prefer to mark their weights on their own paper copy (54.9%) or on an "app" for their hand-held electronic device (31.0%) if they were to use the tool in the future.

Most women (83.8%) reported being given their own copy of the tool, and checked their weight gain on the tool about once a week (4.8%), every two weeks (10.8%), once per month (20.5%), at or before every clinic visit (49.4%).

Discussion

Women in the KT group had better GWG knowledge outcomes compared to women in the control group, even after adjusting for potential confounders. More women in the KT group reported receiving health care provider counseling to gain a specific amount or range and discussing GWG topics with their health care providers, and correctly believed that there were risks to their infants with inadequate GWG. We demonstrated that a simple, sustainable, easily transferable tool improves pregnant women's knowledge of appropriate GWG. However, a substantial proportion of women still did not report receiving any recommendation from the care provider, did not have knowledge about risks with inappropriate GWG, and had not been shown the tool.

A previous study that also measured knowledge outcomes showed that knowledge-based interventions were effective. In a 2012 study, Wilkinson et al. [22] conducted a 60-minute presentation to the intervention group, which included a component of goal-setting and self-monitoring with respect to dietary and physical activity behaviors during pregnancy, and found that the percentage of women with GWG goals within guidelines was significantly greater in the intervention group (8% difference, $p = 0.009$). A systematic review by Brown et al. in 2012 of five randomized trials used goal-setting for GWG alongside modification to diet and/or physical activity [23]. The authors concluded that planning weight gain in conjunction with changes in eating or exercise habits may be effective in lowering excess GWG. Interventions with planned weight gain goals, such as with our study, may be more effective than lifestyle changes alone.

Forty-four percent of women reported that the KT tool could be improved by having more information on

Table 8 Participant's evaluation of knowledge translation tool

Variables	Subcategories (if applicable)	N (%)*, unless otherwise indicated
Would recommend the KT tool to a friend	Definitely not	0 (0.0)
	Probably not	25 (25.3)
	Don't know	25 (25.3)
	Probably yes	42 (42.4)
	Definitely yes	7 (7.1)
Suggested improvements to KT tool	Bigger graph	57 (54.3)
	More information on food servings	46 (43.8)
	More information on exercise	32 (30.5)
	Other	15 (14.3)
	Should remain unchanged	15 (14.3)
HCP showed KT tool	Never	35 (35.4)
	Occasionally	18 (18.2)
	About half the time	9 (9.1)
	Usually	13 (13.1)
	Always	24 (24.2)
Marker of KT tool	Participant (pregnant woman)	40 (40.4)
	Nurse/Nurse Practitioner	15 (15.2)
	Doctor	11 (11.1)
	Midwife	23 (23.2)
	Other	10 (10.1)
Preference if using knowledge KT in the future	Only mark weight on the tool themselves	11 (11.1)
	Only have HCP mark weight on the tool	28 (28.3)
	Have HCP mark their weight on the tool in their chart, and mark their weight on their own copy of the tool themselves	60 (60.6)
Preference in marking weight	On their own paper copy of tool	39 (54.9)
	On an "app" (application) for their hand-held electronic device	22 (31.0)
	Online on a website on a computer	9 (12.7)
	Other	1 (1.4)
Were given a copy of KT tool	No	16 (16.2)
	Yes	83 (83.8)
Checked their weight gain on KT tool	About once a week	4 (4.8)
	About every two weeks	9 (10.8)
	About once per month	17 (20.5)
	Before (or at) every clinic visit	41 (49.4)
	Other	12 (14.5)

Abbreviations: *HCP* health care provider, *KT* knowledge translation, *n* sample size.
*Participants with missing values were discarded from percentage calculations.

food servings. Tanentsapf and colleagues also suggested in a systematic review that interventions that included face-to-face nutritional counseling and recommendations on caloric intake may be more successful at reducing total gestational weight gain than those that do not include these components, and education on appropriate weight gain in early pregnancy may increase the rate of compliancy [24].

More women in the KT group correctly believed that there were risks to themselves with excess GWG, and risks to themselves and their infants with inadequate GWG in the univariate analysis. In contrast, there was no difference between the KT group and control group in the belief that there were risks to their infants with excess GWG, possibly due to the KT tool not specifying risks factors for infants related to excess weight gain.

However, more women in the KT group believed that there were risks to themselves with inadequate GWG despite the tool not stating such risks (Figure 1). Most of the literature suggests there is no increased risk for women who gain below the guidelines, although a study suggests that there may be increased risk of maternal fever, active-phase arrest and the need for episiotomy [25].

Despite the use of the KT tool, only half of women reported that their health care provider counselled them to gain within the IOM guidelines. It is possible that participants are not correctly recalling the amount of weight recommended by their provider [26]. In addition, women may weigh the advice of family or friends, or influences of their culture more heavily, which could be discordant to health care provider recommendations [27,28]. This could explain why 52% of women reported receiving health care provider counselling to gain within the guidelines, but 34% actually planned to gain within. Another explanation is the sensitivity of the topic of GWG. Health care providers may be concerned that women may be offended, angered, saddened or embarrassed when discussing GWG [27], however in previous work, we noted that 84% of women reported being 'comfortable' or 'very comfortable' discussing weight related issues with their care provider [9]. They may also be uncertain of the effectiveness of their counselling [27,28]. These factors coupled with time constraints of the prenatal appointment [10] may cause limited counselling on gaining within the guidelines. To note, over one third of the participants reported that their health care provider "never" showed them the KT tool. A way to address some of these challenges could potentially lie in focusing on the baby's health during counselling. Pregnant women may be more determined to make positive lifestyle changes over the concern of their baby [29]. Change could be easier the greater the perceived risk of the infant [29]. Better awareness the infant risks of excess GWG could make the weight gain recommendations more memorable and impactful to the women, and could address issues of sensitivity, as the focus is away from the women's weight but rather optimizing outcomes for the infant.

We have some limited data from the survey of health care providers, in which 34.8% responded that they or their office staff would refer to the KT graph at about half of the patient's visits, and 30.4% responded 'almost never'. About one quarter of care providers responded that they almost never referred to the graph because it took too much time, while a similar proportion stated because the patient was not interested, and the remainder stated it was due to other issues such as the graph being too small, they had referred the patient to a dietician.

The majority (64.6%) of women reported that their health care provider had shown them the KT tool, which presented the range of the recommended GWG and gave the health care provider an opportunity to discuss it. Another study in a similarly predominantly white, middle-class population showed that women who did not receive advice on weight gain were more likely to gain less (AOR 1.8, 95% CI 1.3-2.5) or more (AOR 2.0, 95% CI 1.5-2.7) than recommended, compared to women who were advised according to the recommendations [30]. Women who gained gestational weight above the IOM guidelines had greater than three times the odds of having received a recommendation to gain above [30] and women who gained weight below the guidelines had greater than three times the odds of having received recommendations to gain below [30]. Brawarsky et al. observed that 71% of women who received recommendations above guidelines gained weight above the guidelines [31]. Herring et al. reported that in a sample composed of women of low-socioeconomic status, those who gained weight above guidelines had almost six times the odds of having received a recommendation that was either above or below instead of within guidelines [32].

Strengths of our study include the longitudinal nature of the study, as we followed the same women throughout their pregnancies to use their evaluation of the KT tool at the end of pregnancy. Although we used historical controls from the year before, they were from the same prenatal clinics and had the same health care providers. Physicians and midwives involved in the development of the tool were knowledge users, and therefore had an understanding of how to utilize the tool in their prenatal care appointments.

Limitations of our study include the relatively small sample size, although it was powered for our primary outcome. The use of historical controls also presented differences between the KT and the control groups, including gestational age, education level, and chronic health conditions. The gestational age at recruitment of the intervention group was earlier than the control group due to the eligibility criteria, and thus could lead to recall bias and bias the results in favor of the intervention group. However it might have also led to bias in the opposite direction, given that women in the control group had had many more opportunities to have discussion about GWG with their care providers. Knowledge was assessed in the KT tool group at a mean of 17 weeks just after recruitment, and in the control group at a mean of 31 weeks. The women in the KT tool group would have typically had 2 regularly scheduled visits before being recruited, approximately four weeks apart (e.g. 12 and 16 weeks). At 32 weeks, the standard visit schedule includes 8 visits.

It is possible that the publication of the results of the historical control survey may have resulted in clinical practice change, so that the difference in knowledge that we found may have been due to factors other than the intervention. However, given that the publication of clinical practice guidelines has been proven to be relatively ineffective at changing practice [33], it is not clear that the publication of a single paper would have done so.

Another potential limitation is that prepregnancy weight was self-reported. However, this is what is done in clinical settings, in which the patients provide their prepregnancy weight. Also, this occurred in *both* the intervention and the control groups. Hence whatever bias might occur had the potential to do so equally in both groups.

We had some missing data, which was addressed through complete case analysis, but there were differences in income in those who responded compared to those who did not respond. Our study population was limited to English-speaking women with singletons and the results are generalizable only to this group. In addition, the majority of women were well-educated and of higher socioeconomic status.

Conclusion

Pregnant women who received a simple knowledge translation tool reported higher rates of counseling on GWG and were more aware of the risks of gaining outside the appropriate range. This pilot study demonstrated that knowledge interventions for GWG may be effective. Further research is needed on the association between GWG education and GWG.

Abbreviations

AOR: Adjusted odds ratio; BMI: Body mass index; CI: Confidence interval; GWG: Gestational weight gain; HCP: Health care provider; IOM: Institute of medicine; SD: Standard deviation.

Competing interests

The authors declare that they have no competing interests.

Authors' contributions

SM conceived and coordinated the study. SM, EP, MB, KB, WS and HM participated in its design. BN and JB performed statistical analysis and contributed to the interpretation of the data. CP, EP, KB, WS, VT, VM and MB participated in interpretation. CP drafted the first version of the manuscript. All authors were involved in revising the manuscript it critically for important intellectual content, have given final approval of the version to be published, and agree to be accountable for all aspects of the work in ensuring that questions related to the accuracy or integrity of any part of the work are appropriately investigated and resolved.

Acknowledgements

We are grateful to the Canadian Institutes of Health Research (CIHR) Grant #115437 and the Hamilton Academic Health Sciences Organization Academic Funding Plan (HAHSO AFP) Innovation Fund Grant for funding this research.

Dr. McDonald's and Dr. Pullenaygum's salaries were supported by Canadian Institutes of Health Research (CIHR) New Investigator Salary Awards, Ottawa, Canada. Dr. Beyene holds the John D. Cameron Chair in the Genetic Determinants of Chronic Disease at McMaster University. None of the funding sources had any role in the idea, design, analyses, interpretation of data, writing of the manuscript or decision to submit the manuscript.

Author details

[1]Department of Obstetrics & Gynecology, McMaster University, 1280 Main St. West, Hamilton, ON L8S 4L8, Canada. Department of Radiology, McMaster University, 1280 Main St. West, Hamilton, ON L8S 4L8, Canada. [3]Department of Clinical Epidemiology & Biostatistics, McMaster University, 1280 Main St. West, Hamilton, ON L8S 4L8, Canada. [4]Child Health Evaluative Sciences Program, Hospital for Sick Children, 555 University Avenue, Toronto, ON M5G 1X8, Canada. [5]Department of Family Medicine, McMaster University, 1280 Main St. West, Hamilton, ON L8S 4L8, Canada. [6]School of Nursing, McMaster University, Hamilton, ON L8S 4L8, Canada. [7]Midwifery Education Program, McMaster University, 1280 Main St. West, Hamilton, ON L8S 4L8, Canada. [8]Department of Psychiatry, Women's College Hospital, 76 Grenville St, Toronto, ON M5S 1B1, Canada. [9]Department of Oncology, McMaster University, 1280 Main St. West, Hamilton, ON L8S 4L8, Canada.

References

1. Fraser A, Tilling K, Macdonald-Wallis C, Hughes R, Sattar N, Nelson SM, et al. Associations of gestational weight gain with maternal body mass index, waist circumference, and blood pressure measured 16 y after pregnancy: the Avon Longitudinal Study of Parents and Children (ALSPAC). Am J Clin Nutr. 2011;93:1285–92.
2. Fraser A, Tilling K, Macdonald-Wallis C, Sattar N, Brion MJ, Benfield L, et al. Association of maternal weight gain in pregnancy with offspring obesity and metabolic and vascular traits in childhood. Circulation. 2010;121:2557–64.
3. Ferraro ZM, Barrowman N, Prud'homme D, Walker M, Wen SW, Rodger M, et al. Excessive gestational weight gain predicts large for gestational age neonates independent of maternal body mass index. J Matern Fetal Neonatal Med. 2012;25:538–42.
4. McDonald SD, Han Z, Mulla S, Lutsiv O, Lee T, Beyene J, et al. High gestational weight gain and the risk of preterm birth and low birth weight: a systematic review and meta-analyses. J Obstet Gynaecol Can. 2011;33:1223–33.
5. Nohr EA, Vaeth M, Baker JL, Sorensen TI, Olsen J, Rasmussen KM. Combined associations of prepregnancy body mass index and gestational weight gain with the outcome of pregnancy. Am J Clin Nutr. 2008;87:1750–9.
6. Stotland NE, Hopkins LM, Caughey AB. Gestational weight gain, macrosomia, and risk of cesarean birth in nondiabetic nulliparas. Obstet Gynecol. 2004;104:671–7.
7. Institute of Medicine. Weight gain during pregnancy: reexamining the guidelines. Washington, DC: The National Academies Press; 2009.
8. Dzakpasu S, Fahey J, Kirby RS, Tough SC, Chalmers B, Heaman MI, et al. Contribution of prepregnancy body mass index and gestational weight gain to caesarean birth in Canada. BMC Pregnancy Childbirth. 2014;14:106.
9. McDonald SD, Pullenayegum E, Taylor V, Lutsiv O, Bracken K, Good C, et al. Despite 2009 guidelines few women report being counseled correctly about weight gain during pregnancy. Am J Obstet Gynecol. 2011;205:e1-6 (Editor's Choice).
10. Lutsiv O, Bracken K, Pullenayegum E, Sword W, Taylor VH, McDonald SD. Little congruence between health care provider and patient perceptions of counselling on gestational weight gain. J Obstet Gynaecol Can. 2012;36:518–24.
11. Raynor DK, Blenkinsopp A, Knapp P, Grime J, Nicolson DJ, Pollock K, et al. A systematic review of quantitative and qualitative research on the role and effectiveness of written information available to patients about individual medicines. Health Technol Assess. 2007;11:1–181.
12. Gysels M, Richardson A, Higginson IJ. Does the patient-held record improve continuity and related outcomes in cancer care: a systematic review. Health Expect. 2007;10:75–91.
13. Murray EBJTS, Lai R, Nazareth I. Interactive Health Communication Appliations for people with chronic disease. Cochrane Database Syst Rev. 2005;4, CD004274.
14. Garg AX, Adhikari NK, McDonald H, Rosas-Arellano MP, Devereaux PJ, Beyene J, et al. Effects of computerized clinical decision support systems on practitioner performance and patient outcomes: a systematic review. JAMA. 2005;293:1223–38.
15. Graham ID, Logan J, Harrison MB, Straus SE, Tetroe J, Caswell W, et al. Lost in knowledge translation: time for a map? J Contin Educ Health Prof. 2006;26:13–24.
16. Health Canada. Prenatal nutrition guidelines for health professionals: gestational weight gain [http://www.hc-sc.gc.ca/fn-an/nutrition/prenatal/ewba-mbsa-eng.php]

17. The American College of Obstetricians and Gynecologists. Nutrition During Pregnancy [http://www.acog.org/~/media/For%20Patients/faq001.pdf?dmc=1&ts=20130702T1112568013]
18. Statistics Canada. Census Profile [http://www12.statcan.gc.ca/census-recensement/2011/dp-pd/prof/index.cfm?Lang=E]
19. Dillman DA, Smyth JD, Christian LM. Implementation procedures. In: Internet, mail, and mixed-mode surveys. The tailored design method. 3rd ed. Hoboken, New Jersey, USA: John Wiley & Sons; 2009. p. 234–99.
20. Grimshaw JM, Thomas RE, MacLennan G, Fraser C, Ramsay CR, Vale L, et al. Effectiveness and efficiency of guideline dissemination and implementation strategies. Health Technol Assess. 2004;8:iii-72.
21. Vittinghoff E, McCulloch CE. Relaxing the rule of ten events per variable in logistic and Cox regression. Am J Epidemiol. 2007;165:710–8.
22. Wilkinson SA, McIntyre HD. Evaluation of the'healthy start to pregnancy' early antenatal health promotion workshop: a randomized controlled trial. BMC Pregnancy Childbirth. 2012;12:131.
23. Brown MJ, Sinclair M, Liddle D, Hill AJ, Madden E, Stockdale J. A systematic review investigating healthy lifestyle interventions incorporating goal setting strategies for preventing excess gestational weight gain. PLoS One. 2012;7, e39503.
24. Tanentsapf I, Heitmann BL, Adegboye AR. Systematic review of clinical trials on dietary interventions to prevent excessive weight gain during pregnancy among normal weight, overweight and obese women. BMC Pregnancy Childbirth. 2011;11:81.
25. Ehrenberg HM, Dierker L, Milluzzi C, ercer BM. Low maternal weight, failure to thrive in pregnancy, and adverse pregnancy outcomes. Am J Obstet Gynecol. 2003;189:1726–30.
26. Kessels RP. Patients' memory for medical information. J R Soc Med. 2003;96:219–22.
27. Stotland NE, Gilbert P, Bogetz A, Harper CC, Abrams B, Gerbert B. Preventing excessive weight gain in pregnancy: how do prenatal care providers approach counseling? J Womens Health (Larchmt). 2010;19:807–14.
28. Chang T, Llanes M, Gold KJ, Fetters MD. Perspectives about and approaches to weight gain in pregnancy: a qualitative study of physicians and nurse midwives. BMC Pregnancy Childbirth. 2013;13:47.
29. Edvardsson K, Ivarsson A, Eurenius E, Garvare R, Nystrom ME, Small R, et al. Giving offspring a healthy start: parents' experiences of health promotion and lifestyle change during pregnancy and early parenthood. BMC Public Health. 2011;11:936.
30. Cogswell ME, Scanlon KS, Fein SB, Schieve LA. Medically advised, mother's personal target, and actual weight gain during pregnancy. Obstet Gynecol. 1999;94:616–22.
31. Brawarsky P, Stotland NE, Jackson RA, Fuentes-Afflick E, Escobar GJ, Rubashkin N, et al. Pre-pregnancy and pregnancy-related factors and the risk of excessive or inadequate gestational weight gain. Int J Gynaecol Obstet. 2005;91:125–31.
32. Herring SJ, Nelson DB, Davey A, Klotz AA, Dibble LV, Oken E, et al. Determinants of excessive gestational weight gain in urban, low-income women. Womens Health Issues. 2012;22:e439–46.
33. Grimshaw J, Freemantle N, Wallace S, Russell I, Hurwitz B, Watt I, et al. Developing and implementing clinical practice guidelines. Qual Health Care. 1995;4:55–64.

2

Weighing as a stand-alone intervention does not reduce excessive gestational weight gain compared to routine antenatal care

Shanna M. Fealy[1,2,3*], Rachael M. Taylor[2,4,5], Maralyn Foureur[1,6], John Attia[5,7,8], Lyn Ebert[2], Alessandra Bisquera[5,7] and Alexis J. Hure[2,5]

Abstract

Background: Excessive gestational weight gain is associated with short and long-term adverse maternal and infant health outcomes, independent of pre-pregnancy body mass index. Weighing pregnant women as a stand-alone intervention during antenatal visits is suggested to reduce pregnancy weight gain. In the absence of effective interventions to reduce excessive gestational gain within the real world setting, this study aims to test if routine weighing as a stand-alone intervention can reduce total pregnancy weight gain and, in particular, excessive gestational weight gain.

Methods: A systematic review and meta–analysis of randomised controlled trials (RCTs) was conducted between November 2014 and January 2016, and reported using the Preferred Reporting Items for Systematic Reviews and Meta-Analyses. Seven databases were searched. A priori eligibility criteria were applied to published literature by at least two independent reviewers. Studies considered methodologically rigorous, as per the Academy of Nutrition and Dietetics Quality Criteria Checklist for Primary Research, were included. Meta-analysis was conducted using fixed-effects models.

Results: A total of 5223 (non-duplicated) records were screened, resulting in two RCTs that were pooled for meta-analysis ($n = 1068$ randomised participants; $n = 538$ intervention, $n = 534$ control). No difference in total weight gain per week was observed between intervention and control groups (weighted mean difference (WMD) -0.00 kg/week, 95% confidence interval (CI) -0.03 to 0.02). There was also no reduction in excessive gestational weight gain between intervention and control, according to pre-pregnancy body mass index (BMI). However, total weight gain was lower in underweight women ($n = 23$, BMI <18.5 kg/m^2) in the intervention compared to control group (−0.12 kg/week, 95% CI −0.23 to −0.01). No significant differences were observed for other pregnancy, birth and infant outcomes.

Conclusion: Weighing as a stand-alone intervention is not worse nor better at reducing excessive gestational weight gain than routine antenatal care.

Keywords: Antenatal care, Gestation, Pregnancy, Weighing, Weight gain

* Correspondence: shanna.fealy@newcastle.edu.au
[1]School of Nursing & Midwifery University of Newcastle, Port Macquarie Campus, PO Box 210, Port Macquarie 2444, NSW, Australia
[2]Faculty of Health & Medicine School of Medicine & Public Health, University of Newcastle, Callaghan, NSW, Australia
Full list of author information is available at the end of the article

Background

Obesity has dramatic effects on reproductive health with complications during pregnancy and at birth all the more prevalent in those carrying excess weight [1]. Globally obesity is more prevalent than undernutrition [2]. The World Health Organisation (WHO) estimates that over 1.9 billion adults (≥18 years) are overweight and 600 million obese [3]. In Australia, 63% of adult women (≥18 years) are reported to have a body mass index (BMI) in the overweight (25.0–29.9 kg/m^2) or obese (≥30.0 kg/m^2) categories [4]. For women who gave birth in Australia, the most recent Mothers and Babies report (2013) shows that one-fifth (19%) of pregnant woman were classified as obese at the beginning of pregnancy with one quarter (24%) overweight [5].

The risks of entering pregnancy obese are well documented [1, 6]. Excessive gestational weight gain (EGWG) as defined by the American Academy of Sciences Institute of Medicine (IOM) is also an independent predictor of adverse pregnancy and birth outcomes [6, 7]. The IOM weight gain guidelines devised in 1990 and revised in 2009 are the most widely cited guidelines for gestational weight gain [8, 9]. In the absence of Australian-based gestational weight gain guidelines, the IOM guidelines have been largely adopted as the standard reference [10, 11]. These guidelines recommend that women who are underweight at the beginning of pregnancy gain more weight than women who are overweight or obese [9].

Weight gain in excess of the IOM guidelines has been associated with both short and long term health risks, including pre-eclampsia, gestational diabetes, caesarean section, large for gestational age infants, postpartum weight retention and childhood obesity [12–14]. Evidence suggests that it is more common for women to gain weight above the IOM guidelines than within or below. In a large retrospective cohort study in the United States ($n = 20{,}456$), Stotland et al. [14] observed that more women gained above the IOM guidelines (43%) compared to those that gained within (37%) or below (20%). An Australian prospective cohort study of pregnancy weight gain ($n = 664$) similarly found 38% of women gained in excess of the IOM weight gain ranges [15]. Fifty-six percent of women who were overweight and obese (BMI ≥25 kg/m^2) had EGWG compared to 30% of women with a BMI <25 kg/m^2 [15]. Furthermore, in the majority of studies included in a recent systematic review, 47–72% of obese women had EGWG according to the IOM ranges [16].

Addressing EGWG has become a public health priority. Intervention studies have primarily focused on diet and physical activity either alone or in combination [17]. The most recent Cochrane review identified 65 randomised controlled trials (RCTs) of diet and/or exercise interventions. In an analysis of 24 included trials ($n = 7096$) diet, exercise or both in combination reduced EGWG on average by 20% (average risk ratio (RR) 0.80, 95% confidence intervals (CI) 0.73 to 0.87). However no differences were observed for the adverse outcomes of pre-eclampsia, infant macrosomia (birth weight >90th centile) or caesarean birth [17].

In the real world setting there are substantial barriers to upscaling diet and exercise interventions at the population level. These include limited access to specialist staff, time constraints, financial implications and motivation to engage in such interventions as part of clinical practice [18].

One gestational weight gain intervention that is feasible at a population level (i.e. low cost and easy to administer) is weighing during routine antenatal care. The schedule of antenatal care appointments consisting of 7–12 regular visits for low risk women with maternal health care providers, presents an opportunity for health promotion interventions to be trialled. The visits additionally provide a window of opportunity for potential behaviour change and lifestyle modification [19, 20]. A recent pilot study evaluating the feasibility of regular weighing in the context of routine antenatal care reported that weighing took on average 1–2 min of a midwife's time, was simple to do, and did not significantly add to midwives existing workloads [21]. A qualitative analysis of pregnant women's experience of routine weighing reported that weighing during antenatal appointments was an acceptable intervention that when introduced did not cause distress or anxiety [22].

The stand-alone practice of weighing in the field of weight management has been successful in aiding non-pregnant adults achieve weight loss, weight maintenance and prevent weight gain as a self-monitoring/self-regulation strategy [23–25]. However, this has not been demonstrated in pregnancy. Weighing was originally introduced during the 1940's as a vital sign of pregnancy, considered useful for the detection of low birth weight infants and pre-eclampsia [26]. Weighing declined in practice during the 1990's and ceased to be recommended as a sign for adverse pregnancy outcomes by the British National Institute of Health and Care Excellence (NICE) in 2003, due to a deficit in evidence that it was an effective screening tool [26–29].

The practice of weighing is limited to the first antenatal visit in Australia and the United Kingdom for the purposes of calculating an early pregnancy BMI [11, 30]. The risks and prevalence of women entering pregnancy obese and exceeding the IOM gestational weight gain guidelines have caused health care providers necessary concern and led to develop the development of antenatal care pathways, recommending a return to weighing during all antenatal care visits [6, 31].

Therefore, this systematic review aimed to summarise the body of high quality evidence and determine any effect of routine antenatal weighing as a stand-alone intervention to reduce pregnancy weight gain and, in particular, prevent EGWG.

Methods

This review follows the Preferred Reporting Items for Systematic Reviews and Meta-Analysis (PRISMA) [32].

Search strategy

An a priori review protocol and eligibility criteria were devised, with consideration given to the research question, study design, population, intervention and outcomes (see Additional file 1). An electronic search of seven databases was conducted, including Medline, Embase, Maternal and Infant Care (via Ovid; http://www.ovid.com/), Cumulative Index to Nursing and Allied Health Literature (CINAHL) (via EBSCO http://www.ebsco.com/cinahl), Scopus (via http://www.scopus.com), Web of science (http://apps.webofknowledge.com) and the Cochrane library (via http://www.cochranelibrary.com).

The initial search was conducted in November 2014 with the assistance of a research librarian (DB) using the following keywords and Boolean operators: "pregnant" OR "pregnancy" AND "weight gain" OR "weighing" AND "randomised controlled trial" OR "clinical trial" OR "random*" (see Additional file 2). All searches were limited to English language and to human studies. No date limits were applied. The Cochrane Library was searched separately to identify any previously conducted systematic reviews in the area. The search was updated in January 2016 to ensure recent evidence was captured (see Additional file 3). The database search results were exported into reference management software.

Study selection

In the first round, publication titles and abstracts were screened independently by at least two reviewers (SMF, RMT, AJH) according to inclusion and exclusion criteria outlined in Table 1. Articles not meeting the eligibility criteria were screened out in the order of (i) study design, (ii) population, (iii) intervention, and (iv) outcome. Articles that met the eligibility criteria were retrieved as full texts and further reviewed by SMF and RMT. Any disagreements in the selection of studies were discussed with consensus achieved. The reference lists of retrieved studies and relevant Cochrane systematic reviews were hand searched for any relevant article not detected by the primary electronic search strategy.

Quality assessment

Articles considered eligible for inclusion were assessed for methodological quality using the Academy of Nutrition and Dietetics Quality Criteria Checklist for Primary Research [33]. Cochrane suggests, it is preferable to use simple approaches for assessing validity that can be fully reported (i.e. how each trial was rated on each criterion) [34]. Similar to the Cochrane Collaboration's tool for assessing risk of bias in each included study, the Academy of Nutrition and Dietetics Quality Criteria Checklist for Primary Research tool requires judgement about risk of bias to be made within each domain and support for the judgement with sufficient detail for potential sources of bias [34]. Two independent reviewers (SMF, RMT) undertook the assessments with a third reviewer (AJH) mentoring the reviewers through the process.

The quality checklist for primary research includes ten 'scientific validity' questions; four of which must be satisfactory to gain a positive rating (Q2 - bias, Q3 – comparable groups, Q6 - intervention, Q7 - outcomes) [33]. Answers were supplied as either "YES" meeting the criteria, "No" not meeting the criteria, or "Unclear" if the criteria was not clearly described. Articles were rated as positive (+) if the validity questions 2, 3, 6, 7, and at least one additional question were answered as "YES"; negative (–) if "No" was answered for 6 or more of the validity questions; or neutral ( ) if answers to questions 2, 3, 6, or 7 did not indicate that the study was exceptionally strong [33]. Quality assessments of included studies are presented in the results.

Table 1 Inclusion/Exclusion Criteria

Inclusion criteria	Exclusion criteria
Randomised control trials with the intervention of any weight measurement, self-recorded or recorded by any health professional	Studies published in languages other than English Studies that are not randomised control trials
Studies that included pregnant women with a singleton pregnancy, of any age, weight, body mass index, without date limits	Studies in animals Multiple pregnancies
Studies that used more than one episode of weight measurement during pregnancy	Poor methodological quality studies
Neutral or good methodological quality studies	

Data extraction

Relevant data were extracted by two reviewers (SMF, AJH) and entered into a Microsoft Excel spreadsheet. Data included: authors, year of publication, sample size, population characteristics, intervention and duration of the study, measures of compliance and outcomes. Weight gain outcomes included: total gestational weight gain (kg), gestational weight gain by pre-pregnancy BMI (kg/wk), and EGWG according to IOM guidelines.

Pregnancy, infant and birth outcomes included: infant birth weight, macrosomia (>90th centile), intrauterine growth restriction (<10th centile), instrumental birth, caesarean birth, combined pregnancy induced hypertension (PIH) and pre-eclampsia (PE), gestational diabetes mellitus (GDM), infant hypoglycaemia, and Apgar <7 at 5 min.

Statistical analysis

Meta-analysis was conducted using the mean and standard deviation for continuous outcomes and counts for categorical outcomes. A fixed-effects model using inverse variance weights was conducted. Fixed-effect models weight studies according to the amount of information they contribute, whereas random-effects models incorporate an estimate of between-study variation (heterogeneity) in the weighting. The fixed-effect assumption is that the true treatment effect is the same in each study, despite any differences in study protocols [35]. We believe a fixed effect model is appropriate as larger studies should be given more weight than smaller ones, and as there are few studies used in our meta-analysis, using a random effects model would provide poor estimates of the distribution of the intervention effects.

Forest plots with unstandardised effect size are reported for continuous variables using weighted mean difference (WMD) and 95% confidence intervals. Categorical outcomes are reported as odds ratios (OR). BMI outcomes were combined across studies to form a single outcome. Test of significance were set at the $p < 0.05$ level with all statistical analyses programmed using Stata Statistical Software [36].

Results

Search results

A flowchart detailing the screening and selection of studies is shown in Fig. 1. The broad search identified 6465 articles ($n = 5223$ after removal of duplicates). Initial screening of the title and abstract excluded 4067 articles. Two full text papers were then assessed and both were eligible for quality checking and meta-analysis. Hand searching did not identify any further articles for assessment.

Study characteristics

The characteristics of studies included in this review are outlined in Table 2. Briefly, both studies were conducted in Australia. The study populations were women of any parity with singleton pregnancies enrolled during early pregnancy. Two types of weighing interventions were trialled. Jefferies et al. [37] used a self-weighing regime where women were instructed to record and document their own weight at 16, 20, 24, 28, 30, 32 and 36 week's gestation. The control group were weighed at recruitment (≤14 week's gestation) and at 36 week's gestation. Both groups received standard antenatal care [37]. The second study by Brownfoot et al. [38] trialled the intervention of clinician weighing of pregnant women during scheduled antenatal care visits. The control group were weighed at the time of recruitment into the study (<21 weeks gestation) and again at 36 weeks gestation only [38]. Both groups received standard antenatal care following the participating hospitals guidelines. Both studies used an intention-to-treat analysis but had low loss to follow-up (<9%).

Study quality

A summary of the quality assessment is presented below in Table 3.

Both studies answered "Yes" to all relevance questions. Of the four validity questions, the study by Jefferies et al. [37] received a "NO" for question 6, with reviewers questioning participant compliance with the intervention and validity of instruments within the intervention group. The corresponding author of the paper was contacted seeking additional information and clarification, however, no further information could be provided. This paper received a neutral quality rating with a score of 9 out of a possible 10 [18].

The second study conducted by Brownfoot et al. [38] reported sufficient information within their publication receiving a "YES" for all scientific validity questions. The paper gained a total score of 10 and received a positive quality rating.

Analysis results

Meta-analysis of continuous outcomes is displayed in Fig. 2. There was no difference in total gestational weight gain between the intervention ($n = 494$) and control groups ($n = 483$). In the sub-group analysis of weight gain by BMI category a statistically significant difference was found for underweight women. The amount of weight gained in underweight women was 0.12 kg/week ($n = 23$, $p = 0.040$) less in the intervention group compared to control.

There were no differences in the total proportion of women exceeding the IOM weight gain ranges between intervention ($n = 290$) and control ($n = 230$): OR 1.10 (95%CI, 0.81 to 1.50). Data on EGWG by BMI category are presented in Fig. 3 and show no differences in the intervention and control groups.

For all secondary pregnancy and birth outcomes (including birth weight on Fig. 2) no significant differences were found between intervention and control as per Fig. 4.

We performed a post-hoc power calculation to determine the minimum detectable difference in total gestational weight gain for the pooled total of 977 participants, distributed approximately evenly between intervention

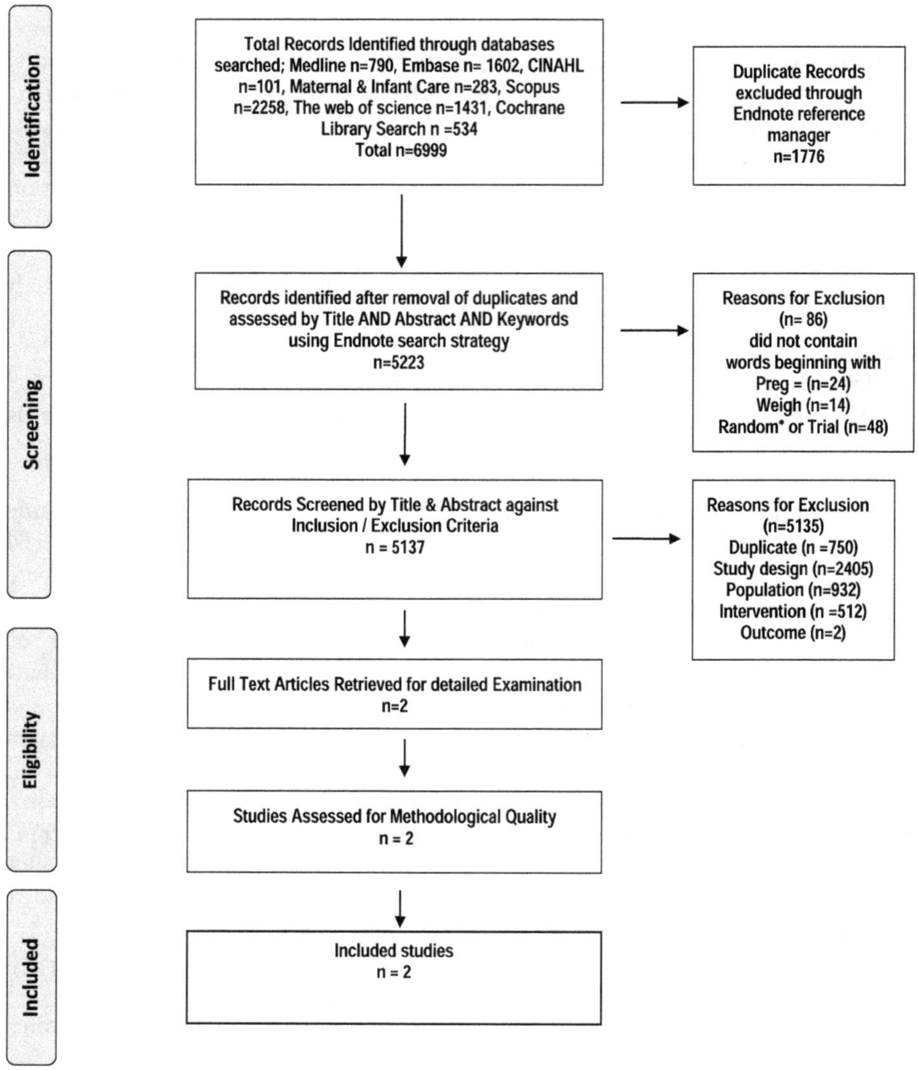

Fig. 1 Study Selection Flowchart. Flow chart adapted from Adapted From: Moher D, Liberati A, Tetzlaff J, Altman DG, The PRISMA Group (2009). Preferred Reporting Items for Systematic Reviews and Meta-Analyses: The PRISMA Statement. PLoS Med 6 (6): e1000097. doi:10.1371/journal.pmed100

and control groups. The minimum detectable difference was approximately 735 g in total gestational weight gain (~20 g per week), with 80% power, $\alpha = 0.05$, and SD ± 4.1 kg [37].

Discussion

This systematic review of RCTs aimed to determine the evidence base for weighing as a stand-alone intervention to reduce pregnancy weight gain and prevent EGWG. Two RCTs were retrieved and meta-analysed. Together they suggest that weighing, as a stand-alone intervention during routine antenatal care, is no better at reducing total pregnancy weight gain or preventing weight gain in excess of the IOM weight gain ranges than routine antenatal care.

A statistically significant lower rate of gain (kg/wk) was observed in women in the underweight BMI category between intervention and control. This finding should be interpreted with caution as it was derived from a BMI group that only included 23 women and due to multiple comparisons across BMI sub-groups could be due to random chance alone. However, it is also plausible that underweight women may be more sensitive to weighing and this practice may have an impact on their rate of weight gain. Nohr et al. [39], in a large Danish birth cohort study ($n = 60{,}892$), determined that women who were categorised as underweight at the beginning of pregnancy (BMI <18.5 kg/m2) who had lower rates of GWG (<10kgs) were found to be more at risk of giving birth to small for gestational age infants (OR 1.9, 95%CI 1.7 to 2.1) [39]. Based on the existing evidence the IOM in 2009 recommended that underweight women should gain towards the upper limits of the weight gain ranges specifically to prevent small for gestational age infants [40].

Table 2 Characteristics of included studies

Author(s), Year Study, Title, Design, & Country	Aim, quality rating	Population characteristics	Intervention, duration of study	Compliance measure(s)	Outcome(s)	Conclusions	Limitations
Jefferies, K., Shub, A., Walker, SP., Hiscock, R & Permezel, M. 2009, Reducing excessive weight gain in pregnancy: a randomised controlled trial. RCT, Melbourne, Australia.	To assess the effect of regular weight measurements and advice about the recommended (IOM 1990) weight ranges on gestational weight gain (GWG). Neutral (–)	Pregnant women recruited before ≤14 week's gestation. Age >18 years.,<45 years., singleton pregnancy. English speaking, no pre-existing Type1 or 2 diabetes Intervention (I_1) $n = 148$ (−23), Control (C) $n = 138$ (−27)	(I_1) Weight measurements + advice compared to standard antenatal care (C). BMI calculated at first antenatal visit and advice on optimal weight gain given as per IOM 1990 guidelines. I_1 self-weighing recorded on participants own antenatal card at first visit, 16, 20, 24, 28, 30, 32, 34 and 36 weeks. (C) Weighed at first visit and at 36 weeks only.	(I_1) Weight self-recorded on personalised measurement card (tabular or graphical), using scales at hospital or participant's home until 34 weeks (I_1) + (C) weighed at recruitment & 36 weeks on hospital scales.	Mean difference in weight gain (Kgs/week) and between BMI subgroups. Total weight gain and proportion gaining in excess of the IOM 1990 weight gain guidelines. Maternal & neonatal pregnancy and birth complications	No difference in total weight gain Kgs/week) between (I_1) and (C). A statistically significant reduction in GWG (Kgs/Week.) between (I_1) and (C) in overweight BMI subgroup only (mean difference of 0.12 kg/week (95% CI, 0.03 to 0.22), $p = 0.01$.	Weight measurements were largely self-reported based on home and hospital scales. There was no measure of participation compliance with the (I_1). A small sample size was used with inadequate power to detect differences between groups for weight gain above IOM 1990 guidelines, pregnancy and neonatal complications.
Brownfoot, FC. Davey, MA. & Kornman, L. 2016 Routine weighing to reduce excessive antenatal weight gain: A randomised controlled trial. RCT Melbourne, Australia.	To assess the effect of clinician weighing at each antenatal visit with advice on a ppropriate GWG using the IOM 2009 weight gain in pregnancy guidelines. Positive (+)	Pregnant women recruited <21 weeks gestation. Age >18 years <45ys, singleton pregnancy. English speaking, no co morbidities or substance abuse identified. Intervention (I_1) $n = 386$ (−17), Control (C) $n = 396$ (−24)	(I_1) Weight recorded by a clinician at each antenatal appointment and documented in hospital antenatal record. The treating clinician encouraged to discuss weight gain (no scripted responses used). (C) Routine antenatal care including advice of appropriate weight gain within the IOM 2009 ranges. Both groups weighed at recruitment with BMI calculated. The (C) weighed again at ≥36 weeks gestation.	(I_1) Weight documented in hospital antenatal records at appointments by attending clinicians. (C) Weighed at recruitment and ≥ 36 weeks only and documented on hospital antenatal record. Data collected from the antenatal hospital record, mean frequency of weight measurements reported for both groups.	Mean difference in weight gain per week (Kgs/week) and between BMI subgroups. Proportion gaining within, less than and more than the IOM 2009 weigh gain ranges. Maternal & neonatal pregnancy and birth complications	No statistically significant differences reported in mean weight gain per week (I_1) 0.54 kg (±0.28) & (C) 0.53 kg (±0.24) $p = 0.63$ ($p = 0.05$). No difference in proportion of women gaining weight within, less than or more than IOM 2009 guidelines. No differences between groups for all neonatal and maternal complications.	Study not powered to detect a between group differences for all maternal and neonatal pregnancy and birth complications reported.

Table 3 Summary of the quality assessment for the included studies

First author, year of publication (reference)	Jefferies et al. 2009 [37]	Brownfoot et al. 2016 [38]
Validity questions		
1. Was the research question clearly stated?	Y	Y
2. Was the selection of study subjects/patients free from bias?	Y	Y
3. Were study groups comparable?	Y	Y
4. Was method of handling withdrawals described?	Y	Y
5. Was blinding used to prevent introduction of bias?	Y	Y
6. Were intervention/exposure factor or procedure and any comparison(s) described in detail?	N	Y
7. Were outcomes clearly defined and the measurements valid and reliable?	Y	Y
8. Was the statistical analysis appropriate for the study design and type of outcome indicators?	Y	Y
9. Were conclusions supported by results with biases and limitations taken into consideration?	Y	Y
10. Is bias due to study's funding or sponsorship unlikely?	Y	Y
Overall quality	N	P

American Dietetic Association Quality Criteria Checklist for Primary Research, *Y* yes, *N* no, *P*, positive rating; *N* neural rating

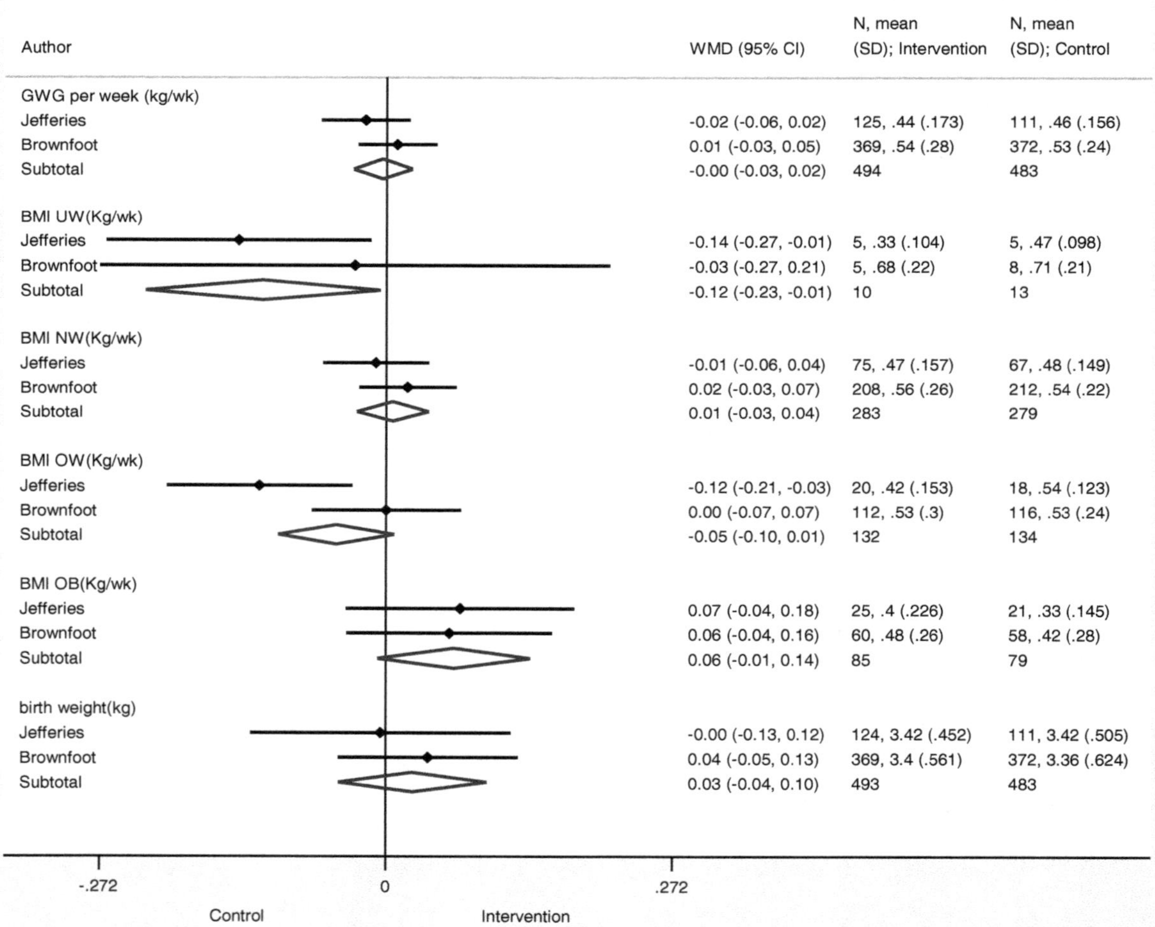

Fig. 2 Results for Continious Variables and Tests of Significance. Significance test(s) of Weighted Mean Difference (WMD = 0), Gestational Weight Gain (GWG) per week (kg/wk) z = 0.23, $p = 0.815$; Body Mass Index (BMI) Underweight (UW) (Kg/wk) z = 2.06, $p = 0.040$; BMI Normal Weight (NW) (Kg/wk) z = 0.36, $p = 0.716$; BMI Overweight (OW) (Kg/wk) z = 1.68, $p = 0.094$; BMI Obese (OB) (Kg/wk) z = 1.74, $p = 0.081$; Birth Weight (kg) z = 0.70, $p = 0.481$

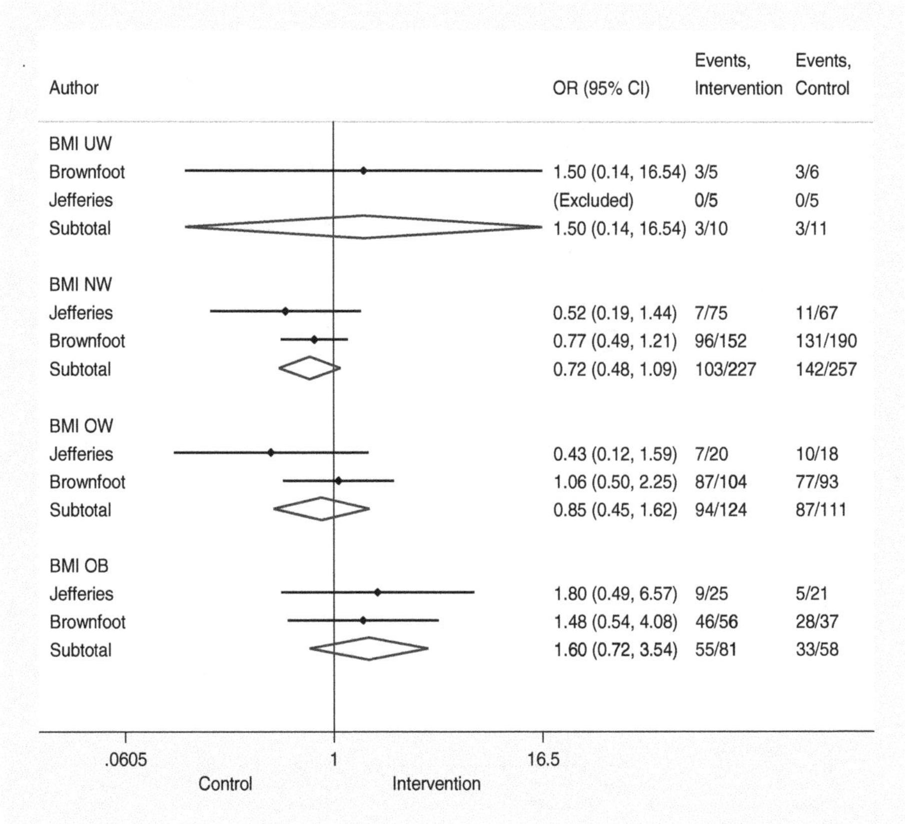

Fig. 3 Proportion of weight gain exceeding the IOM ranges and tests of significance. Significance test(s) of Odds Ratio (OR) =1; Body Mass Index (BMI) Underweight (UW) $z = 0.33$, $p = 0.741$; BMI Normal Weight (NW) $z = 1.55$, $p = 0.122$; BMI Over Weight (OW) $z = 0.50$, $p = 0.617$; BMI Obese (OB) $z = 1.15$, $p = 0.250$

It is extremely interesting that only two recent trials contributed data for this review, given the increased prevalence of obesity and EGWG and changes in practice over time. Additionally, weight gain is characteristic of pregnancy progression and a well-recognised determinant of fetal growth. There is convincing evidence that GWG is associated with infant birth weight: lower GWG is associated with low birth weight and greater GWG is associated with large for gestational age infants [12].

In light of this evidence it is difficult to reasonably explain why antenatal guidelines restrict the practice of routine antenatal weighing and not consider it as an important predictor of pregnancy outcomes, similar to serial measures of blood pressure.

Restricting routine weighing is in direct contrast to the IOM (2009) weight gain guidelines that specifically advise for pregnant women to be weighed at the initial and all subsequent antenatal visits to detect abnormal patterns of pregnancy weight gain [9]. The guidelines recommend that health care providers work in partnership with women to set individual weight gain targets according to their BMI and for weight gains to be graphically documented to enable women to be aware of their weight gains and educate them on the importance of appropriate pregnancy weight gain [9].

Dimperio et al. [41] in response to recommendations that routine weighing should be abandoned, argued that weighing was more than just a stand-alone pregnancy intervention and rather presented health care practitioners with the opportunity to counsel women before weight gains became extreme, advocating that weighing is a valuable screening tool rather than a diagnostic tool for adverse pregnancy outcomes [41].

Weighing as a stand-alone intervention may not be effective for reducing pregnancy weight gain and EGWG under controlled conditions however given the prevalence and risks associated with weight gains outside of the IOM guidelines it is negligent of maternity care providers not to address weight gain in pregnancy. Maternity care providers need to be working in partnership with women to achieve the IOM weight gain in pregnancy targets, monitoring their progress and providing feedback on that progress. Therefore, we recommend further research be undertaken into the impacts and acceptability of this intervention within various

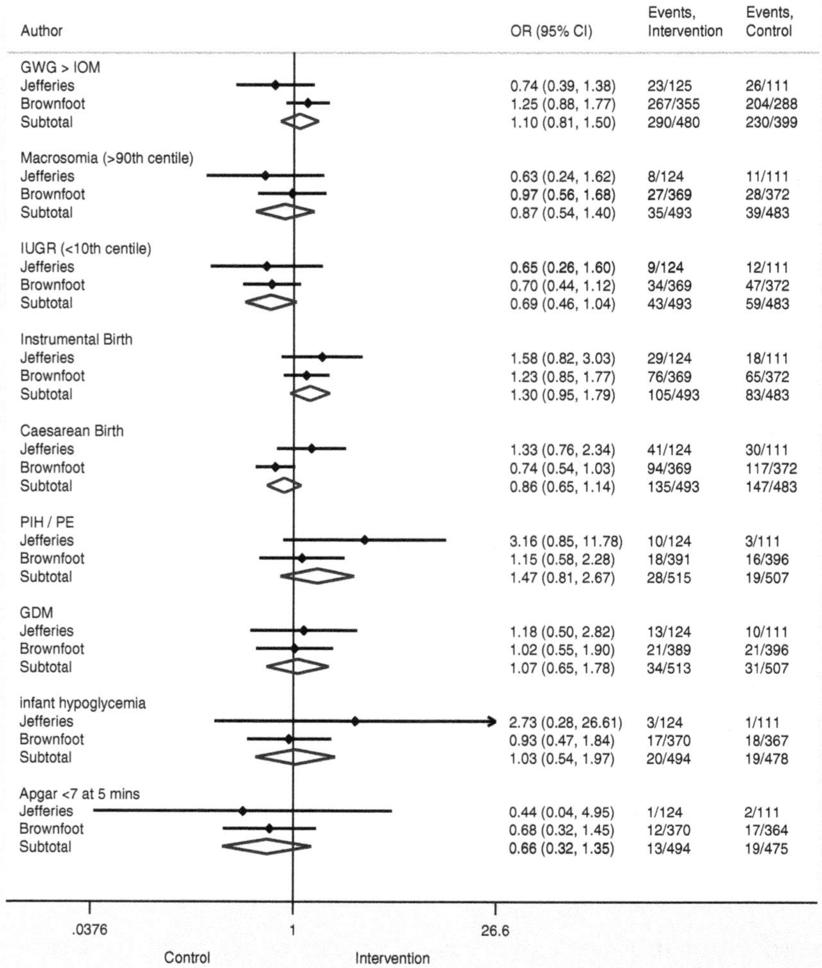

Fig. 4 Pregnancy and Birth Outcomes and Tests of Significance. Significance test(s) of Odds Ratio (OR) =1; Gestational Weight Gain (GWG) > Institute of Medicine (IOM) $z = 0.63$, $p = 0.532$; Macrosomia (>90th centile) $z = 0.58$, $p = 0.560$; Intra Uterine Growth Restriction (IUGR) (<10th centile) $z = 1.76$, $p = 0.079$; Instrumental Birth $z = 1.62$, $p = 0.105$; Caesarean Birth $z = 1.06$, $p = 0.288$; Pregnancy Induced Hypertension (PIH)/Pre-Eclampsia (PE) $z = 1.26$, $p = 0.206$; Gestational Diabetes Mellitus (GDM) $z = 0.27$, $p = 0.787$; Infant hypoglycemia $z = 0.10$, $p = 0.917$; Apgar <7 at 5 mins $z = 1.15$, $p = 0.252$

health care settings and models of pregnancy care, using both experimental and qualitative research methods.

Strengths

We have conducted a methodically rigorous and contemporary search to determine if weighing as a stand-alone intervention can reduce EGWG. All available experimental evidence has been assessed and reported in accordance with the PRISMA guidelines [32] and an appropriate methodological quality checklist [33].

Limitations

Although the included RCTs were deemed good quality, with neutral and positive quality ratings, the following limitations need to be considered. Giving benefit of the doubt, blinding within both studies was rated as adequate, even though neither the participant nor clinicians/researchers (who were also the outcome assessors) were blinded to the intervention. This is because the quality check question is phrased with the qualifier "as appropriate". Jefferies et al. [37] reported that participants were blinded to the purpose of the study, however, discussed that researchers conducting the study were not blinded to treatment groups. No participant blinding was used in the study by Brownfoot et al. [38] because of the nature of the intervention, and this was acknowledged in their limitations. Reviewers gave consideration to each study's methods and concluded that true blinding would be extremely difficult.

Secondary outcomes within both studies including, proportion of women gaining weight above the IOM recommendations, pregnancy birth and neonatal outcomes were not pre specified within each study's statistical analysis plan. These outcomes were not adequately powered to detect a difference between intervention and control limiting the generalisability of these findings.

The decision to exclude studies published in a language other than English was made a priori, for pragmatic reasons. Authors acknowledge that there is potential for this exclusion to have contributed to the low number of included studies.

Conclusion

This systematic review and meta-analysis concludes that weighing, as a stand-alone intervention is neither worse nor better at reducing excessive gestational weight gain than routine antenatal care alone. In light of the presented evidence we recommend that where antenatal guidelines advise women to gain weight within the IOM weight gain ranges that they be enacted in their entirety recommending that women be weighed at the first and all subsequent antenatal visits. We additionally recommend that further research studies be conducted to assess the impact and acceptability of weighing in pregnancy.

Additional files

Additional file 1. Study Protocol. Description of data: Systematic review study protocol.

Additional file 2. Primary Search Strategy November 2014. Description of data: This file contains all details of the primary systematic review search strategy conducted in November 2014. Including databases, search terms and number of citations retrieved.

Additional file 3. Primary Search Strategy (Updated January 2016). Description of data: This file contains all details of the updated primary systematic review search strategy conducted in January 2016. Including databases, search terms and number of citations retrieved.

Additional file 4. Spreadsheet of values used for data analysis.

Abbreviations

BMI: Body mass index; CI: Confidence interval; EGWG: Excessive gestational weight gain; GDM: Gestational diabetes mellitus; IOM: Institute of Medicine; NICE: National Institute of Health and Care Excellence; OR: Odds ratio; PE: Pre-eclampsia; PIH: Pregnancy induced hypertension; PRISMA: Preferred reporting items for systematic reviews and meta – analysis; RCTs: Randomised controlled trials; WMD: Weighted mean difference

Acknowledgements

Research Librarian: Debbie Booth Faculty of Health and Medicine, University of Newcastle, New South Wales, Australia.

Funding

No funding was sought or accepted for this publication.

Authors' contribution

SMF is the primary reviewer and author of this review paper. SMF carried out the initial and final primary and secondary search strategies, undertook screening of citations, quality appraisal; data extraction and the person responsible for managing the study and writing of this review paper. AJH conceived the study and contributed by designing the review protocol and inclusion/exclusion criteria. AJH conducted some initial screening of citations, carried out data extraction and made substantial contributions to the writing of the review paper. RMT is the second reviewer who carried out screening of citations, quality appraisal and editing of manuscript. AB is the statistician who carried out the meta-analysis. JA contributed to the study design and interpretation of data. Both MF and LE have made substantial contributions in the design, drafting and revising this manuscript. All authors have read and have given approval for this manuscript to be published.

Competing interests

The authors declare that they have no competing interests.

Author details

[1]School of Nursing & Midwifery University of Newcastle, Port Macquarie Campus, PO Box 210, Port Macquarie 2444, NSW, Australia. [2]Faculty of Health & Medicine School of Medicine & Public Health, University of Newcastle, Callaghan, NSW, Australia. [3]Maternity Care Services, The Port Macquarie Base Hospital, Port Macquarie, NSW, Australia. [4]Mothers and Babies Research Centre, University of Newcastle, University Drive, Callaghan 2308, NSW, Australia. [5]Hunter Medical Research Institute, Newcastle, NSW, Australia. [6]Centre for Midwifery, Child and Family Health, Faculty of Health, University of Technology Sydney, PO Box 123Broadway, Ultimo, NSW 2007, Australia. [7]Centre for Clinical Epidemiology and Biostatistics, School of Medicine & Public Health, University of Newcastle, Callaghan, NSW, Australia. [8]Division of Medicine, John Hunter Hospital, Newcastle, NSW, Australia.

References

1. Marchi J, Berg M, Dencker A, Olander E, Begley C. Risks associated with obesity in pregnancy, for the mother and baby: a systematic review of reviews. Obes Rev. 2015;16(8):621–38.
2. About Obesity. http://www.worldobesity.org/resources/aboutobesity/. Accessed 29 Nov 2016.
3. Obesity and Overweight Fact sheet No. 311 http://www.who.int/mediacentre/factsheets/fs311/en/. Accessed 29 Nov 2016.
4. Australian Bureau of Statistics. National Health Survey First Results 2014–15. 2015.
5. Australian Institute of Health and Welfare. Australia's mothers and babies 2013—in brief. Perinatal statistics series no. 31. Canberra: AIHW; 2015.
6. Fealy S, Hure A, Browne G, Prince C. Developing a clinical care pathway for obese pregnant women: A quality improvement project. Women Birth. 2014;27(4):e67–71.
7. Cedergren M. Effects of gestational weight gain and body mass index on obstetric outcome in Sweden. Int J Gynaecol Obstet. 2006;93(3):269–74.
8. Institute of Medicine Committee on Nutritional Status During Pregnancy and Lactation: Nutrition During Pregnancy: Part 1 Weight Gain. In.: National Academy of Sciences Institute of Medicine; 1990.
9. Rasmussen KM, Yaktine AL. Nutrition During Pregnancy: Re-Examining the Guidelines. Washington: National Academy of Sciences Institute of Medicine; 2009.
10. The Royal Australian and New Zealand College of Obstetricians and Gynaecologists: Management of Obesity in Pregnancy College Statement: C- OBS 49. In.: The Royal Australian and New Zealand College of Obstetricians and Gynaecologists; 2016.
11. Australian Health Ministers Advisory Council. Clinical Practice Guidelines: Antenatal Care - Module 1. Canberra: Australian Government Department of Health & Ageing; 2012.
12. Johnson J, Clifton RG, Roberts JM, Myatt L, Hauth JC, Spong CY, Varner MW, Wapner RJ, Thorp Jr JM, Mercer BM, et al. Pregnancy outcomes with weight gain above or below the 2009 institute of medicine guidelines. Obstet Gynecol. 2013;121(5):969–75.
13. Oken E, Taveras EM, Kleinman KP, Rich-Edwards JW, Gillman MW.

Gestational weight gain and child adiposity at age 3 years. Am J Obstet Gynecol. 2007;196(4):322 e321–328.
14. Stotland NE, Cheng YW, Hopkins LM, Caughey AB. Gestational weight gain and adverse neonatal outcome among term infants. Obstet Gynecol. 2006;108(3 Pt 1):635–43.
15. de Jersey SJ, Nicholson JM, Callaway LK, Daniels LA. A prospective study of pregnancy weight gain in Australian women. Aust N Z J Obstet Gynaecol. 2012;52(6):545–51.
16. Faucher MA, Barger MK. Gestational weight gain in obese women by class of obesity and select maternal/newborn outcomes: A systematic review. Women Birth. 2015;28(3):e70–9.
17. Muktabhant B, Lawrie TA, Lumbiganon P, Laopaiboon M. Diet or exercise, or both, for preventing excessive weight gain in pregnancy. Cochrane Database Syst Rev. 2015;6:CD007145.
18. Heslehurst N, Newham J, Maniatopoulos G, Fleetwood C, Robalino S, Rankin J. Implementation of pregnancy weight management and obesity guidelines: A meta-synthesis of healthcare professionals' barriers and facilitators using the Theoretical Domains Framework. Pregnancy Hypertens. 2014;4(3):234–5.
19. Harrison CL, Teede HJ, Lombard CB. How effective is self-weighing in the setting of a lifestyle intervention to reduce gestational weight gain and postpartum weight retention? Aust N Z J Obstet Gynaecol. 2014;54(4):382–5.
20. Phelan S, Phipps MG, Abrams B, Darroch F, Grantham K, Schaffner A, Wing RR. Does behavioral intervention in pregnancy reduce postpartum weight retention? Twelve-month outcomes of the Fit for Delivery randomized trial. Am J Clin Nutr. 2014;99(2):302–11.
21. Daley AJ, Jolly K, Jebb S, Roalfe A, Mackillop L, Lewis A, Clifford S, Kenyon S, MacArthur C, Aveyard P. Effectiveness of regular weighing, weight target setting and feedback by community midwives within routine antenatal care in preventing excessive gestational weight gain: randomised controlled trial. BMC Obes. 2016;3(1):1.
22. Brownfoot F, Davey MA, Kornman L. Women's opinions on being weighed at routine antenatal visits. BJOG. 2016;123(2):263–70.
23. Burke LE, Wang J, Sevick MA. Self-monitoring in weight loss: a systematic review of the literature. J Am Diet Assoc. 2011;111(1):92–102.
24. VanWormer JJ, French SA, Pereira MA, Welsh EM. The impact of regular self-weighing on weight management: a systematic literature review. Int J Behav Nutr Phys Act. 2008;5(1):54.
25. Zheng Y, Klem ML, Sereika SM, Danford CA, Ewing LJ, Burke LE. Self-weighing in weight management: A systematic literature review. Obesity. 2015;23(2):256–65.
26. Allen-Walker V, Woodside J, Holmes V, Young I, Cupples ME, Hunter A, McKinley MC: Commentary on Routine weighing of women during pregnancy-is it time to change current practice? BJOG. 2015;123(6):871–74.
27. Dawes M, Grudzinskas J. Patterns of maternal weight gain in pregnancy. BJOG. 1991;98(2):195–201.
28. Dawes MG, Green J, Ashurst H. Routine weighing in pregnancy. BMJ. 1992; 304(6825):487–9.
29. Dawes MG, Grudzinskas JG. Repeated measurement of maternal weight during pregnancy. Is this a useful practice? Br J Obstet Gynaecol. 1991;98(2):189–94.
30. National Institute for Health and Clinical Excellence. Antenatal care for Uncomplicated Pregnancies Guideline CG62. United Kingdom: National Institute of Clinical Excellence; 2008.
31. Queensland Clinical Guidelines: Obesity in Pregnancy Guideline No. MN15. 14-V5-R20. In. Brisbane Queensland Clinical Guidelines; 2015.
32. Moher D, Liberati A, Tetzlaff J, Altman DG. Preferred reporting items for systematic reviews and meta-analyses: the PRISMA statement. Ann Intern Med. 2009;151(4):264–9.
33. Academy of Nutrition and Dietetics. Evidence Analysis Manual: Steps in the Academy Evidence Analysis Process. Chicago: Research and Strategic Business Development Academy of Nutrition and Dietetics; 2012.
34. Higgins JP, Green S: Cochrane handbook for systematic reviews of interventions, vol. 5: Wiley Online Library; 2008.
35. Kontopantelis E, Reeves D. metaan: Random-effects meta-analysis. Stata J. 2010;10(3):395–407.
36. StataCorp. Stata Statistical Software, vol. 143. College Station: StataCorp LP; 2014.
37. Jeffries K, Shub A, Walker SP, Hiscock R, Permezel M. Reducing excessive weight gain in pregnancy: A randomised controlled trial. Med J Aust. 2009; 191(8):429–33.
38. Brownfoot FC, Davey MA, Kornman L. Routine weighing to reduce excessive antenatal weight gain: a randomised controlled trial. BJOG. 2016;123(2):254–61.
39. Nohr EA, Vaeth M, Baker JL, Sorensen T, Olsen J, Rasmussen KM. Combined associations of prepregnancy body mass index and gestational weight gain with the outcome of pregnancy. Am J Clin Nutr. 2008;87(6):1750–9.
40. Rasmussen KM, Yaktine A: Weight Gain During Pregnancy: Reexamining the Guidelines. In.: National Academy of Sciences Institute of Medicine; 2009.
41. Dimperio DL, Frentzen BH, Cruz AC. Routine weighing during antenatal visits. BMJ. 1992;304(6825):460.

3

Is a motivational interviewing based lifestyle intervention for obese pregnant women across Europe implemented as planned? Process evaluation of the DALI study

Judith G. M. Jelsma[1], David Simmons[2,3], Nina Gobat[4], Stephen Rollnick[4], Kinga Blumska[5], Goele Jans[6], Sander Galjaard[6,7], Gernot Desoye[8], Rosa Corcoy[9,10], Fabiola Juarez[9], Alexandra Kautzky-Willer[11], Jürgen Harreiter[11], Andre van Assche[6], Roland Devlieger[6], Dirk Timmerman[6], David Hill[12], Peter Damm[13], Elisabeth R. Mathiesen[13], Ewa Wender-Ożegowska[5], Agnieszka Zawiejska[5], Annunziata Lapolla[14], Maria G. Dalfrà[14], Stefano del Prato[15], Alessandra Bertolotto[15], Fidelma Dunne[16], Dorte M. Jensen[17], Liselotte Andersen[17], Frank J. Snoek[18,19] and Mireille N. M. van Poppel[1,20*]

Abstract

Background: Process evaluation is an essential part of designing and assessing complex interventions. The vitamin D and lifestyle intervention study (DALI) study is testing different strategies to prevent development of gestational diabetes mellitus among European obese pregnant women with a body mass index ≥29 kg/m^2. The intervention includes guidance on physical activity and/or healthy eating by a lifestyle coach trained in motivational interviewing (MI). The aim of this study was to assess the process elements: reach, dose delivered, fidelity and satisfaction and to investigate whether these process elements were associated with changes in gestational weight gain (GWG).

Methods: Data on reach, dose delivered, fidelity, and satisfaction among 144 participants were collected. Weekly recruitment reports, notes from meetings, coach logs and evaluation questionnaires (n = 110) were consulted. Fidelity of eight (out of twelve) lifestyle coach practitioners was assessed by analysing audio recorded counselling sessions using the MI treatment integrity scale. Furthermore, associations between process elements and GWG were assessed with linear regression analyses.

Results: A total of 20% of the possible study population (reach) was included in this analysis. On average 4.0 (of the intended 5) face-to-face sessions were delivered. Mean MI fidelity almost reached 'expert opinion' threshold for the global scores, but was below 'beginning proficiency' for the behavioural counts. High variability in quality of MI between practitioners was identified. Participants were highly satisfied with the intervention, the lifestyle coach and the intervention materials. No significant associations were found between process elements and GWG.
(Continued on next page)

* Correspondence: mnm.vanpoppel@vumc.nl
[1]Department of Public and Occupational Health and, Amsterdam Public Health research institute, VU University Medical Centre, Van der Boechorststraat 7, 1081BT Amsterdam, Amsterdam, The Netherlands
[20]Institute of Sport Science, University of Graz, Graz, Austria
Full list of author information is available at the end of the article

(Continued from previous page)

Conclusion: Overall, the intervention was well delivered and received by the study population, but did not comply with all the principles of MI. Ensuring audio recording of lifestyle sessions throughout the study would facilitate provision of individualized feedback to improve MI skills. A larger sample size is needed to confirm the lack of association between process elements and GWG.

Keywords: Counselling, Fidelity, Dose, Motivational interviewing, Lifestyle behaviour, Process evaluation, Pregnancy

Background

Obesity and excessive gestational weight gain (GWG) are both independent risk factors for adverse outcomes and complications of pregnancy, such as gestational diabetes mellitus (GDM) [1]. The Institute of Medicine (IOM) has developed guidelines for GWG based on the pre-pregnancy body mass index (BMI) [2]. To prevent women from exceeding these recommendations, prevention trials are needed [3]. A number of lifestyle studies have been designed to assist in limiting GWG by providing an intervention focused on healthy eating, physical activity or a combined approach, although so far no definitive answer in favour of any of these interventions has been found [4–6].

Motivational Interviewing (MI) has been shown to be effective in helping persons change their lifestyle behaviours, such as physical activity and diet across different target populations [7–12] and might be an effective counselling technique for professionals to deal with the difficult situations experienced by obese pregnant women [13] and to assist in limiting GWG [14]. MI is a "collaborative, goal-oriented style of communication with particular attention to the language of change. It is designed to strengthen personal motivation for and commitment to a specific goal by eliciting and exploring the person's own reasons for change within an atmosphere of acceptance and compassion" (p.29) [15].

The vitamin D and Lifestyle Intervention (DALI) study aims to investigate across a number of European centres, how effective a behavioural lifestyle intervention is in the prevention of GDM. In these centres, pregnant women with a BMI of ≥29 kg/m^2 receive guidance from a lifestyle coach trained in MI [16]. The pilot study found lowest GWG with a healthy eating (HE) intervention relative to a physical activity (PA) or combined (HE + PA) intervention [17]. While these results seem promising they need to be confirmed in a larger trial including a control group. Furthermore, intervention components are complex in nature, so it is important to evaluate process variables to indicate how a planned intervention was conducted, especially when different persons delivered an intervention across many countries, as is the case in our study.

Process evaluations allow researchers to provide insight into why an intervention has shown positive or negative results [18, 19]. Moreover, in behavioural intervention research it is of utmost importance to report treatment fidelity, which refers to the "methodological strategies used to monitor and enhance the reliability and validity of behavioural interventions" (p.443) [20]. Miller and Rollnick (2014) underscore the importance for assessing the quality of the intervention when delivering MI in order to determine the effect of the quality of MI in the intervention on the results of the study [21]. Another important component is the description of strategies used to acquire a higher treatment fidelity that could be valuable for clinical practice in the actual implementation process [20].

The primary objective of this process evaluation was to assess reach (including recruitment), dose delivered, fidelity and satisfaction of the DALI lifestyle pilot study. The secondary objective was to investigate whether these process elements could explain differential effects of the intervention on changes in GWG.

Methods

There are several approaches for conducting complex process evaluation, with no single best way to design a process evaluation [22]. The current paper uses dimensions from the framework of Linnan and Steckler (2002) [18]. The original framework includes seven dimensions: context, reach, fidelity, dose delivered and received, implementation and recruitment. This has some overlap with the five dimensions of the reach, effectiveness, adoption, implementation, and maintenance (RE-AIM) evaluation framework [23]. In Table 1 an overview of the developed process evaluation plan is presented, with a specification of the research questions, complete and acceptable delivery and used process measure according to Saunders et al. (2005) [24].

DALI study

A detailed description of the cross-national DALI study is provided elsewhere [16]. In short, pregnant women with a body mass index (BMI) ≥ 29 kg/m^2 were recruited between January 2012 and March 2013. All

Table 1 Process evaluation plan

Process evaluation question	Complete and acceptable delivery	Process measure
How many people of the target population took part in the project? (reach)	The intervention group is comparable to the study population	Weekly recruitment report kept by each research centre
What recruitment procedures were used to attract pregnant women? (recruitment)	Strategies on recruitment across multicentre research.	Notes from (telephone) meetings with research nurses, coaches, principal investigators throughout the project
How many participants received 5 face-to-face conversations with a personal lifestyle coach? (dose delivered)	All (100%) received 5 face-to-face conversations with a personal lifestyle coach	Coach logs recorded after a session
To what extend was face-to-face counselling delivered as planned by MI guidelines? (fidelity)	MI was applied to deliver the face-to-face conversations	Recorded conversations assessed using the Motivational Interviewing Treatment Integrity measure (MITI 3.1.1)
How many telephone booster sessions did the participants receive? (dose delivered)	0–4 telephone booster sessions were delivered	Coach logs recorded after a session
How satisfied were participants with the DALI intervention (components)? (dose received: satisfaction)	All participants were satisfied with the DALI intervention	Evaluation questionnaire at 35–37 weeks of gestation

women who agreed to participate in the DALI project underwent a 2 h 75 g oral glucose tolerance test (OGTT) before 20 weeks of gestation, whereby those with GDM according to the International Association of Diabetes in Pregnancy Study Group (IADPSG) criteria were excluded [25]. The pilot lifestyle study was conducted in eleven study centres across nine European countries (Austria (Vienna), Belgium (Leuven), Denmark (Odense and Copenhagen), Ireland (Galway), Italy (Padua and Pisa), Netherlands (Amsterdam), Poland (Poznan), Spain (Barcelona) and the United Kingdom (UK) (Cambridge)). Local medical ethical committees in these countries approved the study and all participants gave written informed consent.

DALI intervention

Women were randomly allocated to one of three intervention arms; either a healthy eating (HE) arm, a physical activity (PA) arm or a combined HE and PA (HE + PA) arm. Between entry and 35 weeks of gestation five face-to-face sessions were planned supplemented with four optional telephone coaching sessions with a personal lifestyle coach, based on the principles of MI. Tools such as a pedometer, a dynaband, a food diary, action goal cards and a manual with information on GDM, appropriate GWG, HE and/or PA were provided to the participants, depending on the intervention randomization arm.

Lifestyle coaches

Key competencies for the lifestyle coach were: being empathic (understanding another person's experience, feeling and behaviour), curious (willingness to explore the person's experience), client focused (primary focus to help another person) and collaborative (equal perception of client and coach). The coach should not be dominant or chaotic (should be able to structure a conversation). In total twelve lifestyle coaches delivered the intervention sessions. In all the individual sites one coach was appointed, except in one site where a coach left the project and was replaced. All coaches were female with various professional backgrounds; most were PhD students with a master's degree in either nutrition or human movement science; one was working as a midwife, one as a registered dietitian and one person had a background in information technology. Three coaches were familiar with MI prior to the start of this study, either by completing a local MI course or by acquiring experience in an earlier intervention study.

Training of the lifestyle coaches

Prior to the start of the pilot study a first 2-day central training was offered to the coaches in Cambridge (UK), and led by experienced MI trainers. The first training included an introduction to MI and its key concepts, followed by role-play exercises and video recordings. These interactive components allowed coaches to play the role of study participant and lifestyle coach to experience the impact of MI. Furthermore, coaches practiced core skills and received individualised feedback on their performance. The training covered the eight stages in learning MI [26], whereby the following skills were taught: 1) spirit of MI; 2) OARS (open questions, affirmations, reflections, summaries): client centred counselling skills; 3) recognizing change talk (desire, ability, need, reason and commitment) and sustain talk; 4) eliciting and strengthening change talk (by the use of OARS); 5) rolling with resistance; 6) developing a change plan/making an action plan (activation, commitment, taking steps); 7) consolidating commitment; and 8) transition and blending with the DALI intervention. A second two day training was delivered a few months later to review the coaches' MI competency, share experiences and receive feedback on a role-play. The DALI coaches received in total 32 h of MI training.

The training was held in English, and it was recommended to non-English practitioners to contact a local and native language speaking MI trainer from the international Motivational Interviewing Network of Trainers (MINT-network) (Virginia, US; http://www.motivationalinterviewing.org) for further feedback based on an actual conversation in their own language.

Reach

Reach is defined as the proportion of participants included in the intervention [24]. The numbers of persons eligible for participation (based on inclusion and exclusion criteria) were recorded in a weekly recruitment sheet at each site. Reasons for (not) participating in the DALI project were recorded. Approaching and attracting participants for a research project can be challenging, especially in a cross-national research project. Therefore, in research meetings with research nurses, coaches and principal investigators, recruitment strategies were discussed and recorded.

Dose delivered

Dose delivered is defined as the amount or number of intended components delivered by the practitioner [24]. The number of face-to-face counselling sessions and telephone booster calls that were delivered to the participants was assessed. The aim was to deliver all (100%) of the five face-to-face conversations, while the telephone booster sessions were optional for the participants. It was preferred to deliver four face-to-face sessions prior to the second measurement at 24–28 weeks of gestation and to deliver the final face-to-face session prior to the last measurement at 35–37 weeks of gestation. Coaches kept information regarding dose delivered on a personal digital assistance (PDA) and uploaded this to a central database. A paper version of the PDA was kept in case of technical problems.

Fidelity

Fidelity is defined as the extent to which the intervention was implemented as intended [24]. To assess fidelity, practitioners were asked to audio record all sessions (with permission of the participant). Fidelity of MI was assessed using the Motivational Interviewing Treatment Integrity (MITI 3.1.1.) scale [27]. The aim was to code at least four sessions of different patients throughout the pilot study of each practitioner to provide a reliable competency score for each practitioner on the MITI [28]. Finally, to assess an overall MI fidelity score for the DALI intervention, the individual scores for each practitioner were weighted for the total number of participants counselled.

Motivational interviewing treatment integrity (MITI 3.1.1)

The MITI 3.1.1. is a behaviour coding system that measures the extent to which a practitioner uses MI skills in a particular session. This instrument is widely used to test MI fidelity and has good reliability and sensitivity [29–32]. The MITI 3.1.1. has two components: global scores and behaviour counts. Coders used two 'passes' through the audiotape. The first pass is used to assess the global scores and the second pass to assign a behaviour count. Global scores were rated on a five point Likert scale for the following five dimensions: Evocation, Collaboration, Autonomy/support, Direction and Empathy. Adding the Evocation, Collaboration, Autonomy/support dimensions forms the global 'spirit' score. Furthermore all utterances were assigned a behaviour count: open and closed questions, simple and complex reflections, giving information, MI adherent (e.g. advise with permission, affirming, emphasizing the client's control, supporting) and MI non adherent (e.g. advice without permission, confronting, directing). It is possible that some utterances remain uncoded (e.g. off-topic talk, self-disclosure statements, facilitative statements, structure statements). The following summary scores of the behaviour counts were formed: Reflection to question ratio; Percent Open questions; Percent Complex reflections; Percent MI-adherent. 'Beginning proficiency' for motivational interviewing is met in the following conditions: global scores ≥3.5, reflection to question ratio in favour of reflection ≥1, percent open questions is ≥50%, percent complex reflection is ≥40% and percent MI-adherent is ≥90% [27]. In Table 2 a more detailed explanation and thresholds of the MITI scores are provided.

Rating procedure

MITI 3.1.1. requires a 20-min randomly selected sample and a clear target behaviour goal. Additional study requirements were that the audio session was delivered prior to the second measurement, making effect correlations possible. Session were chosen randomly from the available recorded sessions (see Table 5). Furthermore the 20-min segment was chosen randomly within each recording, although the segment should start at the beginning of one of the intervention messages (either the discussion of risk factors of GDM, or weight gain targets, or one of the healthy eating or one of the physical activity messages) so off topic talk in the beginning or end, such as discussing time and place for the next appointment was not included in the segment. If off

Table 2 Motivational Interviewing Treatment Integrity 3.1.1 score explanation and threshold [27]

	Explanation	Threshold
Global score		
Evocation	the extent to which the practitioner conveys an understanding that motivation for change and the ability to move toward that change, reside mostly within the client and therefore focuses efforts to elicit and expand it within the therapeutic interaction	3.5
Collaboration	the extent to which the practitioner behaves as if the interview is occurring between two equal partners, both of whom have knowledge that might be useful in the problem under consideration	3.5
Autonomy/Support	the extent to which the practitioner supports and actively fosters client perception of choice as opposed to attempting to control the client's behaviour or choices	3.5
Direction	the degree to which a practitioner maintain appropriate focus on a specific target behaviour or concerns directly tied to it	3.5
Empathy	the extent to which the practitioner understands or makes an effort to grasp the client's perspective and feelings	3.5
Spirit	Average of the Evocation, Collaboration, Autonomy/support dimensions	3.5
Behavioural count		
Reflection: Questions	dividing the total amount of reflections by the total amount of questions	1:1
% Open Questions	dividing the amount of open questions by the total amount of closed and open questions	50%
% Complex Reflections	dividing the amount of complex reflections by the total amount of simple and complex reflections	40%
% MI Adherent	dividing the amount of MI-adherent statements by the total amount of MI adherent and MI non adherent statements combined	90%

topic talk still occurred during the session this remained uncoded, which is according to the MITI 3.1.1.

Coders

The lifestyle coaches delivered the lifestyle intervention in their own language. Therefore the sessions needed to be assessed by different coders proficient in these languages.

The conversations in Belgium, Ireland, The Netherlands and UK were assessed by one of the authors (JJ) and a coder not involved in the study (VM). Both received separately an extensive MITI 3.1.1 training (40 h). Experience with coding according to the MITI 3.1.1 was gained by a supervised coding of 18 samples both in Dutch and English before coding the actual study sample. Global scores of the study sample were discussed to reach consensus, if no consensus was reached the average of both was taken; for behavioural counts, the average of both counts was taken. Inter-rater reliability was assessed on the double coded study sample.

In Spain (PL), Denmark (HFK) and Italy (GP) members from the international MINT network experienced in coding with the MITI 3.1.1 assessed the fidelity of the sessions. Due to pragmatic reasons and costs no second coder was appointed. In Spain the conversations were evaluated according to the MITI 3.0 [33], because a translated Spanish manual for the MITI 3.0 was available. The MITI 3.0 differs from the MITI 3.1.1 in only minor textual revisions.

Satisfaction

In the self-developed evaluation questionnaire (see Additional file 1) the overall participant satisfaction with DALI was measured on a 10 point Likert scale [very negative (1)-very positive (10)]. In addition, participants were asked to rate their satisfaction with the usefulness of the intervention materials (manual, pedometer, dynaband) used in the DALI study on a 10 point Likert scale [not useful at all (1) – very useful (10)]. A satisfaction score for the manual consisted of an averaged score for different parts of the manual (general information, GDM, weight management, healthy eating, physical activity), which was dependent on the intervention arm a woman was allocated to. Satisfaction about the lifestyle coach was assessed with the following six items: overall, overall knowledge, knowledge of the intervention, "helped you rather than told you what to do", attitude, and ability to support. All these items were measured on a 10 point Likert scale [could do a lot better (1) – excellent (10)] and averaged to obtain an overall score. Furthermore, participants could rate both face-to-face and telephone calls on a 10 point Likert scale [not useful at all (1) – very useful (10)].

Effectiveness

We examined the association between trial processes (fidelity, dose, and a composite score of both) and one of the primary outcomes GWG. This can help explain why the interventions did or did not work. To assess GWG, participants were weighed on a weighing scale

(SECA 888; SECA 877) wearing no shoes and light clothes to the nearest 0.1 kg. GWG was calculated by subtracting the baseline weight (before 20 weeks) from the weight measured at the final measurement (35-37 weeks of gestation).

Data analysis

Inter-rater reliability of the MITI 3.1.1 was assessed with intra-class correlation coefficients (ICC) for the behavioural scores and Krippendorf Alpha (KALPHA) [34] for the global scores over the study sample that was double coded (n = 20) [28]. The norm for good reliability is a KALPHA of 0.8 or higher [35]. ICCs were calculated using a two-way mixed model for absolute agreement. The following guidelines for interpretation of ICCs were used: below 0.40 = poor, 0.40–0.59 = fair, 0.60–0.74 = good, 0.75–1.00 = excellent [36].

Linear regression analyses were performed to explore association between process elements (independent variable) and GWG (dependent variable), correcting for baseline BMI and the total number of weeks between measurements. The following independent variables were considered: number of face to face (F2F) conversations, total number of conversations (F2F and phone/email combined), and a dichotomized implementation score for the process element fidelity, which was formed by adding all those MITI 3.1.1 criteria that fulfilled 'beginning proficiency', whereby a score of four or more out of seven elements was considered as 'high' and a score below four as 'low' (in Table 2 those with high MI competency are indicated with an asterisk). An overall score for the variable 'DALI as intended' was scored as 'yes' or 'no' fulfilling the criterion of: "all those who received counselling from a lifestyle coach who fulfilled 'beginning proficiency' in four out of seven elements and who received all five face-to-face sessions". All those participants that lacked follow up data were removed from the sample. $P < 0.05$ was considered to be statistically significant. Analyses were conducted with software IBM Statistical Package for Social Sciences (SPSS) version 20.1.

Results

Reach

In Fig. 1 the flowchart of this study is presented. A total of 144 participants from a total of 733 pregnant women who were invited (19.6%) were included in the DALI project. Of those that declined with a reason 41% reported not to be interested in this project and 36% thought it involved too much of their time to participate in this study. Of the 144 participants randomized to the DALI project, 48 were randomly allocated to the HE intervention, 47 to the PA intervention and 49 to the HE + PA intervention. A total of twenty participants dropped out during the study for various reasons. In one case this was due to the dislike of the HE intervention, the information provided was regarded 'too obvious'.

Some deviations from the inclusion – exclusion criteria led to eight cases with a pre-pregnancy BMI lower than 29 who were randomized (in error) into one of the intervention-groups. Of these, six women had a BMI above 29 at the first DALI visit and are included in the DALI study and will be considered in future analysis. Still, one of these women dropped out of the HE intervention group due to a spontaneous abortion.

Each country applied different recruitment strategies based on differences in the organization of health care services (Table 3). Almost all countries actively invited women based on their BMI from their medical file or from referral from other parties such as obstetrician, midwife or general practitioner. In some cases the research nurse approached women in the waiting room of either the hospital or midwifery centre. Posters and leaflets about this ongoing study were presented, and two centres used TV advertisement in the waiting room. Ultrasound booking scans early in pregnancy were a perfect opportunity in some countries to invite women. In Italy all pregnant women received a booklet with information on all the currently ongoing studies. An advertisement on the hospital website and hosting a website in the local language made DALI visible online. Applied tactics related to pregnancy expositions, newspaper adds, involvement of leaflets in oversized clothes shops and child day care centres led to an extending visibility of DALI, although were less successful in actually recruiting participants. In Table 4, the recruitment numbers for each country are presented separately. The exclusion numbers for GDM were around 22%, although in some countries this was as low as 7% (UK), while in others as high as 44% (Denmark-Odense).

The two most frequently mentioned reasons for participating in this study were the chance to reduce the risk of gestational diabetes (66%) and help society and science (55%). Learning more about lifestyle and pregnancy (36%) and receiving more ultrasound scans than usual (34%) helped subjects as well to decide to participate. Only 11% of the women indicated that more blood tests were a positive reason. A total of 30% of the women took part because someone (e.g. partner, friend, midwife, general practitioner) recommended this study.

Dose delivered

On average 4.0 (SD ± 1.6) F2F conversations and 2.1 (SD ± 1.6) telephone conversations were delivered to the women. In total 63% of the participants received all five F2F sessions. Furthermore, 9% of the participants received a total of four sessions, 13% a total of three

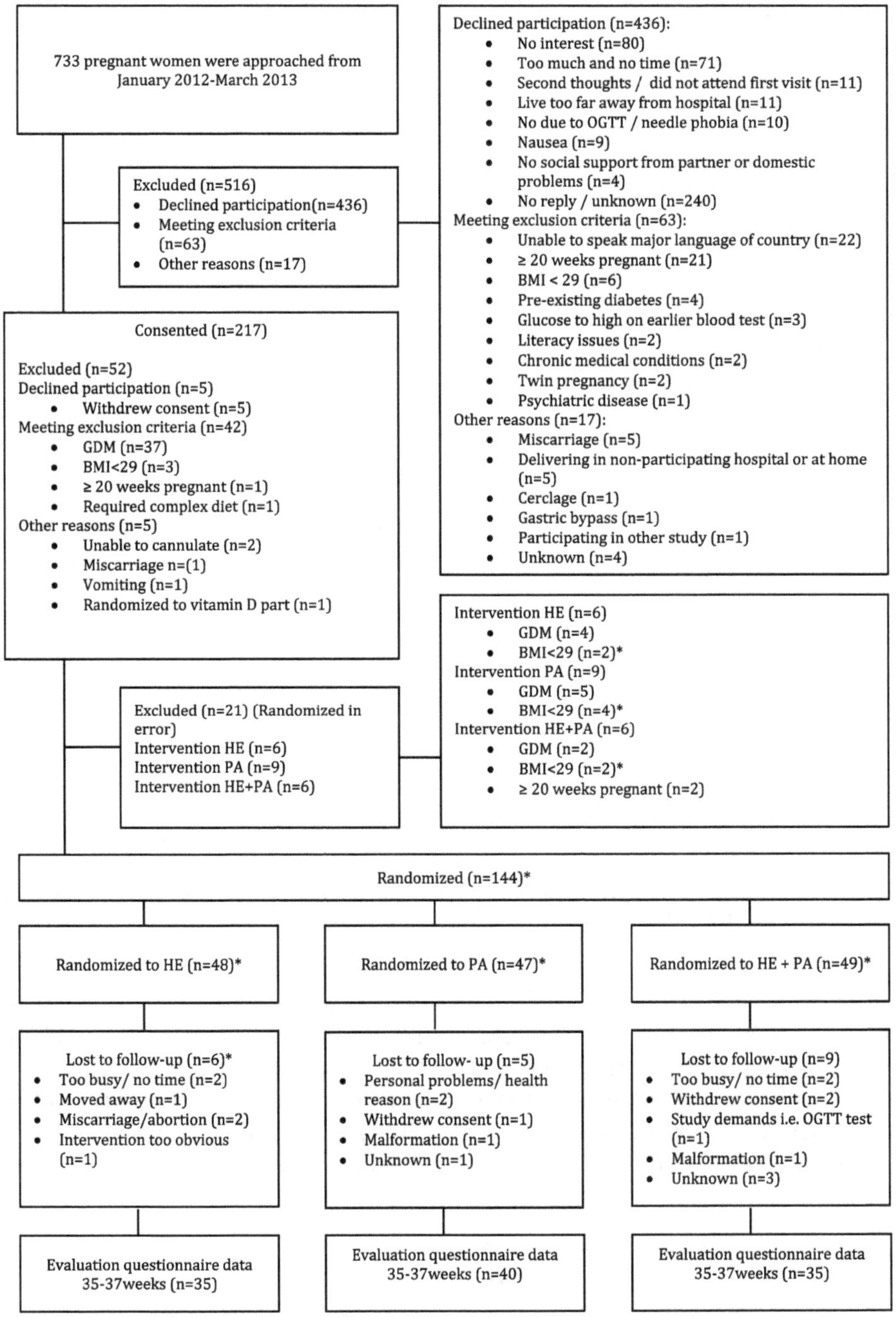

* Six of the eight women with a pre-pregnancy BMI below 29, but with a BMI above 29 at the first DALI visit will be considered included in the study. As a consequence the total number randomized adds to 150, with equal numbers ($n = 50$) in each lifestyle group. In the HE one additional woman dropped out due to an abortion.

Fig. 1 Flowchart of the DALI pilot study

sessions, 3% a total of two sessions and 4% only one session. Directly after randomization 8% of the women dropped out and did not receive any lifestyle intervention. On average the first F2F conversation lasted 52 (SD ± 15) minutes, the second F2F conversation lasted 43 (SD ± 13) minutes, the third F2F conversation lasted 38 (SD ± 11) minutes, the fourth F2F conversation lasted 38 (SD ± 12) minutes and the final F2F conversation lasted 34 (SD ± 12) minutes. The duration of the telephone conversations was on average 14 (SD ± 8) minutes. A total of 42% of the participants received the intended four F2F sessions prior to the second measurement. Twelve Belgium women preferred email support instead of the optional telephone calls.

Table 3 Recruitment strategies applied across Europe

Strategies:	AUT	BEL	DNK- CO	DNK- OD	ESP	GBR	ITA	IRL	NLD	POL
Referral based on BMI:										
Medical file (hospital)	x	x	x	x		x		x	x	x
Early ultrasound	x	x			x	x	x			x
General practitioner			x	x					x	
Obstetrician	x	x			x	x	x	x	x	x
Midwife		x	x	x	x	x	x	x	x	
Community midwife					x	x			x	
Other clinics (e.g. antenatal clinic, endocrinology department, private obstetrician)	x				x		x	x		x
In medical setting:										
Approached by research nurse waiting room	x	x			x	x			x	
Information on all research projects combined							x			
TV advertisement in waiting room		x	x							
poster, leaflets advertisement	x	x	x		x	x	x	x	x	x
Hospital website advertisement					x					
Outside medical setting:										
Advertisement in newspaper					x			x	x	
Advertisement in clothe shops									x	
Advertisement in day-care									x	
Radio								x		
Pregnancy exhibition									x	
QR codes			x							
Website (local language)			x						x	

Abbreviations: *AUT* Austria, *BEL* Belgium, *DNK-CO* Denmark Copenhagen, *DNK-OD* Denmark Odense, *ITA* Italy, *IRL* Ireland, *NLD* The Netherlands, *ESP* Spain, *POL* Poland, *GBR* United Kingdom, *BMI* body mass index

MI Fidelity

No audio records from the pilot study were available from four coaches working in Austria, Denmark (Odense), Italy (Padua) and Poland. In Italy and Poland participants refused consent for recording of the conversations, which made the practitioners reluctant for asking each time. In Austria and Denmark, the practitioners were not aware of the required audio recording. The aim was to select at least four sessions of each practitioners, although due to fewer available recordings (#3, #5, #7) or the exclusion of some recorded session due to recorded time (#2) this was not obtained for certain

Table 4 Recruitment numbers in each site in Europe

	AUT	BEL	DNK-CO	DNK-OD	ESP	GBR	IRL	ITA	NLD	POL	Total
Approached	91	67	84	140	39	118	46	45	71	32	733
Excluded	68	37	62	131	24	90	28	17	48	11	516
Declined	52	30	52	131	20	77	18	12	34	10	436
Excluded meeting exclusion criteria	15	6	5	0	3	9	7	5	13	0	63
Other reason	1	1	5	0	1	4	3	0	1	1	17
Consented	23	30	22	9	15	28	18	28	23	21	217
GDM	6	4	6	4	2	2	2	8	9	5	48
Other reason	1	3	2	2	2	8	5	1	1	0	25
Randomised	16	23	14	3	11	18	11	19	13	16	144

Abbreviations: *AUT* Austria, *BEL* Belgium, *DNK-CO* Denmark Copenhagen, *DNK-OD* Denmark Odense, *ITA* Italy, *IRL* Ireland, *NLD* The Netherlands, *ESP* Spain, *POL* Poland, *GBR* United Kingdom, *BMI* body mass index

Table 5 Fidelity rating on the MITI variables

Overall scores based on n conversations	#1 (n = 4)	#2[a] (n = 3)	#3[a,c] (n = 1)	#4[a] (n = 4)	#5 (n = 3)	#6[a] (n = 8)	#7 (n = 2)	#8 (n = 3)	OVERALL	Inter rater reliability scores[b]
Global scores										*KALPHA*
Evocation (>3.5)	**3.8**	**3.7**	-	**3.8**	1.7	**4.4**	2.0	3.0	3.1	0.76
Collaboration (>3.5)	**3.5**	3.3	-	3.3	1.7	**4.3**	2.5	2.7	3.0	0.75
Autonomy / Support (>3.5)	**4.3**	**4.0**	-	**3.8**	2.3	**4.0**	**3.5**	3.0	**3.5**	0.52
Spirit (>3.5)	**3.6**	**3.7**	-	**3.6**	1.9	**4.2**	2.7	2.9	3.2	0.83
Direction (>3.5)	**5.0**	**5.0**	-	**4.0**	**3.7**	**4.9**	**4.0**	**5.0**	**4.5**	0.86
Empathy (>3.5)	3.3	**3.7**	-	**4.0**	2.7	**4.5**	2.0	3.0	3.3	0.86
Behavioural counts										*ICC*
GI	20.1	30.8	6.0	20.1	10.3	14.9	11.5	16.8	15.9	0.81
MIA	4.9	8.0	4.0	7.3	9.7	4.1	18.5	6.3	7.7	0.80
MINA	0.6	1.0	0.0	1.8	12.0	0.3	14.5	1.3	3.8	0.55
CQ	13.0	18.5	1.0	16.0	8.7	10.2	26.0	12.8	12.8	0.83
OQ	4.9	7.2	5.0	8.3	5.7	6.3	12.0	6.5	6.9	0.71
SR	6.3	13.5	8.0	6.4	2.3	10.1	19.5	7.3	9.0	0.48
CR	0.1	4.7	6.0	5.6	5.7	10.8	4.5	0.5	4.6	0.91
% Open Questions (>50%)	29	28	**83**	36	41	37	31	34	41	0.64
% Complex Reflections (>40%)	2	24	**43**	**44**	**68**	**52**	13	7	31	0.85
Reflections/Questions ratio (>1.0)	0.36	0.71	**2.33**	0.52	0.78	**1.45**	0.76	0.40	0.94	0.58
% MI Adherent (>90%)	87	**90**	**100**	81	52	**95**	49	85	81	0.46
Number of pilot participants	9	11	14	10	12	12	11	18	97	
N recorded conversations/N total conversations	18/47	10/51	1/65	41/42	3/53	44/53	2/44	41/62		

Bold values represent scores are above 'beginning proficiency' according to the MITI 3.1.1. Numbered columns refer to individual coaches
Abbreviations: *GI* giving information, *MIA* MI Adherent, *MINA* MI non Adherent, *CQ* closed question, *OQ* open question, *SR* simple reflection, *CR* complex reflection; [a]Considered high in MI competence; [b]Intraclass reliability scores based on 20 out of the samples of Belgium, Ireland, Netherlands and UK (total of 5 coaches); [c]Only one session was recorded on the behavioural counts

practitioners. Practitioner #3 only had a session recorded on the behavioural counts. The analysed samples comprised 17.5% of the total available audio records. The results of each practitioner are presented in Table 5.

The practitioners had varying levels of MI skilfulness. All coaches had a global Direction score according to 'beginning proficiency'. Three practitioners (#2, #4, #6) reached a 'beginning proficiency' level for the global scores Spirit and Empathy. Two practitioners (#3 and #6) reached almost a 'beginning proficiency' level for all the behavioural counts as well, although most practitioners were far from these required levels. Two practitioners (#5 and #7) scored many MI non adherent statements (12 and 14.5 respectively). These statements were a result of advice giving without (implicit) permission. Overall, after correcting for the number of participants counselled in this study the MI scores reached 'beginning proficiency' for the global scores Direction and Autonomy/support, but scored below the cut off for the behavioural counts.

The inter-class reliability for the English and Dutch conversations on the behaviour counts ranged from fair to excellent (see Table 5). The global ratings Spirit, Empathy and Direction were all in the range for good reliability.

Satisfaction

The overall DALI intervention received an 8.6 (SD ± 1.4) from the participants. The practitioners were rated with a 9.2 (SD ± 1.1). The F2F conversations were rated with an 8.8 (SD ± 1.5) and the phone calls with an 8.2 (SD ± 1.9). The women in the HE + PA group or in the PA group gave a 7.7 (SD ± 2.5) for the exercise dynabands and an 8.4 (SD ± 1.9) for the pedometer. A total of 16% rated the exercise dynabands and 6% the pedometer a 5 or lower (somewhat useful). The received manual was rated in the HE + PA group with an 8.2 (SD ± 0.2) in the HE group with an 8.4 (SD ± 0.3) and in the PA group with a 7.6 (SD ± 0.3). Only 9% of the women rated the manual with a 5 (somewhat useful) or lower.

Table 6 Association for dose and fidelity with change in gestational weight from first to last measurement across the three lifestyle groups

Process elements: dose, context and fidelity	HE Mean (SD) *N*	HE + PA Mean (SD) *N*	PA Mean (SD) *N*	Gestational weight gain (kg) β (95%CI) HE	Gestational weight gain (kg) β (95%CI) HE + PA	Gestational weight gain (kg) β (95%CI) PA
Dose:						
Total number of F2F conversations	4.5 (1.0)	4.7 (0.6)	4.4 (1.2)	1.89	−0.89	−0.21
	34	34	37	(−0.78; 4.55)	(−3.45; 1.67)	(−1.60; 1.18)
Total number of contacts (F2F + phone/email)	7.5 (1.8)	7.1 (1.8)	6.6 (2.1)	0.08	−0.33	0.02
	34	34	37	(−1.41; 1.57)	(−1.23; 0.57)	(−0.75; 0.78)
Fidelity:						
Competence in Motivational Interviewing (high vs. low)[a]	0.50 (0.51)	0.54 (0.51)	0.42 (0.50)	1.11	−0.26	−3.13
	26	24	26	(−4.27; 6.49)	(−5.23; 4.71)	(−7.03; 0.77)
DALI as intended (MI + 5F2F) (yes vs. no)[b]	0.42 (0.50)	0.50 (0.51)	0.42 (0.50)	−0.32	−0.70	−3.13
	26	24	26	(−5.37; 5.09)	(−5.42; 4.02)	(−7.03; 0.77)

F2F face-to-face, *HE* healthy eating, *PA* physical activity, *HE + PA* healthy eating and physical activity, *MI* motivational interviewing. Gestational weight gain was calculated by subtracting the baseline weight from the weight measured at the final measurement and is corrected for BMI at baseline and total weeks between baseline and third measurement. If significant associations ($p < 0.05$) were found these were printed in bold. Significant negative beta's regression coefficients represent a beneficial effect (decline in weight gain) and vice versa

[a]'high' corresponds with four or more out of seven MITI elements according to 'beginning proficiency' on the MITI

[b]'yes' corresponds with a lifestyle coach who was more competent in MI and a participant who received five face-to-face sessions

Effectiveness

Baseline and follow up GWG data was available for a total of 105 participants and was used in the analysis. Table 6 shows no significant associations between process elements and GWG. Although not statistically significant, in the PA group the participants who were counselled by a practitioner who reached 'beginning proficiency' in MI had 3.1 kg less GWG (95%CI: -7.0 to 0.8) compared to those who were counselled by a practitioner who did not reach 'beginning proficiency' in MI. In the HE group those who received more F2F sessions had 1.9 kg (95% CI: -0.8 to 4.6) more GWG, although this was also not statistically significant and partly caused by one outlier who lost 7 kg and attended only one lifestyle session.

Discussion

This process evaluation yields valuable information about the implementation process of the DALI lifestyle pilot study in overweight and obese pregnant women during the course of pregnancy. Delivering an intervention across different countries, with several different languages and various cultures is a real challenge. Evaluation is therefore important and could assist researchers and practitioners in planning future studies. This study reached a subset of the target population and eventually included 20% of the invited women. Overall, the intervention was delivered satisfactorily with 63% of the women receiving all intervention sessions. Furthermore, high variability between practitioners for MI competency resulted in an overall MI score not fulfilling expert opinion. Neither the implementation of MI (fidelity) nor the degree of participation in the intervention (dose delivered) was associated with the primary study outcome GWG.

With regard to reach, one-third of the invited women were willing to participate in this study, which is similar to the response rate of this target population in other intervention studies [37, 38]. The low response rate has implications for the generalizability of the results, as this sample was self-selective and research participants are mostly more motivated to change lifestyle behaviour in comparison to non-responders [39]. The requirement for women to attend three measurement sessions on top of the coaching sessions likely led to lower participation rates, as many women mentioned that the study demanded too much of their time. Additionally, ten women had a previous negative experience with the OGTT and would definitely not undergo this testing once more. On the other hand, the design of the study including individual F2F sessions with delivery at home (if preferred), might have resulted in a higher attractiveness and flexibility for women to participate than studies that require attending group sessions on fixed times and places. Furthermore, the incorporation of healthcare professionals ((community) midwifes, obstetricians, general practitioners) during the recruitment phase definitely led to an extended noticeability.

In comparison to previous studies the dose delivered of the F2F sessions is high, since for example in the UPBEAT pilot study only 6% attended the complete intervention (one F2F session followed by eight weekly group sessions) [37] and in the FitFor2 study only 16.3% attended half of the exercise sessions [38]. Similar attendance rates were found in the LIP study where 92% attended the four dietary counselling sessions and 56% attended half of the intended exercise sessions [40]. Only higher attendance rates were found in a study among Hispanic overweight women, in which 86% received all six prenatal lifestyle sessions [41].

The fidelity of the intervention delivery did not achieve scores above the MITI summary thresholds, although high variance of MI competence was observed between the practitioners. It is very likely that earlier experiences, professional background, personality and culture led to more (or less) skill quality and use of MI principles and as a consequence to a difference in the deliverance of the intervention across sites. This study was not designed to employ already highly skilled coaches. It was designed as a pragmatic trial to relate closely to the situation in actual clinical practice, whereby practitioners were trained in the beginning of this study under ideal training conditions, but needed to deliver their skills in the less predictable field setting. The delivery of this intervention was standardized (e.g. manuals for the coach, manuals for the participant, standardized training) to give practitioners some guidance, but obviously there is an inherent tension between a manualised intervention and the use of MI [42]. So far, the optimum amount of structure to offer practitioners is unclear when wanting them to integrate MI into practice. Certification of practitioners was based on attendance and completion of all requirements, not on quality in using MI skills. Future studies might reconsider this design and build audio recorded supervision into the training process, so coaches receive a mix of workshops and supervision (feedback) of actual practice over a longer time period, which would allow them to develop competence [21, 43–46]. A recent meta-analysis of training studies recommends 3–4 supervision sessions over a six-month period [45]. Supervisors should try to improve the quality of practitioners in evoking change talk (encouraging language about desire, ability, reason and need for behaviour change and commitment to it) and softening sustain talk (avoiding the focus on reasons against changing or maintaining the current situation) [47], since the expression of change talk is directly linked to the practitioners behaviour [48]. In addition, training practitioners in asking permission prior to giving advice is important in research studies were some form of knowledge transfer should harmonize with an MI approach.

The participants were highly satisfied with the intervention and with their lifestyle coach, even though this study was not able to reach a sufficient proficiency level in MI. One of the components in the coach rating was the item 'helped you rather than told you what to do', which is one of the key goals of MI. All participants scored an eight or higher for this item, with the exception of two participants (score of seven and a score of a three) both for a coach considered less skilled in the use of MI.

The secondary aim of this research paper was to investigate the association of dose and fidelity with change in GWG. In the previously published study of Simmons et al. (2015), it was shown that women gained 7.6, 8.5 and 9.6 kg respectively in the HE group, the HE + PA group and the PA group [17]. Purely hypothetical, the non-significant positive association found in the PA group for fidelity and GWG might suggest that the skilfulness of MI is essential when focusing on changing physical activity behaviours. This might suggest a need for training health professionals to a certain skill level of delivering behavioural change interventions, especially since gestational weight gain in the PA group was largest. However the sample size of the current study was probably the foremost reason no significant associations were found between dose, fidelity and GWG. Repeating this analysis in a larger study is needed to confirm the dose-response (more sessions better weight results) relation found in a non-pregnant population [49, 50].

Strength and limitations

One has to balance in conducting a trial such as this between weighing up what is possible to achieve pragmatically and the potential loss of completeness in fidelity data. Not having double coding of the Spanish, Danish and Italian study session due to costs, the use of the Spanish MITI 3.0, and presenting only behavioural count data of #3 are limitations of this study, but the alternative was not to have this data, as was the case in previous MI studies among this target population [51, 52]. We believe these data are of great value for the evaluation process. A lesson learned from the pilot study is that throughout the study the collection of audio recordings should be ensured [28]. In the current study we lacked data from four practitioners, and of the other practitioners not all sessions were audio recorded, which might have led to a biased sample. Another limitation of this study is the gathering of satisfaction data at the end of pregnancy, therefore the response applied only to those who completed the study.

Notwithstanding the previous mentioned limitations, the findings of the present study are important. They provide insight in the 'black box' of the DALI pilot lifestyle intervention and allow for a more in-depth analysis of the outcomes. This study provides useful information across different countries, with its various health services, and is valuable for those planning to use MI in future intervention studies both in research and in practice. Moreover, it is one of the few studies that analysed fidelity of MI. Also, in contrast to other process evaluations, we investigated the association between separate process elements and the primary outcome measure of the study.

Conclusion

Overall, these findings suggest that the DALI intervention with five MI lifestyle sessions was well received across a range of European countries and may even be feasible to implement more widely across Europe. Even though the performance of most of the practitioners in this study left room for improvement, some practitioners did adequately apply certain principles. Key lessons learned from this pilot study include; 1) that more research is needed to investigate which program adaptations are needed to attract the large group of non-responders to participate in a lifestyle intervention during pregnancy; 2) ensuring audio recording of all lifestyle sessions throughout the study; and 3) providing individualized feedback to practitioners throughout the study to increase the chances of achieving MI proficiency. Furthermore, future studies are encouraged to evaluate and report fidelity of MI in their study as to facilitate comparison among trials.

Abbreviations

BMI: Body mass index; F2F: Face-to-face; GDM: Gestational diabetes mellitus; GWG: Gestational weight gain; ICC: Intra-class correlation coefficient; KALPHA: Krippendorff's Alpha; MI: Motivational interviewing; MITI: Motivational Interviewing Treatment Integrity Scale

Acknowledgements

We would like to acknowledge all involved participants and thank them for sharing their experiences and views. Furthermore we would like to acknowledge all lifestyle coaches involved in counselling the participants and all research nurses for the data collection. Additionally, we would like to acknowledge Vera Mertens, Pilar Lusilla, Helene Foss Kjeldsen and Gian Paolo Guelfi for assisting in the MITI codings and providing practitioners with feedback. Furthermore we would like to acknowledge Sarah Donald and Candice Ward for providing the central MI training.
I confirm all patient/personal identifiers have been removed or disguised so the patient/person(s) described are not identifiable and cannot be identified through the details of the story.

Funding

The research leading to these results has received funding from the European Community's 7th Framework Programme (FP7/2007–2013) under Grant Agreement no 242187 and from The Netherlands Organization for Health Research and Development (ZonMw), grant number:200310013. In Poland, additional funding was obtained from Polish Ministry of Science (Grant nr 2203/7. PR/2011/2). In Denmark, additional funding was provided by Odense University Free Research Fund. In the UK, The DALI team acknowledge the support received from the NIHR Clinical Research Network: Eastern, especially the local diabetes clinical & research teams based in Cambridge. In Spain, additional funding was provided by CAIBER 1527-B-226. The funders had no role in any aspect of the study beyond funding.

Authors' contributions

JJ contributed to the data analysis and writing of the manuscript and took the lead in redrafting the script following editorial review. DS coordinated the study. JJ DS SG GD RC AKW JH AA RD DT DH PD EM EWO AZ AL MD SDP AB FD DJ LA FS MP contributed to the conception and design of the study. FJ KB GJ JJ SG JH contributed to the acquisition of data. NG SR MP contributed to the analysis and interpretation of data. All authors read and corrected draft versions of the manuscript and approved the final manuscript. All authors agreed to be accountable for all aspects of the work.

Competing interests

The authors declare that they have no competing interests.

Author details

[1]Department of Public and Occupational Health and, Amsterdam Public Health research institute, VU University Medical Centre, Van der Boechorststraat 7, 1081BT Amsterdam, Amsterdam, The Netherlands. [2]Institute of Metabolic Science, Addenbrookes Hospital, Cambridge, England, UK. [3]Macarthur Clinical School, University of Western Sydney, Campbelltown, NSW, Australia. [4]School of Medicine, Cardiff University, Cardiff, Wales, UK. [5]Medical Faculty I, Poznan University of Medical Sciences, Poznan, Poland. [6]KU Leuven Department of Development and Regeneration: Pregnancy, Fetus and Neonate Gynaecology and Obstetrics, University Hospitals Leuven, Leuven, Belgium. [7]Department of Obstetrics and Gynaecology Division of Obstetrics and Prenatal Medicine Erasmus MC, University Medical Centre Rotterdam, Rotterdam, The Netherlands. [8]Department of Obstetrics and Gynecology, Medizinische Universität Graz, Graz, Austria. [9]Institut de Recerca de L'Hospital de la Santa Creu i Sant Pau, Barcelona, Spain. [10]CIBER Bioengineering, Biomaterials and Nanotechnology, Instituto de Salud Carlos III, Madrid, Spain. [11]Medical University of Vienna, Vienna City, Austria. [12]Recherche en Santé Lawson SA, St. Gallen, Switzerland. [13]Center for Pregnant Women with Diabetes, Departments of Endocrinology and Obstetrics, Rigshospitalet, Faculty of Health Sciences, University of Copenhagen, Copenhagen, Denmark. [14]Universita Degli Studi di Padova, Padova, Italy. [15]Università di Pisa, Pisa, Italy. [16]National University of Ireland, Galway, Ireland. [17]Odense University Hospital, Odense, Denmark. [18]Department of Medical Psychology, Amsterdam Public Health research institute, VU University Medical Centre, Amsterdam, The Netherlands. [19]Department of Medical Psychology, Academic Medical Centre, Amsterdam, The Netherlands. [20]Institute of Sport Science, University of Graz, Graz, Austria.

References

1. O'Reilly JR, Reynolds RM. The risk of maternal obesity to the long-term health of the offspring. Clin Endocrinol. 2013;78:9–16.
2. IOM (Institute of Medicine) and NRC (National Research Council). Weight Gain During Pregnancy: Reexamining the Guidelines. Washington (DC): National Academies Press (US); 2009.
3. Gilmore LA, Klempel-Donchenko M, Redman LM. Pregnancy as a window to future health: excessive gestational weight gain and obesity. Semin Perinatol. 2015;39:296–303.

4. Thangaratinam S, Rogozinska E, Jolly K, Glinkowski S, Roseboom T, Tomlinson JW, et al. Effects of interventions in pregnancy on maternal weight and obstetric outcomes: meta-analysis of randomised evidence. BMJ. 2012;344:e2088.
5. Choi J, Fukuoka Y, Lee JH. The effects of physical activity and physical activity plus diet interventions on body weight in overweight or obese women who are pregnant or in postpartum: a systematic review and meta-analysis of randomized controlled trials. Prev Med. 2013;56:351–64.
6. Sui Z, Grivell RM, Dodd JM. Antenatal exercise to improve outcomes in overweight or obese women: a systematic review. Acta Obstet Gynecol Scand. 2012;91:538–45.
7. Burke BL, Arkowitz H, Menchola M. The efficacy of motivational interviewing: a meta-analysis of controlled clinical trials. J Consult Clin Psychol. 2003;71:843–61.
8. Hettema J, Steele J, Miller WR. Motivational interviewing. Annu Rev Clin Psychol. 2005;1:91–111.
9. Rubak S, Sandbaek A, Lauritzen T, Christensen B. Motivational interviewing: a systematic review and meta-analysis. Br J Gen Pract. 2005;55:305–12.
10. Lundahl BW, Kunz C, Brownell C, Tollefson D, Burke BL. A meta-analysis of motivational interviewing: twenty-five years of empirical studies. Res Soc Work Pract. 2010;20:137–60.
11. Lundahl B, Moleni T, Burke BL, Butters R, Tollefson D, Butler C, et al. Motivational interviewing in medical care settings: a systematic review and meta-analysis of randomized controlled trials. Patient Educ Couns. 2013;93:157–68.
12. Martins RK, McNeil DW. Review of motivational interviewing in promoting health behaviors. Clin Psychol Rev. 2009;29:283–93.
13. Lindhardt CL, Rubak S, Mogensen O, Hansen HP, Goldstein H, Lamont RF, et al. Healthcare professionals experience with motivational interviewing in their encounter with obese pregnant women. Midwifery. 2015;31:678–84.
14. Hill B, Skouteris H, Fuller-Tyszkiewicz M. Interventions designed to limit gestational weight gain: a systematic review of theory and meta-analysis of intervention components. Obes Rev. 2013;14:435–50.
15. Miller WR, Rollnick S: Motivational interviewing: third edition: helping people change. 2013.
16. Jelsma JG, van Poppel MN, Galjaard S, Desoye G, Corcoy R, Devlieger R, et al. DALI: vitamin D and lifestyle intervention for gestational diabetes mellitus (GDM) prevention: an European multicentre, randomised trial – study protocol. BMC Pregnancy Childbirth. 2013;13:142.
17. Simmons D, Jelsma JG, Galjaard S, Devlieger R, Van AA JG, et al. Results from a European multicenter randomized trial of physical activity and/or healthy eating to reduce the risk of gestational diabetes mellitus: the DALI lifestyle pilot. Diabetes Care. 2015;38:1650–6.
18. Linnan L, Steckler A. Process evaluation for public health interventions and research. San Francisco: Jossey-Bass; 2002.
19. Moore GF, Audrey S, Barker M, Bond L, Bonell C, Hardeman W, et al. Process evaluation of complex interventions: Medical Research Council guidance. BMJ. 2015;350:h1258.
20. Bellg AJ, Borrelli B, Resnick B, Hecht J, Minicucci DS, Ory M, et al. Enhancing treatment fidelity in health behavior change studies: best practices and recommendations from the NIH behavior change consortium. Health Psychol. 2004;23:443–51.
21. Miller WR, Rollnick S. The effectiveness and ineffectiveness of complex behavioral interventions: impact of treatment fidelity. Contemp Clin Trials. 2014;37:234–41.
22. Grant A, Treweek S, Dreischulte T, Foy R, Guthrie B. Process evaluations for cluster-randomised trials of complex interventions: a proposed framework for design and reporting. Trials. 2013;14:15.
23. Glasgow RE, Vogt TM, Boles SM. Evaluating the public health impact of health promotion interventions: the RE-AIM framework. Am J Public Health. 1999;89:1322–7.
24. Saunders RP, Evans MH, Joshi P. Developing a process-evaluation plan for assessing health promotion program implementation: a how-to guide. Health Promot Pract. 2005;6:134–47.
25. Metzger BE, Gabbe SG, Persson B, Buchanan TA, Catalano PA, Damm P, et al. International association of diabetes and pregnancy study groups recommendations on the diagnosis and classification of hyperglycemia in pregnancy. Diabetes Care. 2010;33:676–82.
26. Miller WR, Moyers TB. Eight stages of learning motivational interviewing. Journal of Teaching in the Addictions. 2006;5:3–17.
27. Moyers TB, Martin T, Manuel JK, Miller WR, Ernst D. Revised Global Scales: Motivational Interviewing Treatment Integrity 3.1.1 (MITI 3.1.1). 22-1-2010.
28. Jelsma JG, Mertens VC, Forsberg L, Forsberg L. How to measure motivational interviewing Fidelity in randomized controlled trials: practical recommendations. Contemp Clin Trials. 2015;43:93–9.
29. Moyers TB, Martin T, Manuel JK, Hendrickson SM, Miller WR. Assessing competence in the use of motivational interviewing. J Subst Abus Treat. 2005;28:19–26.
30. Forsberg L, Berman AH, Kallmen H, Hermansson U, Helgason AR. A test of the validity of the motivational interviewing treatment integrity code. Cogn Behav Ther. 2008;37:183–91.
31. Forsberg L, Kallmen H, Hermansson U, Berman AH, Helgason AR. Coding counsellor behaviour in motivational interviewing sessions: inter-rater reliability for the Swedish motivational interviewing treatment integrity code (MITI). Cogn Behav Ther. 2007;36:162–9.
32. Pierson HM, Hayes SC, Gifford EV, Roget N, Padilla M, Bissett R, et al. An examination of the motivational interviewing treatment integrity code. J Subst Abus Treat. 2007;32:11–7.
33. Moyers TB, Martin T, Manuel JK, Miller WR, Ernst D. Revised Global Scales: Motivational Interviewing Treatment Integrity 3.0 (MITI 3.0). 25-6-2007.
34. Hayes AF, Krippendorff K. Answering the call for a standard reliability measure for coding data. Communication Methods and Measures. 2007;1:77–89.
35. De Swert K. Calculating inter-coder reliability in media content analysis using Krippendorff's alpha. 2012.
36. Cicchetti DV, Sparrow SA. Developing criteria for establishing interrater reliability of specific items: applications to assessment of adaptive behavior. Am J Ment Defic. 1981;86:127–37.
37. Poston L, Briley AL, Barr S, Bell R, Croker H, Coxon K, et al. Developing a complex intervention for diet and activity behaviour change in obese pregnant women (the UPBEAT trial); assessment of behavioural change and process evaluation in a pilot randomised controlled trial. BMC Pregnancy Childbirth. 2013;13:148.
38. Oostdam N, van Poppel MN, Wouters MG, Eekhoff EM, Bekedam DJ, Kuchenbecker WK, et al. No effect of the FitFor2 exercise programme on blood glucose, insulin sensitivity, and birthweight in pregnant women who were overweight and at risk for gestational diabetes: results of a randomised controlled trial. BJOG. 2012;119:1098–107.
39. Lakerveld J, Ijzelenberg W, van Tulder MW, Hellemans IM, Rauwerda JA, van Rossum AC, et al. Motives for (not) participating in a lifestyle intervention trial. BMC Med Res Methodol. 2008;8:17.
40. Vinter CA, Jensen DM, Ovesen P, Beck-Nielsen H, Jorgensen JS. The LiP (lifestyle in pregnancy) study: a randomized controlled trial of lifestyle intervention in 360 obese pregnant women. Diabetes Care. 2011;34:2502–7.
41. Hawkins M, Hosker M, Marcus BH, Rosal MC, Braun B, Stanek EJ III, et al. A pregnancy lifestyle intervention to prevent gestational diabetes risk factors in overweight Hispanic women: a feasibility randomized controlled trial. Diabet Med. 2015;32:108–15.
42. Lundahl B, Burke BL. The effectiveness and applicability of motivational interviewing: a practice-friendly review of four meta-analyses. J Clin Psychol. 2009;65:1232–45.
43. Madson MB, Loignon AC, Lane C. Training in motivational interviewing: a systematic review. J Subst Abus Treat. 2009;36:101–9.
44. Miller WR, Yahne CE, Moyers TB, Martinez J, Pirritano M. A randomized trial of methods to help clinicians learn motivational interviewing. J Consult Clin Psychol. 2004;72:1050–62.
45. Schwalbe CS, Oh HY, Zweben A. Sustaining motivational interviewing: a meta-analysis of training studies. Addiction. 2014;109:1287–94.

46. Walters ST, Matson SA, Baer JS, Ziedonis DM. Effectiveness of workshop training for psychosocial addiction treatments: a systematic review. J Subst Abus Treat. 2005;29:283–93.
47. Moyers TB, Manuel JK, Ernst D. Motivational Interviewing Treatment Integrity Coding Manual 4.1. Unpublished manual. 2014.
48. Glynn LH, Moyers TB. Chasing change talk: the clinician's role in evoking client language about change. J Subst Abus Treat. 2010;39:65–70.
49. Chao D, Farmer D, Sevick M, Espeland M, Vitolins M, Naughton M. The value of session attendance in a weight-loss intervention. Am J Health Behav. 2000;24:413–21.
50. Byrne S, Barry D, Petry NM. Predictors of weight loss success. Exercise vs. dietary self-efficacy and treatment attendance. Appetite. 2012;58:695–8.
51. Claesson IM, Sydsjo G, Brynhildsen J, Cedergren M, Jeppsson A, Nystrom F, et al. Weight gain restriction for obese pregnant women: a case-control intervention study. BJOG. 2008;115:44–50.
52. Bogaerts AF, Devlieger R, Nuyts E, Witters I, Gyselaers W, Van den Bergh BR. Effects of lifestyle intervention in obese pregnant women on gestational weight gain and mental health: a randomized controlled trial. Int J Obes. 2013;37:814–21.

4

Prevalence and predictors of early gestational weight gain associated with obesity risk in a diverse Australian antenatal population

K. Cheney[1,3*], S. Berkemeier[2], K.A. Sim[4], A. Gordon[3,5] and K. Black[1,3]

Abstract

Background: Excess gestational weight gain (GWG) leads to adverse short- and long-term consequences for women and their offspring. Evidence suggests that excess GWG in early pregnancy may be particularly detrimental, contributing to the intergenerational cycle of obesity. The primary outcome was to investigate the prevalence and predictors of excess GWG in early pregnancy, and if women understand the risks to themselves and their offspring stratified by maternal body mass index (BMI).

Methods: This was a secondary analysis (n = 2131) of a cross-sectional study (n = 2338) conducted over 6 months in 2015 of pregnant women attending antenatal clinics at four maternity hospitals across Sydney, Australia before 22 completed weeks gestation An self-completed questionnaire was used to investigate knowledge of expected weight gain in pregnancy, understanding of risks associated with excess GWG, self-reported anthropometric measures and socio-demographic data.

Results: One third (34.2%) of women gained weight in excess of the recommendations by 22 completed weeks gestation. Women who were overweight (OR: 1.69, 95% CI: 1.33–2.14) or obese (OR: 1.64, 95% CI: 1.20–2.24) pre-pregnancy were more likely to gain excess weight in early pregnancy compared to normal weight women; as were women from lower socio-economic areas (OR: 1.89, 95% CI: 1.49–2.41). Half (51%) the women were unsure about the effect of excess GWG on their baby; 11% did not believe that excess GWG would affect the weight of the baby and 14% did not believe that excess GWG would affect longer term outcomes for their baby. Women who gained weight above the recommendations were significantly more likely to believe that excessive GWG in pregnancy would not have any adverse future effect on health outcomes or weight of their baby.

Conclusions: The women at particular risk of excess early GWG are those who are overweight and obese and/or residing in lower socio-economic areas. These women need to be targeted for appropriate counselling preconception or in early pregnancy. Given the significant adverse outcomes associated with excess GWG in early pregnancy, preconception or early pregnancy counselling with respect to GWG and intervention research regarding best approach remains a public health priority.

Keywords: Early pregnancy, Obesity, Overweight, Gestational weight gain

* Correspondence: kate.cheney@sswahs.nsw.gov.au
[1]Women's and Babies, Royal Prince Alfred Hospital, Missenden Road, Camperdown, Sydney, NSW 2050, Australia
[3]Discipline of Obstetrics, Gynaecology and Neonatology, The University of Sydney, Sydney, NSW 2006, Australia
Full list of author information is available at the end of the article

Background

Excessive gestational weight gain (GWG) is an independent risk factor for a myriad of short and long-term complications for both the mother and her offspring [1–3]. In 2009, the United States Institute of Medicine (IOM) published updated guidelines to provide direction to health professionals around healthy GWG expectations [4]. These guidelines are pre-pregnancy body mass index (BMI) specific and are used to guide clinicians when counselling women regarding weight gain in pregnancy.

While research has focused on overall GWG, trimester specific gains are of growing interest with respect to adverse outcomes. In the short term, excess GWG in the first half of pregnancy irrespective of pre-pregnancy BMI has been shown to increase the risk of gestational diabetes, hypertensive diseases of pregnancy and macrosomia [5–8]. Longer term consequences include greater postpartum weight retention, increased waist circumference and systolic blood pressure in women up to 7 years postpartum [9, 10]. Excess early pregnancy weight gain, in particular, has been shown to be an independent risk factor for development of gestational diabetes and maternal hyperglycaemia [6, 11, 12]. This may be due to the increase in maternal fat mass during early pregnancy which can increase insulin resistance and thus increase the risk of impaired glucose intolerance [11]. Furthermore, while there should be minimal gain physiologically in the first trimester, excess first trimester weight gain has also been shown to increase the risk of overweight and obesity in offspring in the first 4 years of life [13, 14].

A lack of awareness regarding the risk of excess GWG on health outcomes for the mother and her offspring may be an important factor for excessive GWG [15]. Pregnant woman who are already overweight or obese are less likely to be educated about weight gain recommendations than normal weight women, and have been shown to receive information conflicting with the IOM recommendations [16].

Methods

The primary aim of this study was to examine the prevalence and specific health and socio-economic factors which may predict excess early GWG in a diverse early pregnant population. Secondly, we sought to examine the participants understanding of their GWG expectations specific to their BMI and, the significance of GWG on the health outcomes for their baby.

Participants

This was a secondary analysis of a questionnaire (Additional file 1: Table S1) based study examining a relationship between BMI and pregnancy intention. At the second antenatal clinic visit, questionnaires were given to women who then returned them to a collection box. At the Royal Prince Alfred Hospital (RPAH) and Canterbury Hospital, a full-time midwife researcher recruited the women, while at Fairfield and Campbelltown Hospitals midwives in the antenatal clinic recruited on a pragmatic basis. Participants indicated consent by signing g a consent form and ticking a box on the questionnaire and completed it privately. Refusals were recorded at all of recruitment centers. This study was approved by the Human Research Ethics Committees of the participating sites. Ethics approval was obtained from Sydney Local Health District Ethics Review Committee (protocol number X14–0341; HREC/14/RPAH/459) and from the Sydney South West Area Health Service Ethics Review Committee (HREC/14/LPOOL/201).

Study protocol

The original cross sectional analysis of 2313 women was conducted between March and December 2015, using an anonymous, self-completed brief questionnaire including health, socio-demographic data, anthropometry, a self-reported pre-pregnancy weight and weight measured at the second antenatal visit. All women were eligible to complete the survey if they were over 16 years of age, less than 22 weeks pregnant, had a singleton pregnancy and were able to complete the questionnaire in English or one of the other languages the questionnaire was translated into (Mandarin, Vietnamese, Arabic and Korean; the most common language groups at the participating hospitals). The cut-off gestation of 21^{+6} weeks was used as it was the gestation at the second antenatal visit and half way through the second trimester. Women specified their gestational age (by completed weeks) at the time of completion of the survey.

Measurements

GWG was calculated by subtracting their self-reported pre-pregnancy weight from the maternal weight measured at the time of the second visit, allowing for the maximum recommended GWG in the first trimester weight gain of 2 kg [1] and then calculating the mean total weekly weight gain (in grams) by dividing their weight gain beyond the first trimester by the amount of weeks in their second trimester that were completed This was compared with the IOM recommended rate of GWG specific for each BMI category (Table 1). Excess weight gain was defined as greater than the recommended upper limit of weekly weight gain per the IOM guidelines for the specific pre-pregnancy BMI categories. BMI is calculated as weight in kilograms divided by height in metres squared (kg/m^2).

GWG and BMI were also examined with respect to other sociodemographic and health determinants.

Table 1 Institute of Medicine weight gain recommendations for pregnancy by BMI category [1]

Pre-pregnancy body mass index	Body mass index (kg/m^2)	Recommended range of total weight (kg)	Recommended rates of weight gain [a] in the second and third trimesters (kg) (mean range [kg/week])
Underweight	< 18.5	12.5–18	0.51 (0.44–0.58)
Normal weight	18.5–24.9	11.5–16	0.42 (0.35–0.50)
Overweight	25–29.9	7–11.5	0.28 (0.23–0.33)
Obese (includes all classes)	≥ 30	5–9	0.22 (0.17–0.27)

[a]Calculations assume a 0.5–2 kg weight gain in the first trimester

Women were asked to specify their postcode in order to establish their socio-economic status (SES) using the index of relative disadvantage; a low score indicates a comparative lack of social advantage [17]. Ethnicity was self-reported and was categorised into ethnic groups; Caucasian, Asian (including Southern Asian), Middle Eastern/African, Pacific Islander/Maori, South American and Aboriginal/Torres Strait Islander. Women were also asked to complete questions regarding how much weight they expected to gain during the pregnancy and their understanding of the effect of excessive GWG on their pregnancy, the weight of their baby and their knowledge of longer term outcomes.

Statistical analysis

Univariate and multivariable logistic regression was used to examine the association between excess maternal GWG, sociodemographic characteristics as well as expected GWG and understanding of GWG on outcomes. The variables included in the multivariable logistic regression model were those that had significance with a p value <0.25 in the univariate analysis as well as those considered relevant to the research question which was informed by the literature, for example, age group. Chi-squared significance tests were performed to establish whether there was an association with excess weight gain in the specific BMI categories, excess weight gain and understanding of the effect of weight gain on outcomes for the baby. Statistical analysis was performed using IBM© Statistical Package for the Social Sciences (SPSS) version 23.0 (Armonk, NY: IBM Corp).

Results

A total of 2313 women completed the questionnaire, of these 2021 were included in this study. Those excluded (n = 292, 12.6%) had missing anthropometry data necessary to enable analysis of GWG or BMI. There were 14 refusals at RPA and Canterbury Hospitals (0.6%), 40 (15.7%) refusals at Campbelltown and 12 (0.3%) from Fairfield. The mean gestational age at recruitment was 19.4 weeks. Maternal socio-demographic characteristics and related variables are shown in Table 2. Underweight women comprised 6.4% (n = 129), normal weight 60.7% (n = 1227), overweight 21.1% (n = 427) and 11.8% (n = 238) obese.

Gestational weight gain

One third (34.2%; n = 692) of women in the study gained weight in excess of the IOM recommendations by 21 weeks and six days. Of the women who were in the normal weight range, 29.7% (n = 365) had an excessive rate of weight gain, compared with 43.1% (n = 184) of overweight and 45.8% (n = 109) of obese women. The distribution of weekly weight gain per BMI group is demonstrated in Table 3. Compared to women with a healthy pre-pregnancy BMI, overweight (odds ratio [OR] 1.79; 95% confidence interval [95% CI] 1.42–2.25; p < 0.005) and obese women (OR 2.0, 95% CI, 1.50–2.65; p < 0.005) were significantly more likely to gain excess weight.

Predictors of excess gestational weight gain

Univariate analysis of excess GWG (specific to BMI) and sociodemographic predictor variables are shown in Table 4. This demonstrated a significant association of excess weight gain with Middle Eastern/African ethnicity (OR 1.72; 95% CI: 1.28–2.31; p < 0.005) and Pacific Islander/Maori background (OR 1.69, 95% CI: 1.07–2.65; p = 0.023). Women of Muslim faith were more likely to have excess early GWG compared with women from Christian faith (OR 1.45, 95% CI: 1.09–1.93; p = 0.011). Women from a low SES were twice as likely to gain excess weight compared with women from a higher SES (OR 2.07; 95% CI: 1.69–2.54; p < 0.005).

In a multivariate analysis (Table 5), women who were overweight (OR 1.69, 95% CI: 1.33–2.14, p < 0.005) or obese (OR 1.64, 95% CI: 1.20–2.24, p = 0.002) at booking visit were significantly more likely to have excess GWG compared to normal weight women. Low SES background remained a significant independent factor in predicting excess GWG (OR 1.89; 95% CI: 1.49–2.41; p < 0.005). However, there was no significant association seen between ethnicity and excess GWG after adjusting for confounders using multivariate analysis. There were also no significant associations between excessive early GWG with age group, religion, smoking, education or employment.

Table 2 Frequency distribution of maternal sociodemographic characteristics

	Frequency (%)
Age (years)	
16–24 years	353 (17.1%)
25–34 years	1279 (61.9%)
≥ 35	424 (20.5%)
Maternal body mass index (kg/m^2)	
Underweight (< 18.5)	129 (6.4%)
Normal weight (18.5–24.9)	1227 (60.7%)
Overweight (25–29.9)	427 (21.1%)
Obese (> 30)	238 (11.8%)
Relationship status	
Married/de-facto	1859 (89.9%)
Single/widowed/separated	192 (9.3%)
Smoking	
Non-smoker	1974 (95.6%)
Smoker	87 (4.2%)
Maternal ethnicity	
Caucasian	824 (40%)
Asian	815 (39.5%)
Middle Eastern/Africa	237 (11.5%)
Aboriginal or Torres Strait Islander	32 (1/6%)
Pacific Islander/Maori	85 (4.1%)
South American (Latino)	28 (1.4%)
Maternal religion	
Christian	735 (35.6%)
Hindu	143 (6.9%)
Buddhist	104 (5%)
Muslim	270 (13.1%)
No religion	724 (35%)
Other	91 (4.4%)
Maternal education	
Tertiary	1090 (52.7%)
High school	525 (25.4%)
Other (nil, primary)	412 (19.9%)
Socio-economic status	
Low	611 (29.6%)
Medium	243 (11.8%)
High	1165 (56.4%)
Employment	
Working	1220 (59%)
Studying	148 (7.2%)
Unemployed/disability	661 (32%)
Pregnancy loss	
No loss	1312 (80%)
Previous miscarriage, termination or stillbirth	328 (20%)
Medical conditions in pregnancy	
Type 1 diabetes	12 (0.6%)
Type 2 diabetes	32 (1.5%)
Hypertension	82 (4%)
High cholesterol	28 (1.4%)

Knowledge regarding GWG

Chi-squared analysis was performed on a relationship between baseline BMI and women's estimation of weight gain in their pregnancy. Overweight and obese women were significantly more likely to estimate a higher weight than what is recommended for their BMI ($\chi^2 = 922.38$; $p < 0.005$). The proportion of women who overestimated the amount of weight gain they should gain during pregnancy was, respectively, overweight women 73.5% and obese 85.8%.

Half (51.0%; $n = 1057$) the cohort were unsure about whether excess GWG would affect outcomes for their baby; 10.8% ($n = 223$) did not believe that excess GWG would affect the weight of the baby and 13.7% ($n = 283$) of women did not believe that excess GWG would affect longer term outcomes for their baby. Women who gained weight above the IOM recommendations were more likely to believe that excessive GWG in pregnancy would not have any adverse future effect on health outcomes of their baby ($\chi^2 = 6.949$; $p < 0.05$) or the weight of the baby ($\chi^2 = 16.54$; $p < 0.005$) (Table 6).

Discussion

This is the largest Australian survey examining health and sociodemographic factors associated with early GWG and women's understanding of the importance of healthy GWG in pregnancy. We found that in the first half of their pregnancy, more than one third of the cohort (32.4%) gained gestational weight outside the IOM recommendations for their BMI category and the overweight and obese women were more likely to overestimate the appropriate GWG for their baseline BMI. The most significant predictors of excess early GWG were pre-pregnancy BMI and SES status. It is of concern that only half the cohort (51.0%) understood the potential impact of excess GWG on their baby and furthermore, the women who gained the most weight outside the IOM guideline were less likely to believe that excess GWG would impact negatively on their baby. These findings make it clear that education around GWG is

Table 3 Mean and range of early gestational weight gain by pre-pregnancy BMI and the IOM weight gain recommendations [mean (range) in kg] based on self-reported pre-pregnancy BMI

	Underweight (<18.5 kg/m^2) n = 125	Normal weight (BMI 18.5–24.9 kg/m^2) n = 1209	Overweight (BMI 25.0–29.9 kg/m^2) n = 418	Obese (BMI ≥ 30 kg/m^2) n = 229
IOM weekly weight gain recommendation (kg)	0.51 (0.44–0.58)	0.42 (0.35–0.50)	0.28 (0.23–0.33)	0.22 (0.17–0.27)
Weekly weight gain (kg)	0.41 (−1.00–2.60)	0.38 (−2.00–10.00)	0.45 (−8.00–8.00)	0.46 (−2.00–6.33)

IOM Institute of Medicine; *BMI* Body mass index; *kg* kilograms

required to advise women about what are the expected healthy GWG parameters for their BMI.

Our findings support other studies that have reported women who are overweight and obese women are more likely to gain excess weight as per the IOM guidelines for their BMI category [2, 18, 19]. Recommendations regarding appropriate GWG are particularly relevant to overweight and obese women who are already at risk of complications for their pregnancy and offspring due to their pre-pregnancy weight. Any additional risks that accompany excessive GWG may further complicate their pregnancy, their future health and the health of their child. There are limited data on how many women are gaining excessive weight in early pregnancy in Australia. Only one Australian study (n = 664) has examined early gestational weight gain, in the context of overall weight gain in pregnancy. This study reported that by 16 weeks of pregnancy, 8% of women had already reached their recommended weight for the total pregnancy, and 2% had exceeded their total weight gain recommended for the pregnancy. [20] The authors also noted that total gestational weight gain correlated with weight gain in early pregnancy. The LIMIT trial found that delivery of advice about diet, exercise and behavioural changes, to women who are already overweight or obese during pregnancy did not reduce the primary outcome (large for gestational age), nor did it influence GWG despite recruiting between 10 and 20 weeks gestation (intervention 9.39 ± 5.74 kg; standard care 9.44 ± 5.77 kg; p = 0.89) [21].

Even though pre-pregnancy BMI is a significant predictor of early excess GWG in our study, up to a third of normal weight women also gained weight in excess of that recommended by the IOM. This is of concern because even women with a healthy weight are at risk, because early excess GWG significantly increases the risk of gestational diabetes, particularly amongst normal weight women [6, 22].

We found women from lower SES backgrounds were more likely to gain weight in early pregnancy in excess of the IOM recommendations. This finding aligns with previous studies which have consistently shown an association between lower SES background and excess GWG [23, 24]. Women who are socio-economically disadvantaged are likely to have greater psychosocial risks such as stress, depression, poor social supports and unplanned pregnancy, which may contribute to poor dietary choices and minimal physical activity [25]. Furthermore, women from higher SES areas tend to be more proactive with seeking information regarding weight gain recommendations, healthy eating and exercise during pregnancy [25].

Our cohort of overweight and obese women was more likely to overestimate their appropriate GWG suggesting that there is a lack of knowledge regarding healthy GWG by women, especially those most at risk – the overweight and the obese. Our findings validate findings from a smaller Australian study (n = 364) that examined pregnant women's knowledge of GWG expectations and their awareness of complications associated with obesity and excess GWG [26]. A second small Australian study recruited pregnant women at 16–18 weeks gestations (n = 166), comparing GWG expectations over reported GWG. A significant risk factor for excess GWG was mothers overestimating the minimum amount of GWG needed [15]. Our study differed from these; it was confined to early pregnancy, had a much larger sample size and included women from diverse ethnic and cultural backgrounds.

We have demonstrated the paucity of knowledge by pregnant women regarding the importance of optimal GWG. Preconception care has been shown to be effective with reducing the amount of gain pregnant women gain up until their first booking visit at hospital [27, 28]. Our results call for counselling and discussion regarding both expectations about optimal GWG and consequences of excess GWG. The Cochrane Review of directed preconception health programs and interventions for improving pregnancy outcomes for women who are overweight or obese was unable to include any studies for meta-analysis [29]. These conversations should be initiated preconception or at the very least in early pregnancy with their healthcare practitioner. Despite this being good practice, international studies suggest that few women receive such advice [30–32]. Research exploring reasons for this lack of counselling from healthcare professionals [30, 31] has found the reasons to be limited awareness of current pregnancy weight gain guidelines, belief that such counselling is ineffective, or awkwardness about raising the issue of weight and weight gain

Table 4 Univariate analysis of the sociodemographic factors of women who gained excess weight in early pregnancy

	Odds ratio	95% CI	*p* value
Age (years)			
16–24 years	1.04	0.81–1.33	0.75
25–34 years	Ref		
≥ 35	0.86	0.68–1.09	0.22
Maternal body mass index (kg/m^2)			
Normal weight (18.5–24.9)	Ref		
Underweight (< 18.5)	0.85	0.56–1.27	0.42
Overweight (25–29.9)	1.79	1.42–2.25	< 0.005
Obese (> 30)	2.00	1.50–2.65	< 0.005
Relationship status			
Married/de-facto	Ref		
Single/widowed/separated	0.95	0.69–1.30	0.73
Smoking			
Non-smoker	Ref		
Current smoker	0.77	0.50–1.20	0.26
Maternal ethnicity			
Caucasian	Ref		
Asian	0.87	0.71–1.07	0.196
Middle Eastern/Africa	1.72	1.28–2.31	< 0.005
Aboriginal or Torres Strait Islander	1.25	0.60–2.60	0.55
Pacific Islander/Maori	1.69	1.07–2.65	0.023
South American (Latino)	0.70	0.29–1.66	0.41
Maternal religion			
Christian	Ref		
Other (Hindu, Buddhist, Jewish)	0.81	0.61–1.07	0.31
Muslim	1.45	1.09–1.93	0.011
No religion	0.83	0.66–1.03	0.09
Maternal education			
Tertiary	Ref		
High school	1.23	0.99–1.54	0.06
Other (nil, primary)	1.06	0.83–1.35	0.65
Not answered	0.93	0.46–1.92	0.85
Socio-economic status			
High	Ref		
Medium	1.31	0.97–1.76	0.075
Low	2.07	1.69–2.54	< 0.005
Employment			
Employed	Ref		
Unemployed	0.85	0.70–1.02	0.07
Pregnancy loss			
Previous pregnancy loss	Ref		
No pregnancy loss	1.15	0.90–1.49	0.26
Medical conditions in pregnancy			
No diabetes	Ref		
Pre-existing diabetes	0.89	0.46–1.72	0.73
No hypertension	Ref		
Hypertension	0.87	0.54–1.40	0.56

with women. If healthcare providers do counsel women and outline expected GWG recommendations, encouragingly there is an increased likelihood of appropriate GWG, particularly when additionally offered lifestyle coaching [33]. The timing of an intervention or patient education is however important. Our study shows women are already gaining excessive weight in early

Table 5 Multivariate analysis of maternal sociodemographic factors and excess gestational weight gain

	Odds ratio	95% CI	*p* value
Age (years)			
16–24 years	0.91	0.70–1.19	0.50
25–34 years	Ref		
≥ 35	0.85	0.67–1.09	0.20
Maternal body mass index (kg/m^2)			
Normal weight (18.5–24.9)	Ref		
Underweight (< 18.5)	0.77	0.50–1.20	0.26
Overweight (25–29.9)	1.69	1.33–2.14	< 0.005
Obese (> 30)	1.64	1.20–2.24	0.002
Smoking			
Non-smoker	Ref		
Current smoker	0.96	0.60–1.53	0.86
Maternal ethnicity			
Caucasian	Ref		
Asian	0.90	0.70–1.15	0.40
Middle Eastern/Africa	1.26	0.89–1.80	0.20
Aboriginal or Torres Strait Islander	1.0	0.47–2.12	0.99
Pacific Islander/Maori	1.13	0.68–1.87	0.65
South American (Latino)	0.62	0.26–1.49	0.28
Maternal religion			
Christian	Ref		
Other (Hindu, Buddhist, Jewish)	0.79	0.57–1.12	0.18
Muslim	1.02	0.72–1.42	0.92
No religion	1.01	0.79–1.27	0.97
Socio-economic status			
High	Ref		
Medium	1.17	0.86–1.59	0.32
Low	1.89	1.49–2.41	< 0.005

Table 6 Excess gestational weight gain and maternal understanding of the effect on health and weight of the baby

	No excess GWG[a] (%)	Excess GWG (%)	*p* value
Will excess gestational weight gain affect the weight of the baby?			
Yes	71.7	28.3	< 0.005
No	59.6	40.4	< 0.005
Will excess gestational weight gain affect health outcomes for my baby?			
Yes	72.5	27.5	< 0.005
No	63.3	36.7	< 0.005

[a]GWG: gestational weight gain

pregnancy and remain at risk of adverse outcomes independent of total GWG and pre-pregnancy BMI.

Our finding that Middle Eastern and Pacific Islander/ Maori women were more likely to have excess GWG compared with other ethnic backgrounds was not sustained in the multivariate analysis but warrants further investigation as the evidence is inconclusive around ethnicity as a risk factor for excess GWG [34–38]. Research from New Zealand in the early pregnancy period has reported that Pacific Islander and Maori women women's knowledge of their BMI and recommended GWG to be inaccurate, irrespective of BMI [39]. There are only a few studies investigating cultural background and GWG and they are commonly from the United States comparing racial differences between Hispanic, white and black women [40, 41]. The recent series in the Lancet on maternal obesity has called for more ethnic and culturally specific research [42]. Cultural background may be an important determinant for GWG, and due to increasing globalisation and migration, it is difficult to ascertain whether any relationship is due to cultural background per se or the result of assimilation into a new environment and culture. Furthermore, there are no current ethnic specific guidelines with regards to healthy GWG. A recent study from Singapore showed that there may be a variation in terms of weight gain recommendations and adverse outcomes specific to those of an Asian ethnicity [43]. Further research is needed to examine whether ethnic specific recommendations for GWG need to be developed and whether there are any specific cultural beliefs that may influence GWG for different ethnic groups.

The strengths of this study is the large number of participants, the inclusion of participants from a number of hospitals (both secondary and tertiary) and the diverse ethnic and cultural backgrounds making these results generalisable to the diverse multicultural Australian population [44]. The inclusion of a multivariable regression analysis assesses a significant association between obese, low SES and excess early gestational weight gain.

A limitation of this study was the use of self-reported pre-pregnancy weight and height, although this has been shown to have adequate correlation with measured height and weight [45]. These results may not be generalisable to other perinatal centres with a distribution of maternal ethnic representation in Australia. There are no current ethnic specific guidelines with respect to ideal weight gain in pregnancy. We could not be certain of specifically when women gained significant weight, whether it be in their first trimester or second trimester therefore we assumed that women gained up to 2 kg in their first trimester and then the weight beyond that can be calculated to be their weekly weight gain.

Conclusion

Women are gaining weight in early pregnancy outside the recommendations of the IOM, which have been accepted in Australia as the guideline for healthcare professionals to use when counselling women. The women at particular risk of excess early GWG are those who are overweight and obese and women residing in lower SES areas. These women need to be targeted for appropriate counselling preconception or in early pregnancy. This study also suggests that their remains a lack of understanding of healthy weight gain recommendations in early pregnancy, where weight gain has a significant impact on short-term pregnancy outcomes and also long-term consequences for both the mother and child. Given the significant adverse outcomes associated with excess GWG in early pregnancy, preconception or early pregnancy counselling with respect to GWG and intervention research regarding best approach remains a public health priority.

Abbreviations

95% CI: 95% confidence interval; BMI: body mass index; GWG: gestational weight gain; IOM: Institute of Medicine; OR: odds ratio; RPAH: Royal Prince Alfred Hospital; SES: socio-economic status; SPSS: Statistical Package for the Social Sciences

Acknowledgements

Not applicable.

Funding

This research did not receive any specific grant from funding agencies in the public, commercial, or not-for-profit sectors.

Authors' contributions

Kate Cheney (KC), Sophia Berkemeier (SB), Kyra Sim (KS), Adrienne Gordon (AG), Kirsten Black (KB). Conceptualisation: KC, KS, SB, AG, KB. Data curation: KC, SB. Formal analysis: AG, KC, KB. Writing – original draft: KC. Writing – review and editing: KC, KS, SB, AG,KB. All authors read and approved the final manuscript.

Competing interests

The authors declare that they have no competing interests.

Author details

[1]Women's and Babies, Royal Prince Alfred Hospital, Missenden Road, Camperdown, Sydney, NSW 2050, Australia. [2]Division of Obstetrics and Gynaecology, Campbelltown Hospital, Sydney, NSW 2560, Australia. [3]Discipline of Obstetrics, Gynaecology and Neonatology, The University of Sydney, Sydney, NSW 2006, Australia. [4]The Boden Institute, Charles Perkins Centre, The University of Sydney, Sydney, NSW 2006, Australia. [5]Charles Perkins Centre, The University of Sydney, Sydney, NSW 2006, Australia.

References

1. Deputy NPSA, Kim SY, Hinkle SN. Prevalence and characteristics associated with gestational weight gain adequacy. Obstet Gynecol. 2015;125(4):773–81.
2. Johnson J, Clifton RG, Roberts JM, Myatt L, Haunth JC, Spong CY, et al. Pregnancy outcomes with weight gain above or below the 2009 Institute of Medicine Guidelines. Obstet Gynecol. 2013;121(5):969–75.
3. Truong YNYL, Caughey AB, Cheng YW. Weight gain in pregnancy: does the Institute of Medicine have it right? Am J Obstet Gynecol. 2015; 212(362):e1–8.
4. Rasmussen KM, Yaktine AL, editors. Weight gain during pregnancy: reexamining the guidelines. Washington, DC: National Academies Press; 2009.
5. Brunner S, Stecher L, Ziebarth S, Nehring I, Rifas-Shiman SL, Sommer C, et al. Excessive gestational weight gain prior to glucose screening and the risk of gestational diabetes: a meta-analysis. Diabetologia. 2015;58:2229–37.
6. Cho EH, Hur J, Lee KJ. Early gestational weight gain rate and adverse pregnancy outcomes in Korean women. PLoS One. 2015;10(10):e0140376.
7. Macdonald-Wallis C, Tilling K, Fraser A, Nelson SM, Lawlor DA.. Gestational weight gain as a risk factor for hypertensive disorders of pregnancy. Am J Obstet Gynecol. 2013;209:327.e1–17.
8. Ferraro ZM, Barrowman N, Prud'homme D, Walker M, Wen SW, Rodger M, et al. Excessive gestational weight gain predicts large for gestational age neonates independent of maternal body mass index. J Matern Fetal Neonatal Med. 2012;25(5):538–42.
9. Walter JR, Perng W, Kleinman KP, Rifas-Shiman SL, Rich-Edwards JW, Oken E. Associations of trimester-specific gestational weight gain with maternal adiposity and systolic blood pressure at 3 and 7 years postpartum. Am J Obstet Gynecol. 2015;212:499.e1–12.
10. Blencowe H, Cousens S, Oestergaard MZ, Chou D, Moller A-B, Narwal R, et al. National, regional, and worldwide estimates of preterm birth rates in the year 2010 with time trends since 1990 for selected countries: a systematic analysis and implications. Lancet. 2012;379(9832):2162–72.
11. Herring SJ, Oken E, Rifas-Shiman SL, Rich-Edwards JW, Stuebe AM, Kleinman KP, et al. Weight gain in pregnancy and risk of maternal hyperglycemia. Am J Obstet Gynecol. 2009;201(61):e1–7.
12. National Institute for Health and Care Excellence. Antenatal care: routine care for healthy pregnant women. London: National Institute for Health and Care Excellence; 2008.
13. Karachaliou M, Georgiou V, Roumeliotaki T, Chalkiadaki G, Daraki V, Koinaki S, et al. Association of trimester-specific gestational weight gain with fetal growth, offspring obesity, and cardiometabolic traits in early childhood. Am J Obstet Gynecol. 2015;212:502.e1–14.
14. Mamun AA, Mannan M, Doi SA. Gestational weight gain in relation to offspring obesity over the life course: a systematic review and bias-adjusted meta-analysis. Obes Rev. 2014;15:338–47.
15. McPhie S, Skouteris H, Hill B, Hayden M. Understanding gestational weight gain: the role of weight-related expectations and knowledge. Aust N Z J Obstet Gynaecol. 2015;55(1):21–6.
16. Wrotniak BH, Dentice S, Mariano K, Salaam EM, Cowley AE, Mauro EM. Counseling about weight gain guidelines and subsequent gestational weight gain. J Women's Health. 2015;24(10):819–24.
17. Australian Bureau of Statistics. Census of population and housing: socio-economic indexes for areas (SEIFA), Australia 2011. Canberra: Australian Bureau of Statistics; 2011.
18. Tanaka T, Ashihara K, Nakamura M, Kanda T, Fujita D, Yamashita Y, et al. Associations between the pre-pregnancy body mass index and gestational weight gain with pregnancy outcomes in Japanese women. J Obstet Gynaecol Res. 2014;40(5):1296–303.
19. Haugen M, Brantsæter AL, Winkvist A, Lissner L, Alexander J, Oftedal B, et al. Associations of pre-pregnancy body mass index and gestational weight gain with pregnancy otucome and postpartum weight retention: a prospective observational cohort study. BMC Pregnancy Childbirth. 2014;14:201.
20. de Jersey SJ, Nicholson JM, Callaway LK, Daniels LA. A prospective study of pregnancy weight gain in Australian women. Aust N Z J Obstet Gynaecol. 2012;52(6):545–51.
21. Dodd JM, Turnbull D, McPhee AJ, Deussen AR, Grivell RM, Yelland LN, et al. Antenatal lifestyle advice for women who are overweight or obese: LIMIT randomised trial. BMJ. 2014;348:g1285.
22. Carreno CA, Clifton RG, Hauth JC, Myatt L, Roberts JM, Spong CY, et al. Excessive early gestational weight gain and risk of gestational diabetes mellitus in nulliparous women. Obstet Gynecol. 2012;119(6):1227–33.
23. Heery E, Kelleher CC, Wall PG, McAuliffe FM. Prediction of gestational weight gain - a biopsychosocial model. Public Health Nutr. 2015;18(08): 1488–98.
24. Huynh M, Borrell LN, Chambers EC. Maternal education and excessive gestational weight gain in New York City, 1999–2001: The effect of race/ ethnicity and neighbourhood socioeconomic status. Matern Child Health J 2014;18:138–145.
25. Paul KH, Graham ML, Olson CM. The web of risk factors for excessive gestational weight gain in low income women. Matern Child Health J. 2013; 17:344–51.
26. Shub A, Huning EY, Campbell KJ, McCarthy EA. Pregnant women's knowledge of weight, weight gain, complications of obesity and weight management strategies in pregnancy. BMC Res Notes. 2013;6:278.
27. Beckmann MM, Widmer T, Bolton E. Does preconception care work? Aust N Z J Obstet Gynaecol. 2014;54:510–4.
28. Weisman CS, Hillemeier MM, Downs DS, Feinberg ME, Chuang CH, Botti JJ, et al. Improving women's preconceptional health: long term effects of the strong healthy women behaviour change intervention in central Pennsylvania Women's health study. Womens Health Issues. 2011;21(4): 265–71.
29. Opray N, Grivell RM, Deussen AR, Dodd JM. Directed preconception health programs and interventions for improving pregnancy outcomes for women who are overweight or obese. Cochrane Database Syst Rev. 2015;7: CD010932.
30. Moore Simas TA, Waring ME, Sullivan GM, Liao X, Rosal MC, Hardy JR, et al. Institute of Medicine 2009 gestational weight gain knowledge: survey of obstetrics/gynecology residents and family medicine residents of the United States. Birth. 2013;40(4):237–46.
31. Stotland NE, Gilbert P, Bogetz A, Harper CC, Abrams B, Gerbert B. Preventing excessive weight gain in pregnancy: how do prenatal care providers approach counselling? J Women's Health. 2010;19(4):807–14.
32. Stengel MR, Kraschnewski JL, Hwang SW, Kjerulff KH, Chuang CH. "What my doctor didn't tell me": examining health care provider advice to overweight and obese pregnant women on gestational weight gain and physcial activity. Womens Health Issues. 2012;22(6):e535–40.
33. Harris ST, Liu J, Wilcox S, Moran R, Gallagher A. Exercise during pregnancy and its association with gestational weight gain. Matern Child Health J. 2015;19:528.
34. Gunderson EP, Abrams B, Selvin S. The relative importance of gestational gain and maternal characteristics associated with the risk of becoming overweight after pregnancy. Int J Obes. 2000;24(12):1660–8.
35. Brawarsky P, Stotland NE, Jackson RA, Fuentes-Afflick E, Escobar GJ, Rubashkin N, et al. Pre-pregnancy and pregnancy-related factors and the risk of excessive or inadequate gestational weight gain. Int J Gynaecol Obstet. 2005;91(2):125–31.
36. Gunderson EP, Abrams B. Epidemiology of gestational weight gain and body weight changes after pregnancy. Epidemiol Rev. 1999;21(2):261–75.
37. Hivert MF, Rifas-Shiman SL, Gillman MW, Oken E. Greater early and mid-pregnancy gestational weight gains are associated with excess adiposity in mid-childhood. Obesity. 2016;24(7):1546–53.
38. Waage C, Falk R, Sommer C, Mørkrid K, Richardsen K, Baerug A, et al. Ethnic differences in postpartum weight retention: a Norwegian cohort study. BJOG. 2016;123(5):699–708.
39. Jeffs E, Haszard J, Sharp B, Gullam J, Paterson H. Pregnant women lack

accurate knowledge of their BMI and recommended gestational weight gain. N Z Med J. 2016;129(1439):37.

40. Vahratian A. Prevalence of overweight and obesity among women of childbearing age: results from the 2002 National Survey of family growth. Matern Child Health J. 2009;13(2):268–73.
41. Hanson M, Barker M, Dodd JM, Kumanyika S, Norris S, Steegers E, et al. Interventions to prevent maternal obesity before conception, during pregnancy, and post partum. Lancet Diabetes Endocrinol. 2017;5(1):65–76.
42. Poston L, Caleyachetty R, Cnattingius S, Corvalán C, Uauy R, Herring S, et al. Preconceptional and maternal obesity: epidemiology and health consequences. Lancet Diabetes Endocrinol. 2016;4(12):1025–36.
43. Ee TX, Allen JC, Malhotra R, Koh H, Østbye T, Tan TC. Determining optimal gestational weight gain in a multiethnic Asian population. J Obstet Gynaecol Res. 2014;40(4):1002–8.
44. Australian Institute of Health and Welfare. Australia's Mothers and babies 2013 -in brief. Canberra: Australian Institute of Health and Welfare; 2015.
45. Holland E, Moore Simas T, Doyle Curiale DK, Liao X, Waring ME. Self reported pre-pregnancy weight versus weight measured at first prenatal visit: effects on catergorisation of pre-pregnancy body mass index. Matern Child Health J. 2013;17:1872–8.

5

Weight management during pregnancy: a qualitative study of women's and care providers' experiences and perspectives

Sara Holton[1*], Christine East[2] and Jane Fisher[1]

Abstract

Background: Obesity during pregnancy is a serious health problem for women and their children. Despite the high prevalence of high body mass index (BMI) among women of reproductive age in high-income countries, there is insufficient evidence to inform practice and policy about weight management for women with high BMI who are pregnant. The aim of this project was to describe women's and midwives' experiences and perspectives of care for weight management during pregnancy in Melbourne, Australia.

Methods: A qualitative study. Semi-structured interviews were conducted with pregnant women and midwives. Transcripts were analysed thematically.

Results: A total of 17 women and 2 midwives were interviewed. Five themes were identified: 1. Reluctance to and difficulties discussing weight and its implications; 2. Barriers to providing appropriate pregnancy care for women with high BMI; 3. Inconsistent weighing practices; 4. Beliefs about the causes of obesity; and 5. Opportunities to assist women to manage their weight. Although most women were satisfied with the pregnancy care they had received, both women and midwives expressed concerns about effective weight management during pregnancy. These included constraints on discussing weight, difficulties accessing appropriate resources and additional support from other health care providers, and inconsistent weighing practices.

Conclusions: The findings suggest that women with high BMI would benefit from additional information and support about weight management prior to conception, during pregnancy, and postnatally.

Keywords: Obesity, Prenatal care, Australia, Pregnant women, Midwives

Background

In Australia, it is estimated that almost two-thirds (62.8%) of the population aged 18 years and over are overweight or obese [1]. Almost half the women of reproductive age have a body mass index (BMI) of ≥25 kg/m^2 [2] which is classified by the World Health Organization as overweight or obese, and up to 43% of women who are pregnant are overweight or obese.

Women who are pregnant and have a high BMI are at elevated risk of obstetric complications including gestational diabetes, preeclampsia, caesarean birth and postoperative infections, and they require longer postpartum hospital stays [3], are less likely to initiate and maintain breastfeeding [4], and may be at greater risk of postnatal depression than women of normal BMI [5]. Their babies are also significantly more likely to be large for gestational age and require neonatal intensive care [3, 6]. Pregnancy care for women with a high BMI is therefore complex and resource-intensive, requires specialist skills, and incurs substantial costs to health services and systems.

There is considerable variation in clinicians' knowledge of obesity in pregnancy and their education, training and skills for obesity counselling. Many have pejorative views about women in this predicament [7, 8]. National and international guidelines for weight management in pregnancy are focused on diet and exercise recommendations, sometimes coupled with specific information about risks to maternal or fetal health [9–11]. Although such

* Correspondence: sara.holton@monash.edu
[1]Jean Hailes Research Unit, Monash University, Level 4/553 St Kilda Road, Melbourne, Victoria 3004, Australia
Full list of author information is available at the end of the article

guidelines are important in ensuring a consistent approach to weight management during pregnancy, subjective accounts suggest that current weight management practices can be experienced as shaming, lacking in empathy and generally unhelpful [12].

There is increasing evidence that people with high BMI experience stigma and discrimination in their day-to-day lives [13–15] including in health care-settings [16]. Pregnant women with high BMI report feeling humiliation, discomfort and anxiety during medical examinations and fears that gowns and equipment may not accommodate their bodies [12, 14, 17], but less is known about their overall experiences of and satisfaction with pregnancy care. Very little is known about clinicians' experiences of providing care for women with high BMI in Australia.

Strategies are required to ensure that women with a high BMI receive evidence-informed, effective, acceptable, supportive clinical care that assists them to manage pregnancy weight gain, and that practitioners and health services are able to provide it.

The aim of this project was to describe women's and midwives' experiences and perspectives of care for weight management during pregnancy in Melbourne, Australia.

Methods

Study design

Qualitative methods are used to answer questions about experience, meaning and perspective, most often from the standpoint of the participant [18]. This study used individual semi-structured interviews, an established qualitative approach when exploring topics about which little is known [19]. Semi-structured interviews were conducted with two groups: 1. Pregnant women with and without a high BMI; and 2. Midwives providing pregnancy care.

Setting

Participants were recruited from Monash Medical Centre (MMC), a large tertiary teaching hospital in metropolitan Melbourne, Australia. More than 3600 women give birth at the MMC annually, of whom 44% are overweight and 18% are obese [20]. Women who develop complications during pregnancy and require a higher level of pregnancy care, including women with a BMI > 43 kg/m^2, are also referred to the MMC for specialist care from other primary and secondary level maternity care services. Standard pregnancy care at MMC includes the provision of a table of recommended weight gain during pregnancy (within the pregnancy booklet given to all women attending the MMC for their pregnancy care) and a Monash Health guideline that recommends regular weighing when attending for pregnancy care clinic visits. In addition to the usual standard of care, the hospital provides a specialised clinic for women with high BMI.

Sample and recruitment

Inclusion criteria for Group 1 participants were to be an English-speaking woman aged more than 18 years, with or without a high BMI and receiving pregnancy care at the MMC. Women were recruited using purposive recruitment strategies, including via flyers and direct approaches from members of the research team in the hospital waiting room. We aimed to recruit a similar number of women who were receiving standard care and care from the specialised clinic. It was anticipated that an approximate sample of 15–20 women would provide sufficient information power for descriptions of different pregnancy care experiences and contribute new knowledge [21].

Inclusion criteria for Group 2 were to be a midwife practising in pregnancy care clinics at MMC. They were invited to participate by researchers during regular staff meetings. As the midwives invited to participate in the study would have specific experiences and knowledge of pregnancy care for women with high BMI, a sample of 3–5 midwives was considered to offer adequate information power [21].

Participants for both groups were recruited between March and November 2016, and interviews were conducted between March 2016 and March 2017.

Data source

Interview guides were developed, informed by the investigators' clinical and research expertise, the published literature relating to weight management in pregnancy, and the research questions. The interviews with women in late pregnancy sought their reflections on experiences of receiving pregnancy care as women with and without high BMI, including experiences of stigma or discrimination, beliefs about causes of high BMI, and the most effective ways to assist women manage weight during pregnancy. Women were also asked about their childbearing experiences including their ideal number of children; number of pregnancies, live births and unintended pregnancies; fertility problems, and age at first birth. At the end of the interview, participants were asked for sociodemographic and other information, including age, country of birth, relationship status, highest level of education, health insurance status, and their pre-pregnancy height (cms) and weight (kgs). In the postnatal interview, details about women's most recent birth experience including mode of delivery, the baby's weight, and women's weight at the end of pregnancy were sought.

The semi-structured interview guide for midwives elicited participants' reflections on their experiences of providing care for pregnant women with and without high BMI, beliefs about causes of high BMI, the most effective ways to assist women to manage weight during pregnancy, and the interaction between optimal care provision and contextual factors. Sociodemographic and employment details sought at the end of the interview included country of birth, number of years practised, and the number of women with high BMI they cared for each year.

Procedure

Women were invited to participate in a telephone interview in late pregnancy (≥ 28 weeks gestation) and 4–6 weeks after giving birth. Midwives were invited to participate in an in-person or telephone interview. All participants were given printed information in plain language about the study and provided either written consent or audio-recorded verbal consent at the beginning of the interview. All interviews were conducted by the first author, audio-recorded with permission, and transcribed verbatim.

Data management and analysis

Group 1 participants were invited to choose a pseudonym. Those who did not were assigned one from the list of the top 20 baby girl names in Australia in 2016. Participants were identified in the analysis by pseudonym only. In order to distinguish the midwives from the women, midwives were not given a pseudonym but identified as "Midwife 1" or "Midwife 2".

Self-reported weight and height were used to calculate BMI according to the World Health Organization's classification of underweight and normal weight (BMI <18.5–24.9 kg/m^2), overweight (BMI of 25–29.9 kg/m^2) and obese (BMI ≥30 kg/m^2) [22]. Transcripts were analysed using thematic analysis techniques commonly practised in qualitative research [23]. As identified by Braun and Clarke [23] this consisted of six phases. Phases 1 and 2: Transcripts were repeatedly read and reread, and coded. Phases 3–5: Codes were grouped into meaningful categories that described how participants talked about the topics, including contradictions and exceptions. Themes were created, named and defined in order to explain and interpret the content. The overall "story" identified by the analysis was established. Examples of the identified themes were selected in the final phase (phase 6) and related back to the research objective. The analysis was conducted by the first author and interpretations discussed within the research team until consensus was reached. Quotes have been used in the text to illustrate the findings.

Results

Interviews were conducted with 17 women and two midwives. Among the pregnant women, 15 chose to be interviewed by telephone, two in person. All women who participated in a pregnancy interview, except for one who could not be contacted, also completed an interview 4–6 weeks after giving birth. The characteristics of the participants are shown in Tables 1 and 2. Most were aged in their early thirties, born outside Australia, had a postsecondary school qualification, and just over half were overweight or obese. Seven of the women were receiving standard pregnancy care whilst nine attended a speciality pregnancy clinic for women with high BMI (>43 kg/m^2).

Two midwives were interviewed, both by telephone. Both were female midwives who practised mostly in the speciality pregnancy care clinic at the MMC for women with a BMI more than 43 kg/m^2. Each had practised as a midwife for at least 3 years.

Key themes

Five themes about women's and midwives' experiences and perspectives of pregnancy care for pregnant women with high BMI were identified.

Theme 1: Reluctance to and difficulties discussing weight and its implications

The midwives reported that many women with high BMI are reluctant to discuss their weight during pregnancy care appointments. They also commented that it can often be difficult to discuss weight with women and many women become defensive if care providers attempt to discuss their weight. Nevertheless, midwives thought it was important that women were aware of the maternal and fetal implications of high BMI during pregnancy, and tried not to make women feel like they were "attacking" them when providing weight management advice.

> *Most women we see with high BMI* [in the pregnancy clinic] *don't want to discuss the weight issue. (Midwife #1)*

> *Midwives don't want to 'lecture' women about their weight, they just want to talk about the implications of high weight for pregnancy and the baby. (Midwife #1)*

> *We talk to every women in the booking appointment about their BMI and optimal weight for pregnancy so I take that as an opportunity to determine how receptive they would be to a discussion about diet but I make sure I include it in every appointment* [not just for women with high BMI] *... and make sure women are aware that we are not telling them they need to go on a crazy diet but it is about making small changes ... I try not to make them feel like I am attacking them ... and that any changes they make will benefit them and their baby ... and acknowledge any changes that they make. (Midwife #2)*

Table 1 Women's sociodemographic characteristics and childbearing experiences

Characteristic	Women (n = 17)	Women giving birth in Australia[a]
Average age (years) (range)	32.6 (24–43)	30.4
Country of birth		
Born in Australia	7 (41.2%)	67%
Born overseas	10 (58.8%)	33%
Highest level of education		
Post-secondary school qualification	15 (88.2%)	
No post-secondary school qualification	2 (11.8%)	
Relationship status		
Partnered	17 (100%)	
Not partnered	0 (0.0%)	
Healthcare concession card		
Yes	2 (11.8%)	
No	15 (88.2%)	
Private health insurance		
Yes	9 (52.9%)	
No	8 (47.1%)	
BMI		
Normal weight (<24.9 kg/m^2)	8 (47.1%)	54%
Overweight (25–29.9 kg/m^2)	3 (17.6%)	26%
Obese (≥30 kg/m^2)	6 (35.3%)	20%
Fertility problems		
Yes	5 (29.4%)	
No	12 (70.6%)	
Average ideal number of children (range)	2.6 (2–4)	
Average number of pregnancies (range)	2.3 (1–6)	
Average number of live births (range)	0.8 (0–2)	
Average number of unintended pregnancies (range)	0.2 (0–2)	
Average age at first birth (years) (range)	30.0 (19–41)	
Mode of delivery (index pregnancy)		
Vaginal	9 (56.3%)	67%
Caesarean section	7 (43.8%)	33%
Average baby birth weight (kgs) (range)	3.3 (2.4–4.1)	3.335
Baby admitted to NICU or SCU		
Yes	6 (40.0%)	15%
No	9 (60.0%)	
Infant feeding		
Breastfeeding	16 (100%)	96%
Average weight at end of pregnancy (kgs) (range)	93.5 (65–150)[b]	
Average weight gain during pregnancy (kgs) (range)	12.8 (−5.5–23)[b]	

[a]Women giving birth in Australia in 2014 [41]
[b]data unavailable from 4 participants

Table 2 Women's individual weight characteristics

Participant	Pre-pregnancy BMI (kg/m^2)	WHO weight classification
Isla	21	Normal
Ivy	21	Normal
Matilda	21	Normal
Amelia	22	Normal
Chloe	22	Normal
Olivia	22	Normal
Emily	24	Normal
Isabella	24	Normal
Mia	25	Overweight
Zoe	25	Overweight
Charlotte	27	Overweight
Lily	41	Obese
Grace	43	Obese
Ruby	46	Obese
Sophia	47	Obese
Ella	55	Obese
Evie	58	Obese

> *Although it can be frustrating caring for women with high BMI, I don't want to belittle them in any way ... I want to make sure they are supported. (Midwife #2)*

Although most women reported positive pregnancy care experiences, were satisfied with the care they received, and perceived that the response from care providers about their weight was appropriate, they felt that care providers should not "criticise" pregnant women who have a high BMI.

> *I think women may be hesitant to bring up the issue of weight with the midwives and doctors so they need to be approachable and provide advice. (Zoe, BMI 25-29.9 kg/m^2)*

> *I think that the midwives and doctors at* [the hospital] *don't make a huge deal about weight ... they don't emphasise your weight but they do tell you the risks. (Ruby, BMI ≥ 30 kg/m^2)*

> *I feel very insecure about my weight ...* [the midwives] *really tried not to mention it or make me feel uncomfortable. (Evie, BMI ≥ 30 kg/m^2)*

Most women had received some dietary advice and information from their care provider but this was mainly about foods that should be avoided during pregnancy such as those that may contain harmful bacteria such as *Listeria*. However, women, both with and without a high BMI, also wanted their care provider to give them advice and information about managing weight and appropriate weight gain during pregnancy, and have opportunities to discuss these with them.

I asked my doctor for advice about my weight ... I have put on 15kgs and would like to know if this is normal and get some tips about what I should eat. (Ivy, BMI < 24.9 kg/m²)

The two midwives stated that they were often guided by women's individual level of interest in weight management when determining how much information to provide but felt they needed to be "blunt" with women who were at high risk of maternal and foetal complications such as women with a BMI > 40 kg/m^2. They also thought it was important to manage the expectations of women with a high BMI about the most appropriate settings for labour and delivery. For example, that home or water births are not usually recommended for women with a high BMI. Midwives also tried to focus on discussing establishing better health habits such as regular exercise and healthy eating but reported becoming frustrated if women did not follow their advice.

It is frustrating to give women advice and information during pregnancy about healthy eating and then see them in the postnatal ward eating McDonald's ... it feels like you are wasting your time. (Midwife #1)

The midwives felt that women "normalised" obesity and this was especially true for women attending the speciality pregnancy care clinic for women with high BMI.

Theme 2: Barriers to providing appropriate pregnancy care for women with high BMI

Several barriers were identified to providing appropriate pregnancy care for women with a high BMI by the midwives, including a lack of suitable equipment, few resources to assist women manage their weight, and limited formal training for midwives about caring for pregnant women with high BMI.

The midwives reported difficulties sourcing suitable equipment and facilities for women with high BMI given the hospital's limited supply including wide wheelchairs, large blood pressure cuffs, bariatric beds, and wards with appropriate toilet facilities, and felt this affected their ability to provide effective care. Despite midwives' concerns about sourcing appropriate equipment, most women reported that the equipment used during pregnancy care, labour and birth was suitable for their needs.

I didn't have to worry about my weight ... [the hospital] *had all the equipment I needed and it was appropriate for me ... everything was organised before my appointments so I wasn't inconvenienced. This was much better than other hospitals I have gone to which were not prepared for caring for someone* [of my weight]. *... I didn't have to apologise for being overweight. (Evie, BMI ≥ 30 kg/m²)*

Midwives commented that although they attempted to "treat all women the same" regardless of their weight, some women required or would benefit from additional support particularly from other care providers such as dieticians. However, opportunities for additional support were limited and midwives expressed frustration in not being able to refer women easily, especially those who expressed concern about their weight and wanted to take action for individual appointments or group sessions with dieticians.

Although the midwives felt confident about and well-supported in providing pregnancy care for women with a high BMI, they commented that they had received little or no formal training about the care and management of such women and that they had mostly "learnt on the job".

Theme 3: Inconsistent weight management/weighing practices

Many women had expected to be weighed at every visit especially those who had pregnancy-related conditions such as gestational diabetes. However, both midwives and women described inconsistent weighing practices. Women reported not being weighed at all, weighed only at their first pregnancy care appointment, weighed inconsistently during pregnancy, or weighed at every pregnancy care appointment.

I have never been weighed in the pregnancy clinic (Olivia, BMI < 24.9 kg/m²).

I have only been weighed at the pre-pregnancy clinic for women with diabetes. I haven't been weighed at any of my routine hospital visits. (Zoe, BMI 25-29.9 kg/m²)

I have been weighed by the midwife at every visit. I've also been weighed by my diabetes educator at the hospital. (Sophia, BMI ≥ 30 kg/m²)

Several women commented that whether or not they were weighed appeared to be inconsistent and when they sought clarification from their care provider about whether they should weigh themselves were told it was not necessary.

I have been weighed twice by the midwives. First when I was diagnosed with diabetes and then at another midwife visit but it seems a bit random. I thought I would be weighed at every visit given that I have gestational diabetes. (Emily, BMI < 24.9 kg/m²)

I was only weighed at my first clinic visit. I asked the doctor if I should weigh myself and was told not to bother. (Lily, BMI ≥ 30 kg/m²)

Some women who were not weighed regularly by their care providers weighed themselves.

I haven't been weighed at any of my pregnancy clinic visits ... but I weigh myself at home. (Mia, BMI 25-29.9 kg/m²)

Midwives stated reasons for not weighing women including not always having time (especially if the woman was late to her appointment) as they had to prioritise other care activities, and trying to avoid women feeling that they were focused on their weight.

Theme 4: Beliefs about the causes of obesity

Midwives and women expressed consistent views about the causes of obesity, and identified time, cost, and psychological and cultural barriers to women being able to manage their weight effectively during pregnancy. Women reported that fast food, soft drinks, and sedentary lifestyles or a lack of exercise were the main reasons people were overweight. Midwives believed that women with high BMI often ate too much food and the "wrong" types of food, lacked nutritional knowledge and motivation to effectively manage their weight, and were time poor. Women had similar beliefs, as well as suggesting that hormones caused weight gain during pregnancy. Several women also commented that some women "use pregnancy as an excuse to eat" and gained weight during pregnancy due to misperceptions such as "eating for two".

Although few women reported personal experiences of stigma or discrimination due to their weight, both midwives and women identified negative societal stereotypes about people who are obese. Women felt that "*everyone has an opinion on pregnant women's weight*" (Charlotte, BMI 25–29.9 kg/m²) and pregnant women who have a high BMI often receive negative comments from a range of people including strangers and care providers. Concerns for the health of the baby were often the main focus of such comments with women told that their weight would have detrimental effects for their baby. Women also thought that because women with a high BMI may not look pregnant, especially at the beginning of pregnancy, they were often treated differently to other women who are pregnant.

People question whether women who are overweight during pregnancy are really pregnant ... no-one gives up their seat on the train for them ... and people stare. (Lily, BMI ≥ 30 kg/m²)

When I was in the [hospital] *waiting room, people looked at me differently ... people think that you don't look after yourself or take care of yourself when you are overweight. (Evie, BMI ≥ 30 kg/m²)*

Women also felt that negative societal perceptions and comments about pregnant women who have a high BMI may result in women becoming distressed and eating for emotion regulation or self-soothing. Midwives also believed that women who had a high BMI often lacked self-esteem and self-confidence.

Most women were able to identify a number of strategies to assist with weight management during pregnancy even if they did not implement or practice these themselves. These included eating healthy foods, reducing portion sizes, and regular exercise.

Although most women reported being satisfied with their body weight and shape during pregnancy, several had concerns about the amount of weight they had gained and felt "miserable" or that they had gained too much weight. Some women expressed concern about their ability to manage their weight given their pregnancy, especially in the first trimester if they had morning sickness and struggled to find suitable food to eat.

I think I gained weight due to severe morning sickness. The only thing I could eat was bread which helped to stop the nausea and heartburn. I ate bread even when I wasn't hungry as it alleviated the alkaline taste on my tongue. (Ivy, BMI < 24.9 kg/m²)

I have found it difficult to feel full whilst I have been pregnant so have eaten a lot more than I usually would. (Isabella, BMI < 24.9 kg/m²)

Theme 5: Opportunities to assist women manage their weight during pregnancy and postnatally

Women expressed concern about managing their weight during pregnancy and losing excess weight after the birth. Women and midwives identified several possible interventions to assist women manage their weight. They recommended that women with high BMI be offered specialised services and support similar to that which pregnant women with other conditions such as gestational diabetes or women having multiple pregnancies/births currently receive. For example, group information sessions about weight management offered as part of routine pregnancy care supported with printed or web-based information and individualised appointments with allied health care providers as is done with women with gestational diabetes. It was suggested that midwife-led, non-judgemental group sessions would provide a safe place for women to talk and receive information about weight management.

> *I saw a dietician at the pre-pregnancy clinic* [due to diabetes]. *She gave me useful information about food groups and healthy eating during pregnancy. I think other women would benefit from similar information. (Zoe, BMI 25-29.9 kg/m^2)*

> *When we have women who are diagnosed with gestational diabetes they have an education session, I think something like that is needed for women with a high BMI ... a group session. (Midwife #1)*

> *I think the midwives could offer a group information session like what the twin clinic does for women having twins ... they could talk about nutrition and engage women with a high BMI in a group ... it could be a safe place ... where women could ask questions ... and where we could also address all the risks of high BMI in labour. (Midwife #2)*

> *I think midwives should give women information about managing their weight during pregnancy and this could include pamphlets or free seminars or groups sessions like mothers' groups. (Emily, BMI < 24.9 kg/m^2)*

> *I think midwives should speak to women at antenatal classes and at individual appointments about managing their weight, particularly if the midwife has concerns about a woman's weight or weight gain. (Isla, BMI < 24.9 kg/m^2)*

Women reported positive experiences with online pregnancy support groups, smartphone apps, and web-based tools in seeking and obtaining weight management information. Midwives were identified as the most appropriate people to talk to about managing their pregnancy weight. Women thought that care providers should discuss weight management with women and suggested that women should be given information about healthy eating, a diet plan, and recommendations about appropriate exercise. Women also thought it would be useful for care providers to regularly check women's weight and that women could also use smartphone apps to track their weight during pregnancy. As well as web-based resources women also identified written information such as pamphlets as useful and thought any information provided should focus on why it is important to manage weight during pregnancy and how to do this, and be framed positively.

During the postnatal interviews participants reported that primary or routine care is mostly focused on the baby not the mother, and it would be useful for care during the postnatal period to include information on the best ways to lose weight. Maternal child and health care nurses who see women regularly after birth in Australia were also perceived as having a role in providing women with information about weight management and losing weight after pregnancy.

Midwives felt that weight management programs or interventions should not just be focused on pregnancy but also on making lifelong changes. Midwives believed that women with high BMI often lacked motivation about making changes during pregnancy so it would be beneficial for programs to be targeted at women prior to pregnancy and given that this may not always be possible then during the postnatal period before future pregnancies.

Discussion

Being overweight or obese has become more common in countries such as Australia, and the proportion of pregnant women with a high BMI is increasing. Pregnancy care provides an opportunity to assist women to control weight gain and reduce perinatal morbidities. This study provides an important insight into contemporary weight management experiences and perspectives of pregnant women and midwives. Although most women in this study were satisfied with the pregnancy care they had received, both women (with normal and high BMI) and midwives expressed concerns about effective weight management and identified that women would benefit from additional information and support in managing their weight both during pregnancy and postnatally.

Similar to other studies [24–28], we found that both women and midwives find it difficult and are reluctant to discuss weight and weight management during pregnancy care. Having a high BMI is a source of shame and these data suggest that it can be intensified in pregnancy with the awareness that there are risks to the foetus as well as the self. Avoidance is a common (but ineffective) psychological mechanism to reduce embarrassment, awkwardness and shame and it appears that women, especially those with a high BMI, are unlikely to initiate discussion about weight and weight management with pregnancy care providers. Although care providers acknowledge that women need to be informed about the implications of high BMI during pregnancy, it appears that they might avoid or delay discussing weight management because they are unsure about how to communicate effectively without offending, shaming, stigmatising, discouraging, or causing anxiety [29].

As found in other studies [28], most women in this study understood that eating and activity were related to weight but midwives felt that some women lacked the knowledge and skills to effectively manage their weight. Nevertheless, many women expressed dissatisfaction about the amount or lack of information they received from pregnancy care providers about weight management, wanted more weight management information and support during pregnancy and postnatally, and felt that this should be incorporated into routine care. These findings are consistent with others that have highlighted the lack of consistent and reliable information women receive from pregnancy and postnatal care providers about weight management [25, 26, 30].

There is a trend for greater social acceptance of obesity in some social settings [25, 28, 31]. Midwives in this study, similar to those in other studies [24, 28, 31, 32], perceived that women often 'normalised' their weight and believed that this may result in less motivation to implement weight management changes measures.

Routine weighing of women at every pregnancy care visit is no longer routine practice in countries such as Australia, the UK and the US. Instead it is recommended that women be weighed at their first pregnancy care appointment and that only women with risk factors for pregnancy complications such as women with high BMI be weighed at every appointment [9, 33, 34]. At Monash Health, however, recognition of the importance of weight management during pregnancy and of Australia's obesity epidemic has prompted a recommendation to weigh women when they attend for each clinic visit. Nonetheless, weighing practices revealed in this study were inconsistent and many women reported that they had expected to be weighed throughout their pregnancy. This is consistent with other studies where women have expressed a preference for more frequent weighing and believe that it should be part of standard pregnancy care as it would provide reassurance and motivation for weight management in pregnancy and postnatally [26, 35]. Furthermore, pregnancy care providers in a recent Australian study suggested that weighing all women would avoid stigmatising those who are overweight or obese [31].

Strengths and limitations

This was a small study that recruited participants exclusively from one large teaching hospital located in a metropolitan area. Many of the women were receiving pregnancy care from a speciality clinic for women with high BMI and therefore, their pregnancy care experiences may not reflect those of women with high BMI in general or women receiving standard pregnancy care.

A strength of this study is that is investigated both women's and midwives' experiences and perspectives of pregnancy care for women with high BMI assisting to identify possible interventions that will be effective and acceptable to those who use them. Additionally, women who had a BMI within the normal range were also included in the study enabling the perspectives of women of all BMI categories to be considered. This is important given that women with a normal BMI may gain weight after pregnancy and may also benefit from weight management advice and support during pregnancy and prior to their next pregnancy.

Nevertheless, the results are limited by the participation of only two midwives. It was not possible to interview other pregnancy care providers such as obstetricians for this study. Accordingly, the perspectives and experiences of the participants may not reflect those of other pregnancy care providers nor of women and pregnancy care providers in other settings, although similar findings have been found in recent Australian studies [27, 31].

Implications for health policy and practice

Effective weight management strategies are required in order to reduce the likelihood of maternal and foetal complications, and reduce the risk of future maternal obesity. Pregnancy care provides an opportunity to offer interventions to assist women to manage weight gain and reduce perinatal morbidities.

The findings of this study suggest that effective pregnancy weight management for women with high BMI requires interventions that address the barriers to weight-management during pregnancy, offer clear advice and non-judgemental support, and are provided during both routine pregnancy care (weight-management) and the postnatal period (weight-optimisation prior to conception). Interventions such as these will contribute substantially to enhanced clinical services, and improved weight management, wellbeing, and health outcomes for pregnant women with high BMI.

The reluctance of pregnancy care providers to discuss weight and weight management with women with a high BMI may be due to a lack of confidence in discussing these matters without upsetting women [7, 32]. Taken together, findings of this and other studies [7, 25] suggest that pregnancy care providers may benefit from specific training in counselling women about weight management during pregnancy, and highlight the importance of care providers discussing weight and weight management with women with a high BMI in non-judgemental ways. This will assist in ensuring that women are comfortable and do not perceive their care experiences as humiliating or their care providers as holding pejorative views which may result in women being psychologically harmed, avoiding care, and increasing comfort eating [36].

During pregnancy and the postnatal period, women have regular and frequent consultations with health care providers, and are often motivated to health behavioural changes that may optimise the outcome of their pregnancy [37] and losing gestational weight gain [25]. Australian, UK and US guidelines recommend that weight management during pregnancy requires the input of dieticians or other appropriate health care providers [9, 11, 34]. Many women in this study and others [27] felt that there was currently a lack of specialist nutritional support available to them and believed that support from dieticians during routine pregnancy care would be beneficial to their weight management. Women with gestational diabetes in this study who had consulted a dietician reported positive experiences. This is consistent with the findings of other studies [25, 35] which found that women who were diagnosed with a co-morbidity such as gestational diabetes appreciated the additional support and educational sessions from health care providers including dieticians.

Future research

There is a lack of research on weight management in women before pregnancy or between pregnancies [38, 39]. Future research in this area would assist in developing interventions to optimise maternal health and weight before future pregnancies.

Previous research has indicated the potential for innovative weight loss interventions that use technology platforms such as Facebook and text messaging in non-pregnant populations [40]. Further research is also needed to investigate the effectiveness of such technologies in weight management during pregnancy.

Conclusion

As obesity in pregnancy has significant health implications for mothers and their babies, it is important that women receive appropriate and effective pregnancy care. This study indicates that many women would benefit from additional weight management information and support prior to conception, during pregnancy, and postnatally.

Acknowledgements
The authors are most grateful to the women and midwives who participated in the interviews, and to Monash Health for allowing access to its Maternity Services.

Funding
Not applicable.

Authors' contributions
All authors contributed to the study design. SH contributed to participant recruitment and interviews, data analysis, interpretation of results, manuscript write-up and management of the study. CE and JF contributed to manuscript write-up and revisions of the manuscript. All authors read and approved the final manuscript.

Competing interests
The authors declare that they have no competing interests.

Author details
[1]Jean Hailes Research Unit, Monash University, Level 4/553 St Kilda Road, Melbourne, Victoria 3004, Australia. [2]Maternity Services, Monash Health and Monash University, Monash Medical Centre, 246 Clayton Rd, Clayton, Victoria 3168, Australia.

References
1. Australian Bureau of Statistics. 4338.0 - Profiles of Health, Australia, 2011–13. Canberra: ABS; 2013.
2. Australian Institute of Health and Welfare. Who is overweight?: AIHW; 2013 [cited 2017 13 March 2017]; Available from: https://www.aihw.gov.au/reports/biomedical-risk-factors/risk-factors-to-health/contents/overweight-and-obesity/who-is-overweight.
3. Athukorala C, Rumbold AR, Willson KJ, Crowther CA. The risk of adverse pregnancy outcomes in women who are overweight or obese. BMC Pregnancy Childbirth. 2010;10:56.
4. Amir L, Donath S. A systematic review of maternal obesity and breastfeeding intention, initiation and duration. BMC Pregnancy Childbirth. 2007;7:9.
5. Milgrom J, Skouteris H, Worotniuk T, Henwood A, Bruce L. The association between ante- and postnatal depressive symptoms and obesity in both mother and child: a systematic review of the literature. Womens Health Issues. 2012;22(3):e319–e28.
6. Hildingsson I, Thomas J. Perinatal outcomes and satisfaction with care in women with high body mass index. J Midwifery Womens Health. 2012; 57(4):336–44.
7. Biro M, Cant R, Hall H, Bailey C, Sinni S, East C. How effectively do midwives manage the care of obese pregnant women? A cross-sectional survey of Australian midwives. Women Birth. 2013;26:119–24.
8. Stewart ZA, Wallace E, Allan C. Weight gain in pregnancy: a survey of current practices in a teaching hospital. Aust N Z J Obstet Gynaecol. 2012; 52(2):208–10.
9. Institute of Medicine. Weight gain during pregnancy: reexamining the guidelines. Washington, DC: The National Academies Press; 2009.
10. National Health and Medical Research Council. Australian dietary guidelines. Canberra: National Health and Medical Research Council; 2013.
11. The Royal Australian and New Zealand College of Obstetricians and Gynaecologists. Management of obesity in pregnancy. 2013 Contract No.: C-Obs 49.
12. Mulherin K, Miller YD, Barlow FK, Diedrichs PC, Thompson R. Weight stigma in maternity care: women's experiences and care providers' attitudes. BMC Pregnancy Childbirth. 2013;13:19.
13. Ni Mhurchu C, Bennett D, Lin R, Hackett M, Jull A, Rodgers A. Obesity and health-related quality of life: results from a weight loss trial. N Z Med J. 2004;117(1207):U1211.
14. Nyman VMK, Prebensen AK, Flensner GEM. Obese women's experiences of encounters with midwives and physicians during pregnancy and childbirth. Midwifery. 2010;26:424–9.
15. Brewis AA. Stigma and the perpetuation of obesity. Soc Sci Med. 2014;118:152–8.
16. Ingraham N, Roberts SC, Weitz TA. Prior family planning experiences of obese women seeking abortion care. Womens Health Issues. 2014;24(1): e125–e30.
17. Dotlic J, Terzic M, Babic D, Vasiljevic N, Janosevic S, Janosevic L, et al. The influence of body mass index on the perceived quality of life during pregnancy. Appl Res Qual Life. 2013;9(2):387–99.
18. Hammarberg K, Kirkman M, De Lacey S. Qualitative research methods: when to use them and how to judge them. Hum Reprod. 2016;31(3):498–501.
19. Cohen D, Crabtree B. Qualitative research guidelines project. July 2006. Robert Wood Johnson Foundation; 2006 [cited 2017 22 May 2017]; Available from: http://www.qualres.org/HomeSemi-3629.html.
20. East C. In: Holton DS, editor. Women giving birth at the Monash Medical Centre; 2014.

21. Malterud K, Siersma VD, Guassora AD. Sample size in qualitative interview studies: guided by information power. Qual Health Res. 2016;26(13):1753–60.
22. World Health Organization. Physical status: the use and interpretation of anthropometry. Report of a WHO expert committee. Geneva: World Health Organization; 1995 [cited 2017 10 March 2017]; Available from: http://www.who.int/entity/childgrowth/publications/physical_status/en/index.html.
23. Braun V, Clarke V. Using thematic analysis in psychology. Qual Res Psychol. 2006;3:77–101.
24. Foster CE, Hirst J. Midwives' attitudes towards giving weight-related advice to obese pregnant women. Br J Midwifery. 2014;22(4):254–62.
25. Atkinson S, McNamara PM. Unconscious collusion: an interpretative phenomenological analysis of the maternity care experiences of women with obesity (BMI≥30 kg/m^2). Midwifery. 2017;49:54–64.
26. Allen-Walker V, Mullaney L, Turner MJ, Woodside JV, Holmes VA, McCartney DMA, et al. How do women feel about being weighed during pregnancy? A qualitative exploration of the opinions and experiences of postnatal women. Midwifery. 2017;49:95–101.
27. Knight-Agarwal CR, Williams LT, Davis D, Davey R, Shepherd R, Downing A, et al. The perspectives of obese women receiving antenatal care: a qualitative study of women's experiences. Women Birth. 2016;29(2):189–95.
28. Furness PJ, McSeveny K, Arden MA, Garland C, Dearden AM, Soltani H. Maternal obesity support services: a qualitative study of the perspectives of women and midwives. BMC Pregnancy Childbirth. 2011;11(1):69.
29. Stotland N, Gilbert P, Bogetz A, Harper C, Abrams B, Gerbert B. Preventing excessive weight gain in pregnancy: how do prenatal care providers approach counseling? J Women's Health. 2010;19(4):807–14.
30. Keely A, Cunningham-Burley S, Elliott L, Sandall J, Whittaker A. "If she wants to eat ...; and eat and eat ...; fine! It's gonna feed the baby": pregnant women and partners' perceptions and experiences of pregnancy with a BMI >40 kg/m2. Midwifery. 2017;49:87–94.
31. Knight-Agarwal CR, Kaur M, Williams LT, Davey R, Davis D. The views and attitudes of health professionals providing antenatal care to women with a high BMI: a qualitative research study. Women and Birth. 2013; http://dx.doi.org/10.1016/j.wombi.2013.11.002
32. Lingetun L, Fungbrant M, Claesson I-M, Baggens C. 'I just want to be normal' – a qualitative study of pregnant women's blogs who present themselves as overweight or obese. Midwifery. 2017;49:65–71.
33. Three Centres Collaboration. Routine weighing at antenatal visits. Melbourne 2006 [cited 2017 3 March 2017]; Available from: http://3centres.com.au/guidelines/low-risk-pregnancy/routine-weighing-at-antenatal-visits.
34. National Institute for Health and Clinical Excellence. NICE public health guidance 27: dietary interventions and physical activity interventions for weight management before, during and after pregnancy. London: NICE; 2010.
35. Heslehurst N, Dinsdale S, Brandon H, Johnston C, Summerbell C, Rankin J. Lived experiences of routine antenatal dietetic services among women with obesity: a qualitative phenomenological study. Midwifery. 2017;49:47–53.
36. Puhl RM, Brownell KD. Confronting and coping with weight stigma: an investigation of overweight and obese adults. Obesity. 2006;14(10):1802–15.
37. O'Brien OA, Lindsay KL, McCarthy M, McGloin AF, Kennelly M, Scully HA, et al. Influences on the food choices and physical activity behaviours of overweight and obese pregnant women: a qualitative study. Midwifery. 2017;47:28–35.
38. Ma RCW, Schmidt MI, Tam WH, McIntyre HD, Catalano PM. Clinical management of pregnancy in the obese mother: before conception, during pregnancy, and post partum. Lancet Diabetes Endocrinol. 2016; 4(12):1037-49. doi:10.1016/S2213-8587(16)30278-9.
39. Hanson M, Barker M, Dodd JM, Kumanyika S, Norris S, Steegers E, et al. Interventions to prevent maternal obesity before conception, during pregnancy, and post partum. Lancet Diabetes Endocrinol. 2017;5:65–76.
40. Napolitano MA, Hayes S, Bennett GG, Ives AK, Foster GD. Using Facebook and text messaging to deliver a weight loss program to college students. Obesity. 2013;21(1):25–31.
41. Australian Institute of Health and Welfare. Australia's mothers and babies 2014 — in brief. Canberra: AIHW; 2016. Contract No.: Cat no. PER 87.

6

Pre-pregnancy BMI, gestational weight gain and risk of preeclampsia: a birth cohort study in Lanzhou, China

Yawen Shao[1], Jie Qiu[1], Huang Huang[2], Baohong Mao[1], Wei Dai[1], Xiaochun He[1], Hongmei Cui[1], Xiaojuan Lin[1], Ling Lv[1], Dennis Wang[2], Zhongfeng Tang[1], Sijuan Xu[1], Nan Zhao[2], Min Zhou[1], Xiaoying Xu[1], Weitao Qiu[1], Qing Liu[1*†] and Yawei Zhang[2,3*†]

Abstract

Background: To evaluate the independent and joint effects of maternal pre-pregnancy BMI and gestational weight gain (GWG) on the risk of preeclampsia and its subtypes.

Methods: A birth cohort study was conducted from 2010 to 2012 in Lanzhou, China. Three hundred fourty seven pregnant women with preeclampsia and 9516 normotensive women at Gansu Provincial Maternity and Child Care Hospital were included in the present study. Unconditional logistic regression models were used to evaluate the associations between pre-pregnancy BMI, GWG, and risk of preeclampsia and its subtypes.

Results: Compared to women with normal pre-pregnancy BMI, those who were overweight/obese had an increased risk of preeclampsia (OR = 1.81; 95%CI: 1.37–2.39). Women with excessive GWG had an increased risk of preeclampsia (OR = 2.28; 95%CI: 1.70–3.05) compared to women with adequate GWG. The observed increased risk was similar for mild-, severe- and late-onset preeclampsia. No association was found for early-onset preeclampsia. Overweight/obese women with excessive GWG had the highest risk of developing preeclampsia compared to normal weight women with no excessive weight gain (OR = 3.78; 95%CI: 2.65–5.41).

Conclusions: Our results suggested that pre-pregnancy BMI and GWG are independent risk factors for preeclampsia and that the risk might vary by preeclampsia subtypes. Our study also proposed a potential synergistic effect of pre-pregnancy BMI and GWG that warrants further investigation.

Keywords: Pre-pregnancy BMI, Gestational weight gain, Preeclampsia, China, Birth cohort

Background

Preeclampsia is defined as the development of hypertension and proteinuria after 20 weeks of gestation [1]. It affects up to 8% of all pregnancies worldwide and increases morbidity and mortality rates among both mothers and infants [2, 3]. Preeclampsia is the leading cause of prematurity and fetal growth restriction [4, 5]. The mortality rate among babies born to mothers with preeclampsia is five times higher than that among babies born to healthy mothers [6]. Preeclampsia is also the second leading cause of pregnancy-related intensive care unit admissions after obstetric hemorrhage [7]. Furthermore, preeclampsia is associated with an elevated risk of cardiovascular disease later in life [8, 9].

Given the known and potential adverse consequences of preeclampsia, an understanding of the risk factors of this condition is warranted. A wide range of pregnancy-specific characteristics (e.g. parity, placental factors, multi-fetal gestation, and excessive weight gain during pregnancy) and pre-existing maternal features (e.g. age, race, pre-pregnancy overweight or obesity, pre-pregnancy diabetes, chronic hypertension etc.) are considered to be associated with preeclampsia [10]. Pre-pregnancy BMI and gestational weight gain (GWG) are two modifiable

* Correspondence: 2305470816@qq.com; yawei.zhang@yale.edu
†Equal contributors
[1]Gansu Provincial Maternity and Child Care Hospital, 143 North Road, Qilihe District, Lanzhou, Gansu Province 730050, China
[2]Yale University School of Public Health, 60 College Street, New Haven, CT 06520, USA
Full list of author information is available at the end of the article

risk factors [11–13]. Both pre-pregnancy BMI and GWG may increase oxidative stress levels, stimulate a systemic inflammatory response, and accelerate damage to vascular endothelial cells, resulting in preeclampsia [14, 15]. Studies from different populations have consistently reported that elevated pre-pregnancy BMI is associated with an increased risk of preeclampsia [16–38]. However, the relationship between GWG and preeclampsia is still inconclusive, with some studies suggesting a positive association [9, 30, 39–49] and others reporting no association [11, 21, 50, 51]. Few studies have examined the relationship between pre-pregnancy BMI, GWG and the risk of preeclampsia by different subtypes [14, 30, 43, 52, 53]. Even fewer studies have investigated the joint effect of pre-pregnancy BMI and GWG on preeclampsia and its subtypes. Here, we analyzed data from a birth cohort study conducted in Lanzhou, China [54, 55] to evaluate the independent and joint effects of maternal pre-pregnancy BMI and GWG on the risk of preeclampsia and its various subtypes.

Methods

A birth cohort study was carried out from 2010 to 2012 at Gansu Provincial Maternity and Child Care Hospital, the largest hospital of its kind in Lanzhou, China. Eligible study participants were pregnant women who came to the hospital for delivery with gestational age ≥ 20 weeks, who had no history of mental illness, and who were 18 years or older. A total of 14,359 eligible women were identified and invited to participate. Of those, 3712 refused to participate and 105 did not complete in-person interviews, yielding 10,542 (73.4%) women with completed interviews. Upon obtaining written consent, a standardized and structured questionnaire was used to collect information on demographic factors, reproductive and medical history, smoking and alcohol consumption, occupational and residential history, physical activity, and diet. Information on pregnancy complications and birth outcomes were abstracted from medical records. After excluding women with pre-existing chronic hypertension before pregnancy and missing values of pre-pregnancy BMI or GWG, the final sample size was 9863. Among these women, 347 were diagnosed with preeclampsia. All study procedures were approved by the Human Investigation Committees at the Gansu Provincial Maternity and Child Care Hospital and Yale University. Additional detailed information on the cohort has previously been published [54, 55].

Preeclampsia was defined as hypertension (two separate blood pressure readings ≥ 140/90 mmHg taken at least 6 h apart) and proteinuria (≥ 1+ on dipstick test in two urine samples or ≥ 300 mg of protein in a 24 h urine sample) after 20 weeks of gestation. Preeclampsia was further subcategorized as mild preeclampsia (M-PE) and severe preeclampsia (S-PE), as well as early-onset preeclampsia (EOPE) and late-onset (LOPE) [54]. M-PE was defined as raised blood pressure (≥ 140/90 mmHg and <160/110 mmHg) and proteinuria (≥ 1+ and <2+ on dipstick test in two urine samples) without symptoms of severity. S-PE was defined as raised blood pressure (≥ 160/110 mmHg) and proteinuria (≥ 2+ on dipstick test in two urine samples) with additional symptoms of severity such as headache, blurred vision, epigastric pain, decreased urine output, and decreased or absent fetal kick. Women with EOPE had preeclampsia before 34 weeks of gestation, while those with LOPE had preeclampsia at or after 34 weeks of gestation.

Pre-pregnancy weight was self-reported during the first prenatal care visit. Pre-pregnancy BMI was calculated as weight (kg) divided by the square of height (m), and then subcategorized as underweight (BMI < 18.5 kg/m^2), normal weight (18.5 kg/m^2 ≤ BMI < 24 kg/m^2), and overweight (BMI≥24 kg/m^2) groups. Since East Asians have a higher body fat percentage than Caucasians [56], the BMI cutoffs for overweight and obesity differ between Eastern and Western populations. The standards used in this study were established by the Working Group of Obesity in China [57]. As only a small number of women were obese, overweight and obese women were combined to increase statistical power.

Gestational weight gain (GWG) in kg was calculated by subtracting pre-pregnancy weight from maternal weight at delivery. Since there were no official recommendations specific to the Chinese population, GWG was categorized based on the US Institute of Medicine (IOM) GWG Guidelines 2009 [58]. Adequate weight gain was defined as 12.5–18.0 kg, 11.5–16.0 kg, and 7.0–11.5 kg for underweight, normal weight, and overweight women, respectively.

Differences in selected characteristics between women with preeclampsia and normotensive women were evaluated using Chi-square tests or Fisher's exact tests if necessary. Unconditional logistic regression was used to determine odds ratios (OR) and 95% confidence intervals (CI) for the associations between pre-pregnancy BMI, GWG, and the risk of preeclampsia and its subtypes. Confounding factors including maternal age, maternal employment during pregnancy, monthly household income, maternal education level, parity, twin status, newborn gender, and family history of hypertension were adjusted for in the unconditional logistic regression models. All statistical tests were two-sided. Analyses were performed using SAS 9.3 (SAS Institute, Inc., Cary, NC, USA).

Results

A total of 9863 women were included in the final analysis of which 347 (3.52%) were diagnosed with preeclampsia. Among those with preeclampsia, 206 (59.4%) had S-PE and

Table 1 Distribution of Selected Characteristics of the Study Population

Characteristics	All participants		Preeclampsia		P-value[a]
	n	(%)	n	(%)	
All	9863	100	347	3.5	
Maternal age					<0.001
< 25y	4780	48.5	131	2.7	
25-29y	1530	15.5	52	3.4	
≥ 30y	3553	36.0	164	4.6	
Employment status					0.0012
Yes	5180	52.5	151	2.9	
Not during pregnancy	1524	15.5	56	3.7	
Never	3159	32.0	140	4.4	
Monthly income (RMB)					<0.0001
< 3000	4995	50.6	227	4.5	
≥ 3000	3998	40.5	84	2.1	
Education level					<0.0001
≥ college	3734	37.9	83	2.2	
< college	5878	59.6	250	4.3	
Parity					0.0035
Multifarious	2679	27.2	118	4.4	
Primiparous	7184	72.8	229	3.2	
Newborn gender					0.0073
Male	5200	52.7	159	3.1	
Female	4633	47.0	188	4.1	
Twin					<0.0001
Yes	284	2.9	58	20.4	
No	9579	97.1	289	3.0	
Family history of hypertension					<0.0001
Yes	1510	15.3	91	6.0	
No	8353	84.7	256	3.1	
Pre-pregnancy BMI[b]					
Normal weight	6699	67.9	221	3.3	<0.0001
Underweight	2104	21.3	46	2.2	
Overweight	1060	10.7	80	7.5	
Gestational weight gain(GWG)					<0.0001
Inadequate	1323	13.4	33	2.5	
Adequate	3279	33.2	62	1.9	
Excessive	5261	53.3	252	4.8	
Maternal diabetes					
Yes	97	1.0	7	7.2	0.085*
No	9766	99.0	340	3.5	
Smoking (passive and active) during pregnancy					0.323
Yes	1928	19.5	75	3.9	
No	7935	80.5	272	3.4	

Table 1 Distribution of Selected Characteristics of the Study Population *(Continued)*

Characteristics	All participants		Preeclampsia		P-value[a]
	n	(%)	n	(%)	
Alcohol consumption during pregnancy					1*
Yes	17	0.2	0		
No	9846	99.8	347	3.5	
Physical activity during pregnancy					0.796
Yes	8250	83.6	292	3.5	
No	1613	16.4	55	3.4	

[a]The analysis did not account for missing data. For variable Monthly income (RMB), data was missing for 870 participants, for variable Education level, data was missing for 251 participants, for variable Newborn gender, data was missing for 30 participants
[b]Weight(kg) / height^2 (m^2)
*Fisher's exact test, for all other variables Chi-square test

141 (40.6%) had M-PE, while 304 (87.6%) had LOPE, and 43 (12.4%) had EOPE. The prevalence of pre-pregnancy underweight, normal weight and overweight (including obesity) were 21.33%, 67.92%, and 10.75%, respectively.

Table 1 shows general characteristics of the study population. Compared to normotensive women, women with preeclampsia were more likely to be older, unemployed, less educated, multiparous, pregnant with a female fetus or multiple fetuses, had lower monthly household income and a family history of hypertension. The distributions of maternal diabetes, smoking (active and passive) during pregnancy, alcohol consumption during pregnancy, and physical activity during pregnancy were similar between women with and without preeclampsia.

Pre-pregnancy overweight or obesity was associated with an increased risk of preeclampsia (OR = 1.81, 95%CI: 1.37–2.39), M-PE (OR = 1.76, 95%CI: 1.14–2.71), S-PE (OR = 1.79, 95%CI: 1.26–2.54), and LOPE (OR = 1.79, 95%CI: 1.33–2.41) compared to normal weight (Table 2). Underweight was associated with a reduced risk of S-PE (OR = 0.60, 95%CI: 0.38–0.95) compared to normal weight. Compared to women with adequate GWG, women with excessive GWG had more than a two-fold increased risk of preeclampsia (OR = 2.28, 95%CI: 1.70–3.05), M-PE (OR = 2.79, 95%CI: 1.74–4.47), S-PE (OR = 2.03, 95%CI: 1.41–2.92), and LOPE (OR = 2.53, 95%CI: 1.84–3.48). Inadequate GWG was not associated with the risk of preeclampsia and its subtypes. We further analyzed GWG using the quartiles of GWG among normotensive women. Compared to the lowest GWG quartile, the highest quartile was associated with an increased risk of preeclampsia (OR = 2.59, 95%CI: 1.90–3.53), M-PE (OR = 3.55, 95%CI: 2.13–5.92), S-PE (OR = 2.17, 95%CI: 1.48–3.19), and LOPE (OR = 2.95, 95%CI: 2.10–4.13). The second highest GWG quartile was associated with an increased risk of preeclampsia (OR = 1.66, 95%CI: 1.18–2.33), M-PE (OR = 2.17, 95%CI: 1.25–3.78), and

Table 2 Associations of Pre-pregnancy BMI, Total GWG with the Risk of Preeclampsia and Subtypes ($N = 9863$)[a,b]

	Control	PE		M-PE		S-PE		EOPE		LOPE	
	$n = 9516$	Cases $n = 347$	OR (95% CI)	Cases $n = 141$	OR (95% CI)	Case $n = 206$	OR (95% CI)	Case n = 43	OR (95% CI)	Case $n = 304$	OR (95% CI)
Pre-pregnancy BMI (kg/m^2)											
Normal weight	6478	221	1.00	86	1.00	135	1.00	29	1.00	192	1.00
Underweight	2058	46	0.76 (0.54–1.06)	24	1.00 (0.62–1.59)	22	0.60 (0.38–0.95)	4	0.49 (0.17–1.42)	42	0.80 (0.57–1.14)
Overweight/obese	980	80	1.81 (1.37–2.39)	31	1.76 (1.14–2.71)	49	1.79 (1.26–2.54)	10	1.84 (0.87–3.90)	70	1.79 (1.33–2.41)
Total GWG (kg) by IOM Guidelines											
Adequate	3217	62	1.00	22	1.00	40	1.00	12	1.00	50	1.00
Inadequate	1290	33	1.27 (0.82–1.96)	11	1.24 (0.59–2.57)	22	1.29 (0.75–2.19)	5	0.99 (0.34–2.85)	28	1.34 (0.83–2.15)
Excessive	5009	252	2.28 (1.70–3.05)	108	2.79 (1.74–4.47)	144	2.03 (1.41–2.92)	26	1.23 (0.61–2.50)	226	2.53 (1.84–3.48)
Total GWG (kg) Change by quartile[c]											
GWG ≤ 13.5	2500	68	1.00	21	1.00	47	1.00	14	1.00	54	1.00
13.5 < GWG ≤ 17	2711	55	0.85 (0.59–1.23)	21	1.03 (0.56–1.89)	34	0.78 (0.49–1.22)	4	0.30 (0.10–0.92)	51	0.99 (0.67–1.47)
17 < GWG ≤ 20	2101	81	1.66 (1.18–2.33)	35	2.17 (1.25–3.78)	46	1.44 (0.94–2.20)	13	1.35 (0.62–2.93)	68	1.74 (1.20–2.52)
20 < GWG	2204	143	2.59 (1.90–3.53)	64	3.55 (2.13–5.92)	79	2.17 (1.48–3.19)	12	1.17 (0.53–2.59)	131	2.95 (2.10–4.13)
P_{trend}			<0.0001		<0.0001		<0.0001		0.357		<0.0001

[a]Pre-pregnancy BMI, total GWG and total GWG change were evaluated in separate models
[b]Adjusted for maternal age, maternal employment during pregnancy, education level, monthly household income, newborn gender, parity, twin status, family history of hypertension; pre-pregnancy BMI and total GWG were mutually adjusted
[c]Distribution of GWG based on quartile

LOPE (OR = 1.74, 95%CI: 1.20–2.52). A significant P trend was observed for preeclampsia, M-PE, S-PE, and LOPE. We also found a decreased risk of EOPE associated with the second GWG quartile (OR = 0.30, 95%CI: 0.10–0.92), but this association was based on four exposed cases.

Joint effects between pre-pregnancy BMI and GWG on the risk of preeclampsia and its subtypes are presented in Table 3. Women with both pre-pregnancy overweight (including obesity) and excessive GWG had the highest risk of preeclampsia (OR = 3.78, 95%CI: 2.65–5.41), M-PE (OR = 4.82, 95%CI: 2.71–8.59), S-PE (OR = 3.22, 95%CI: 2.06–5.03), and LOPE (OR = 4.11, 95%CI: 2.81–6.03), although there was no statistically significant interaction between pre-pregnancy BMI and GWG ($P_{interaction} > 0.05$).

Discussion

Our study supported that pre-pregnancy overweight and excessive GWG were independently associated with an increased risk of preeclampsia and that the risk might vary by its clinical subtypes. Higher BMI is associated with a risk of preeclampsia in a dose-dependent manner. The present study also found that the positive association between pre-pregnancy BMI and preeclampsia was similar for S-PE and M-PE, but different for LOPE and EOPE, as pre-pregnancy BMI had a positive association with LOPE but no association with EOPE.

Excessive GWG is associated with an increased risk of preeclampsia. Our study also found that the association between GWG and preeclampsia varied by subtype. We observed an increased risk of M-PE, S-PE, and LOPE, but not EOPE, associated with excessive GWG.

In our study, the highest risk for preeclampsia, S-PE, M-PE, and LOPE was observed among women who were overweight/obese and had an excessive GWG, although the interactions between pre-pregnancy BMI and GWG were not statistically significant. A potential synergistic effect between pre-pregnancy BMI and GWG warrants further investigation.

The classic concept suggests that preeclampsia is a two-stage disorder [59, 60]. The first stage involves abnormal implantation, including shallow trophoblastic invasion and insufficient spiral artery remodeling or other pathological disorders leading to decreased placental

Table 3 Joint Effects of Pre-pregnancy Maternal BMI and GWG on Preeclampsia and Subtypes in Different Groups (N=9863)

Pre-pregnancy BMI	Weight Gain During Pregnancy (GWG) by IOM Guidelines						$P_{interaction}$
	Not Excessive			Excessive[a]			
	Cases	Controls	OR[b] (95%CI)	Cases	Controls	OR[b] (95% CI)	
Preeclampsia							0.69
Underweight	19	1234	0.75 (0.44-1.27)	27	824	1.65 (1.03-2.64)	
Normal weight	65	3054	1.00	156	3424	2.16 (1.60-2.92)	
Overweight/obese	11	219	2.10 (1.08-4.06)	69	761	3.78 (2.65-5.41)	
M-PE							0.87
Underweight	10	1234	1.16 (0.54-2.49)	14	824	2.42 (1.21-4.84)	
Normal weight	21	3054	1.00	65	3424	2.68 (1.62-4.42)	
Overweight/obese	2	219	1.22 (0.28-5.27)	29	761	4.82 (2.71-8.59)	
S-PE							0.47
Underweight	9	1234	0.55 (0.26-1.13)	13	824	1.26 (0.66-2.38)	
Normal weight	44	3054	1.00	91	3424	1.94 (1.34-2.82)	
Overweight/obese	9	219	2.45 (1.17-5.13)	40	761	3.22 (2.06-5.03)	
EOPE							0.11
Underweight	2	1234	0.51 (0.11-2.31)	2	824	0.81 (0.18-3.73)	
Normal weight	11	3054	1.00	18	3424	1.61 (0.75-3.45)	
Overweight/obese	4	219	4.48 (1.40-14.31)	6	761	1.97 (0.72-5.37)	
LOPE							0.80
Underweight	17	1234	0.80 (0.46-1.40)	25	824	1.81 (1.10-2.97)	
Normal weight	54	3054	1.00	138	3424	2.27 (1.64-3.15)	
Overweight/obese	7	219	1.59 (0.71-3.56)	63	761	4.11 (2.81-6.03)	

[a]Excessive weight gain: weight gain above the IOM recommendations, defined as weight gain during pregnancy over 18 kg, 16 kg, and 11.5 kg for underweight, normal weight, and overweight women, respectively

[b]Adjusted for maternal age, maternal employment during pregnancy, education level, monthly household income, newborn gender, parity, twin status, family history of hypertension

perfusion. During the second stage, maternal systemic inflammatory response and oxidative stress converge to alter vascular endothelium function, ultimately leading to multi-organ damage [10, 59–62]. The metabolic and biochemical disturbances associated with overweight and obesity may provide the maternal milieu associated with the second stage of preeclampsia [33]. Overweight/obesity, which is considered a chronic inflammatory condition, increases the levels of plasma C-reactive protein and certain inflammatory cytokines [63–65]. This leads to a systemic inflammatory response, resulting in an increase in neutrophils that release toxic compounds (i.e. reactive oxygen species and myeloperoxidase), capable of attacking and destroying vascular endothelium cell integrity. This mechanism ultimately causes the clinical symptoms of preeclampsia [66].

The association between higher BMI and risk of preeclampsia reported in our study is consistent with that of previous studies based on both Western populations [17–21, 23, 26, 28–30, 32–36, 38], and Asian populations [16, 22, 24, 25, 27, 31, 37, 67, 68]. Among the few previous studies that investigated the association between pre-pregnancy BMI and preeclampsia subtypes [14, 19, 30, 38], their results suggested that overweight/obesity before pregnancy increased the risk of S-PE [14, 19], M-PE [30], LOPE [30, 38], but not EOPE [14, 19, 30, 38]. This finding was supported in our study. The lack of a significant association between pre-pregnancy BMI and EOPE in our study could be due to the small number of EOPE cases ($n = 43$). The consistency of this finding with others suggest that EOPE and LOPE are two different diseases associated with different biochemical markers, risk factors, clinical features, and hemodynamic states [69]. For example, EOPE is typically associated with fetal growth restriction, reduction in placental volume [69], abnormal uterine and umbilical artery Doppler evaluation [70], as well as adverse maternal and neonatal outcomes — maternal mortality is approximately 20-folds higher for preeclampsia cases that manifest at less than 32 weeks' gestation compared to those that occur at term [71]. In contrast, LOPE often involves normal fetal growth, larger placental volume, normal birth weight and favorable maternal and neonatal outcomes [72].

Our results supported those of previous studies showing that excessive GWG is associated with an increased risk of preeclampsia [9, 30, 39–49], and contrary to those of other studies [11, 21, 50, 51]. Differences in results could be due to the heterogeneity of study designs and methods. Some studies [9, 11, 21, 30, 39, 40, 44, 45] adopted 2009 IOM GWG Guidelines to classify GWG according to pre-pregnancy BMI categories as defined by the WHO, others [41, 42, 48, 50] used the 1990 IOM GWG Guidelines to categorize GWG according to pre-pregnancy BMI categories based on Metropolitan Life Insurance Company's weight-for-height standards, and the rest [43, 46, 47, 49] did not use the US IOM GWG Guidelines. In addition to differences in GWG categorization, variations in study population (different ethnic/race distribution) and sources of GWG data (self-reported vs medical record) might also contribute to the inconsistency of the study results.

Previous studies suggested that different preeclampsia subtypes may have different features [69], potentially accounting for varying synergistic effects between pre-pregnancy BMI and GWG with different preeclampsia subtypes. However, studies on synergistic effect between pre-pregnancy BMI and GWG with preeclampsia are scarce: only two previous studies [13, 49] evaluated the combined effects of pre-pregnancy BMI and GWG on preeclampsia. Both of the studies were based on Western populations, and neither of them examined potential associations with different preeclampsia subtypes. To address the literature gap, our study sought to analyze these joined effects on Asian populations. According to our results, women who were overweight/obese before pregnancy and had an excessive GWG had the highest risk for preeclampsia, S-PE, M-PE, and LOPE. Interestingly, the interaction between pre-pregnancy BMI and GWG was not statistically significant. The potential combined effects of pre-pregnancy BMI and GWG on different preeclampsia subtypes require further investigation.

There were several strengths and limitations to our study. Detailed information on demographic factors, medical histories, and lifestyle factors allowed us to control for important confounding factors. Diagnoses of preeclampsia and its subtypes based on medical records rather than self-reports, minimized potential disease misclassification. In terms of pre-pregnancy weight, such data was self-reported, potentially resulting in unavoidable recall bias. Based on previous literature, pre-gravid overweight/obese women are more likely to underreport pre-pregnancy weight than normal weight women [73]. As information on GWG by trimester was unavailable, we were not able to distinguish between weight gain from adiposity (early weight gain) and that from edema (later weight gain). Previous studies have shown that greater weight gain in early pregnancy led to an elevated risk of future gestational hypertension [74, 75], proposing that adipose tissue rather than edema is part of the etiology of pregnancy-induced hypertension. Further investigations focusing on weight gain trajectory during pregnancy and disease progression are necessary to better understand the effect of pre-pregnancy BMI and GWG on preeclampsia and its subtypes.

Conclusions

In conclusion, our study results support that pre-pregnancy overweight (including obesity) and excessive

GWG are independently associated with an increased risk of preeclampsia and the risk may vary by its clinical subtypes. A potential synergistic effect between pre-pregnancy BMI and GWG warrants further investigation. Consequently, future preventive strategies are needed to address pre-pregnancy overweight and obesity and to limit gestational weight gain in order to prevent preeclampsia.

Funding
The study was supported by internal funding from the Gansu Provincial Maternity and Child Care Hospital, Gansu Provincial Science and Technology Department Grant (1204WCGA021) and the National Institutes of Health Grants (K02HD70324, R01ES016317, and R01ES019587). The funding bodies did not play any role in study design, data collection, data analysis, data interpretation, or writing and revising of the manuscript.

Authors' contributions
JQ, QL, and YZ designed the research; YS, HH, BM, WD, XH, HC, XL, LL, ZT, SX, MZ, XX, and WQ performed statistical analysis. YS, JQ, NZ, DW, and YZ collected data and drafted the manuscript. All authors contributed to the final draft and approved the manuscript.

Competing interests
The authors declare that they have no competing interests.

Author details
[1]Gansu Provincial Maternity and Child Care Hospital, 143 North Road, Qilihe District, Lanzhou, Gansu Province 730050, China. [2]Yale University School of Public Health, 60 College Street, New Haven, CT 06520, USA. [3]Yale School of Medicine, New Haven, CT, USA.

References

1. Hutcheon JA, Lisonkova S, Joseph KS. Epidemiology of pre-eclampsia and the other hypertensive disorders of pregnancy. Best prac res Clin obstet gynaecol. 2011;25(4):391–403.
2. Lenfant C. National Education Program Working Group on high blood pressure in pregnancy: working group report on high blood pressure in pregnancy. J Clin Hypertens (Greenwich). 2001;3(2):75–88.
3. Roberts JM, Cooper DW. Pathogenesis and genetics of pre-eclampsia. Lancet. 2001;357(9249):53–6.
4. Redman CW, Sargent IL: Latest advances in understanding preeclampsia. *Science* 2005, (308(5728)):1592–1594.
5. Xiao R, Sorensen TK, Williams MA, Luthy DA. Influence of pre-eclampsia on fetal growth. The journal of maternal-fetal & neonatal medicine : the official journal of the European Association of Perinatal Medicine, the Federation of Asia and Oceania Perinatal Societies. Int Perinatal Obstet. 2003;13(3):157–62.
6. Roberts JM, Pearson G, Cutler J, Lindheimer M. Pregnancy NWGoRoHD: summary of the NHLBI working group on research on hypertension during pregnancy. Hypertension. 2003;41(3):437–45.
7. Porreco RP, Barkey R. Peripartum intensive care. The journal of maternal-fetal & neonatal medicine : the official journal of the European Association of Perinatal Medicine, the Federation of Asia and Oceania Perinatal societies. Int Perinatal Obstet. 2010;23(10):1136–8.
8. Irgens HU, Reisaeter L, Irgens LM, Lie RT. Long term mortality of mothers and fathers after preeclampsia population based cohort study. BMJ. 2001; 323(7323):1213–7.
9. Haugen M, Brantsaeter AL, Winkvist A, Lissner L, Alexander J, Oftedal B, Magnus P, Meltzer HM. Associations of pre-pregnancy body mass index and gestational weight gain with pregnancy outcome and postpartum weight retention: a prospective observational cohort study. Bmc Pregnancy and Childbirth. 2014;14
10. Jeyabalan A. Epidemiology of preeclampsia: impact of obesity. Nutr Rev. 2013;71(Suppl 1):S18–25.
11. O'Dwyer V, O'Toole F, Darcy S, Farah N, Kennelly MM, Turner MJ. Maternal obesity and gestational weight gain. J obstet gynaecol: J Inst of Obstet Gynaecol. 2013;33(7):671–4.
12. Swank ML, Caughey AB, Farineli CK, Main EK, Melsop KA, Gilbert WM, Chung JH. The impact of change in pregnancy body mass index on the development of gestational hypertensive disorders. J Perinatol. 2014;34(3):181–5.
13. Barton JR, Joy SD, Rhea DJ, Sibai AJ, Sibai BM. The influence of gestational weight gain on the development of gestational hypertension in obese women. Am J Perinatol. 2015;32(7):615–9.
14. Ornaghi S, Tyurmorezova A, Algeri P, Giardini V, Ceruti P, Vertemati E, Vergani P. Influencing factors for late-onset preeclampsia. J Matern-Fetal Neonatal Med. 2013;26(13):1299–302.
15. Redman CWG, Sacks GP, Sargent IL. Preeclampsia: an excessive maternal inflammatory response to pregnancy. Am J Obstet Gynecol. 1999;180(2): 499–506.
16. Wei YM, Yang HX, Zhu WW, Liu XY, Meng WY, Wang YQ, Shang LX, Cai ZY, Ji LP, Wang YF, et al. Risk of adverse pregnancy outcomes stratified for pre-pregnancy body mass index. J Matern Fetal Neonatal Med. 2015:1–5.
17. Vinturache A, Moledina N, McDonald S, Slater D, Tough S. Pre-pregnancy body mass index (BMI) and delivery outcomes in a Canadian population. BMC Pregnancy Childbirth. 2014;14:422.
18. Fox NS, Roman AS, Saltzman DH, Klauser CK, Rebarber A. Obesity and adverse pregnancy outcomes in twin pregnancies. J Matern Fetal Neonatal Med. 2014;27(4):355–9.
19. Pare E, Parry S, McElrath TF, Pucci D, Newton A, Lim KH. Clinical risk factors for preeclampsia in the 21st century. Obstet Gynecol. 2014;124(4):763–70.
20. Magann EF, Doherty DA, Sandlin AT, Chauhan SP, Morrison JC. The effects of an increasing gradient of maternal obesity on pregnancy outcomes. Aust N Z J Obstet Gynaecol. 2013;53(3):250–7.
21. Gaillard R, Durmus B, Hofman A, Mackenbach JP, Steegers EAP, Jaddoe VWV. Risk factors and outcomes of maternal obesity and excessive weight gain during pregnancy. Obesity. 2013;21(5):1046–55.
22. Tsai IH, Chen CP, Sun FJ, Wu CH, Yeh SL. Associations of the pre-pregnancy body mass index and gestational weight gain with pregnancy outcomes in Taiwanese women. Asia Pac J Clin Nutr. 2012;21(1):82–7.
23. Persson M, Pasupathy D, Hanson U, Westgren M, Norman M. Pre-pregnancy body mass index and the risk of adverse outcome in type 1 diabetic pregnancies: a population-based cohort study. BMJ Open. 2012;2(1):e000601.
24. Liu X, Du J, Wang G, Chen Z, Wang W, Xi Q. Effect of pre-pregnancy body mass index on adverse pregnancy outcome in north of China. Arch Gynecol Obstet. 2011;283(1):65–70.
25. Chen Z, Du J, Shao L, Zheng L, Wu M, Ai M, Zhang Y. Prepregnancy body mass index, gestational weight gain, and pregnancy outcomes in China. Int J Gynaecol Obstet. 2010;109(1):41–4.
26. Stone CD, Diallo O, Shyken J, Leet T. The combined effect of maternal smoking and obesity on the risk of preeclampsia. J Perinat Med. 2007;35(1):28–31.
27. Khader Y, Jibreal M, Burgan S, Amarin Z. Risk indicators of pre-eclampsia in north Jordan: is dental caries involved? Gynecol Obstet Investig. 2007;63(4):181–7.
28. Doherty DA, Magann EF, Francis J, Morrison JC, Newnham JP. Pre-pregnancy body mass index and pregnancy outcomes. Int J Gynaecol Obstet. 2006;95(3):242–7.
29. Arbour NC, Lorenz E, Schutte BC, Zabner J, Kline JN, Jones M, Frees K, Watt JL, Schwartz DA. TLR4 mutations are associated with endotoxin hyporesponsiveness in humans. Nat Genet. 2000;25(2):187–91.
30. Baker AM, Haeri S. Estimating risk factors for development of preeclampsia in teen mothers. Arch Gynecol Obstet. 2012;286(5):1093–6.
31. Nanjundan P, Bagga R, Kalra JK, Thakur JS, Raveendran A. Risk factors for early onset severe pre-eclampsia and eclampsia among north Indian women. J Obstet Gynaecol. 2011;31(5):384–9.
32. O'Brien TE, Ray JG, Chan WS. Maternal body mass index and the risk of preeclampsia: a systematic overview. Epidemiology. 2003;14(3):368–74.
33. Bodnar LM, Ness RB, Markovic N, Roberts JM. The risk of preeclampsia rises with increasing prepregnancy body mass index. Ann Epidemiol. 2005;15(7):475–82.
34. Catov JM, Ness RB, Kip KE, Olsen J. Risk of early or severe preeclampsia related to pre-existing conditions. Int J Epidemiol. 2007;36(2):412–9.
35. Sibai BM, Ewell M, Levine RJ, Klebanoff MA, Esterlitz J, Catalano PM,

Goldenberg RL, Joffe G. Risk factors associated with preeclampsia in healthy nulliparous women. Am J Obstet Gynecol. 1997;177(5):1003–10.
36. Baeten JM, Bukusi EA, Lambe M. Pregnancy complications and outcomes among overweight and obese nulliparous women. Am J Public Health. 2001;91(3):436–40.
37. Leung TY, Leung TN, Sahota DS, Chan OK, Chan LW, Fung TY, Lau TK. Trends in maternal obesity and associated risks of adverse pregnancy outcomes in a population of Chinese women. Bjog-an Int J Obstet Gynaecol. 2008;115(12):1529–37.
38. Fang R, Dawson A, Lohsoonthorn V, Williams M. Risk factors of early and late onset preeclampsia among Thai women. Asian Biomed (Res Rev News). 2009;3(5):477–186.
39. Swank ML, Marshall NE, Caughey AB, Main EK, Gilbert WM, Melsop KA, Chung JH. Pregnancy outcomes in the super obese, stratified by weight gain above and below Institute of Medicine Guidelines. Obstet Gynecol. 2014;124(6):1105–10.
40. Truong YN, Yee LM, Caughey AB, Cheng YW. Weight gain in pregnancy: does the Institute of Medicine have it right? Am J Obstet Gynecol. 2015; 212(3):362.e1–8.
41. DeVader SR, Neeley HL, Myles TD, Leet TL. Evaluation of gestational weight gain guidelines for women with normal prepregnancy body mass index. Obstet Gynecol. 2007;110(4):745–51.
42. Flick AA, Brookfield KF, de la Torre L, Tudela CM, Duthely L, Gonzalez-Quintero VH. Excessive weight gain among obese women and pregnancy outcomes. Am J Perinatol. 2010;27(4):333–8.
43. Aksornphusitaphong A, Phupong V. Risk factors of early and late onset pre-eclampsia. J Obstet Gynaecol Res. 2013;39(3):627–31.
44. Harper LM, Tita A, Biggio JR. The Institute of Medicine Guidelines for gestational weight gain after a diagnosis of gestational diabetes and pregnancy outcomes. Am J Perinatol. 2015;32(3):239–45.
45. Liu L, Hong Z, Zhang L. Associations of prepregnancy body mass index and gestational weight gain with pregnancy outcomes in nulliparous women delivering single live babies. Sci Rep. 2015;5:12863.
46. Gavard JA, Artal R. GestationalWeight gain and maternal and neonatal outcomes in term twin pregnancies in ObeseWomen. Twin Res Hum Genet. 2014;17(2):127–33.
47. Tabatabaei M. Gestational weight gain, prepregnancy body mass index related to pregnancy outcomes in KAZERUN, FARS, IRAN. J oprenatal med. 2011;5(2):35–40.
48. Langford A, Joshu C, Chang JJ, Myles T, Leet T. Does gestational weight gain affect the risk of adverse maternal and infant outcomes in overweight women? Matern Child Health J. 2011;15(7):860–5.
49. Cedergren M. Effects of gestational weight gain and body mass index on obstetric outcome in Sweden. Int J Gynecol Obstet. 2006;93(3):269–74.
50. Shirazian T, Monteith S, Friedman F, Rebarber A. Lifestyle modification program decreases pregnancy weight gain in obese women. Am J Perinatol. 2010;27(5):411–4.
51. Tanentsapf I, Heitmann BL, Adegboye AR. Systematic review of clinical trials on dietary interventions to prevent excessive weight gain during pregnancy among normal weight, overweight and obese women. BMC Pregnancy Childbirth. 2011;11:81.
52. Mbah AK, Kornosky JL, Kristensen S, August EM, Alio AP, Marty PJ, Belogolovkin V, Bruder K, Salihu HM. Super-obesity and risk for early and late pre-eclampsia. BJOG. 2010;117(8):997–1004.
53. Chandrasekaran S, Levine LD, Durnwald CP, Elovitz MA, Srinivas SK. Excessive weight gain and hypertensive disorders of pregnancy in the obese patient. J Matern Fetal Neonatal Med. 2015;28(8):964–8.
54. Wang Y, Zhao N, Qiu J, He X, Zhou M, Cui H, Lv L, Lin X, Zhang C, Zhang H, et al. Folic acid supplementation and dietary folate intake, and risk of preeclampsia. Eur J Clin Nutr. 2015;69(10):1145–50.
55. Qiu J, He X, Cui H, Zhang C, Zhang H, Dang Y, Han X, Chen Y, Tang Z, Zhang H, et al. Passive smoking and preterm birth in urban China. Am J Epidemiol. 2014;180(1):94–102.
56. Wang J, Thornton J, Russell M, Burastero S. S H, Jr PR: Asians have lower body mass index but higher percent body fat than do whites comparions of anthropometric measurements. Am J Clin Nutr. 1994;60(1):23–8.
57. Zhou B. Cooperative meta-analysis Group of the Working Group on obesity in China: predictive values of body mass index and waist circumference for risk factors of certain related diseases in Chinese adults–study on optimal cut-off points of body mass index and waist circumference in Chinese adults. Asia Pac J Clin Nutr. 2002;11(Suppl):S685–93.
58. Medicine lo: Weight gain during pregnancy: reexamining the guidelines. 2009.
59. Ness RB, Roberts JM. Heterogeneous causes constituting the single syndrome of preeclampsia: a hypothesis and its implications. Am J Obstet Gynecol. 1996;175(5):1360–70.
60. Roberts JM, Hubel CA. Is oxidative stress the link in the two-stage model of pre-eclampsia? Lancet. 1999;354(9181):788–9.
61. Roberts JM, Bodnar LM, Patrick TE, Powers RW. The role of obesity in preeclampsia. Pregnancy Hypertens. 2011;1(1):6–16.
62. Metzger BE, Lowe LP, Dyer AR, Trimble ER, Sheridan B, Hod M, Chen R, Yogev Y, Coustan DR, Catalano PM, et al. Hyperglycemia and adverse pregnancy outcome (HAPO) study associations with neonatal anthropometrics. Diabetes. 2009;58(2):453–9.
63. Esposito K, Nicoletti G. Giugliano D: cytokines and endothelial dysfunction a link for the raised cardiovascular risk associated with visceral obesity. J Endocrinol Investig. 2002;25(7):646–9.
64. Ziccardi P. Reduction of inflammatory cytokine concentrations and improvement of endothelial functions in obese women after weight loss over one year. Circulation. 2002;105(7):804–9.
65. Straczkowski M, Dzienis-Straczkowska S, Stepien A, Kowalska I, Szelachowska M, Kinalska I. Plasma interleukin-8 concentrations are increased in obese subjects and related to fat mass and tumor necrosis factor-alpha system. J Clin Endocrinol Metab. 2002;87(10):4602–6.
66. Walsh SW. Obesity: a risk factor for preeclampsia. Trends Endocrinol Metab. 2007;18(10):365–70.
67. Tanaka T, Ashihara K, Nakamura M, Kanda T, Fujita D, Yamashita Y, Terai Y, Kamegai H, Ohmichi M. Associations between the pre-pregnancy body mass index and gestational weight gain with pregnancy outcomes in Japanese women. J Obstet Gynaecol Res. 2014;40(5):1296–303.
68. Kazemian E, Sotoudeh G, Dorosty-Motlagh AR, Eshraghian MR, Bagheri M. Maternal obesity and energy intake as risk factors of pregnancy-induced hypertension among Iranian women. J Health Popul Nutri. 2014;32(3):486–93.
69. Raymond D, Peterson E. A critical review of early-onset and late-onset preeclampsia. Obstet Gynecol Surv. 2011;66(8):497–506.
70. Crispi F, Llurba E, Dominguez C, Martin-Gallan P, Cabero L, Gratacos E. Predictive value of angiogenic factors and uterine artery Doppler for early-versus late-onset pre-eclampsia and intrauterine growth restriction. Ultrasound Obstet Gynecol. 2008;31(3):303–9.
71. MacKay AP, Berg CJ, Atrash HK. Pregnancy-related mortality from preeclampsia and eclampsia. Obstet Gynecol. 2001;97(4):533–8.
72. Obed S, Patience A. Birth weight and ponderal index in pre-eclampsia: a comparative study. Ghana Med J. 2006;40(1):8–13.
73. Mandujano A, Huston-Presley L, Waters TP, Catalano PM. Women's reported weight: is there a discrepancy? J Matern Fetal Neonatal Med. 2012;25(8):1395–8.
74. Macdonald-Wallis C, Tilling K, Fraser A, Nelson SM, Lawlor DA. Gestational weight gain as a risk factor for hypertensive disorders of pregnancy. Am J Obstet Gynecol. 2013;209(4):327 e1–317.
75. Zhou A, Xiong C, Hu R, Zhang Y, Bassig BA, Triche E, Yang S, Qiu L, Zhang Y, Yao C, et al. Pre-Pregnancy BMI, Gestational Weight Gain, and the Risk of Hypertensive Disorders of Pregnancy: A Cohort Study in Wuhan, China. PLoS One. 2015;10(8):e0136291.

7

The mindful moms training: development of a mindfulness-based intervention to reduce stress and overeating during pregnancy

Cassandra Vieten[1,2*], Barbara A. Laraia[3,4], Jean Kristeller[5], Nancy Adler[3,5], Kimberly Coleman-Phox[3], Nicole R. Bush[3,6], Helané Wahbeh[2], Larissa G. Duncan[7] and Elissa Epel[3]

Abstract

Background: Pregnancy is a time of high risk for excessive weight gain, leading to health-related consequences for mothers and offspring. Theory-based obesity interventions that target proposed mechanisms of biobehavioral change are needed, in addition to simply providing nutritional and weight gain directives. Mindfulness training is hypothesized to reduce stress and non-homeostatic eating behaviors – or eating for reasons other than hunger or caloric need. We developed a mindfulness-based intervention for high-risk, low-income overweight pregnant women over a series of iterative waves using the Obesity-Related Behavioral Intervention Trials (ORBIT) model of intervention development, and tested its effects on stress and eating behaviors.

Methods: Overweight pregnant women ($n = 110$) in their second trimester were enrolled in an 8-week group intervention. Feasibility, acceptability, and facilitator fidelity were assessed, as well as stress, depression and eating behaviors before and after the intervention. We also examined whether pre-to-post intervention changes in outcomes of well-being and eating behaviors were associated with changes in proposed mechanisms of mindfulness, acceptance, and emotion regulation.

Results: Participants attended a mean of 5.7 sessions (median = 7) out of 8 sessions total, and facilitator fidelity was very good. Of the women who completed class evaluations, at least half reported that each of the three class components (mindful breathing, mindful eating, and mindful movement) were "very useful," and that they used them on most days at least once a day or more. Women improved in reported levels of mindfulness, acceptance, and emotion regulation, and these increases were correlated with reductions in stress, depression, and overeating.

Conclusions: These findings suggest that in pregnant women at high risk for excessive weight gain, it is both feasible and effective to use mindfulness strategies taught in a group format. Further, increases in certain mindfulness skills may help with better management of stress and overeating during pregnancy.

Keywords: Pregnancy, Obesity, Stress, Depression, Acceptance-based coping, Emotion regulation, Gestational weight gain, Behavioral intervention, Mindfulness, Mindful motherhood training

* Correspondence: cvieten@noetic.org

[1]California Pacific Medical Center Research Institute, 475 Brannan Street, San Francisco, CA 94120, USA

[2]Institute of Noetic Sciences, 625 Second Street, # 200, Petaluma, CA 94952, USA

Full list of author information is available at the end of the article

Background

Obesity is a leading public health concern in the United States [1]. In 2013–2014, the prevalence of overall obesity (body mass index [BMI] ≥30) was 40.4% among adult women, and 9.9% for class 3 obesity (BMI ≥40), with a significant linear increase over time between 2005 and 2013–2014 [2]. The prevalence of obesity for black (57.2%) and Latina/Hispanic (46.9%) women far exceeds that of white women (38.7%). Women who are already overweight or obese before pregnancy have greater risk for gestational weight gain greater than the recommended 15–25 pounds, or 11–20 pounds, respectively [3].

Both pre-pregnancy obesity and excessive maternal weight gain during pregnancy are associated with a number of unfavorable outcomes. Obesity during pregnancy increases risks of antenatal obstetric problems, caesarean delivery, and fetal risks [4] and gestational weight gain in excess of IOM guidelines has been linked to neonatal complications [5, 6]. Excessive weight gain during pregnancy is also directly associated with increased BMI and risk of obesity in offspring into adolescence [7]. Current studies suggest that obese women gaining no or low gestational weight have better health outcomes [8]. Pregnancy may be a unique opportunity to positively influence a woman's weight gain trajectory by offering low-cost, feasible, and effective interventions that could reduce health risks for both mother and child.

Obesity and weight gain cannot be remedied through a simplistic approach to reducing caloric intake. Food, medications, physical inactivity, toxins, and viruses interact with genetics to interfere with energy balance and contribute to obesity [9]. Weight gain is fostered in some by non-homeostatic eating (defined as eating reflexively in response to factors other than caloric need or hunger), and includes mindless eating, reward-based eating, and stress eating [10–12], which are especially common during periods of chronic stress [13–15]. The drive to eat non-homeostatically is primed by strong neurobiological signals involving reward and stress systems [10]. For example, palatability of high fat and sweet foods is heightened with stress [16] by increasing cortisol, which in turn stimulates dopamine activity. Secretion of stress-related glucocorticoids also increases motivation for food and secretion of insulin, which promotes food intake and obesity [17]. This pattern is reflects what has been observed in animal studies on the neurobiology of addiction and drug abuse [18, 19].

Maternal obesity during pregnancy confers increased risk of her child becoming overweight through a number of biopsychosocial mechanisms such as maternal and fetal hyperglycemia and hyperinsulinemia [20], stress-induced excessive gestational weight gain [21, 22], and stress-induced epigenetic changes leading to offspring fat storage and obesity [23].

Current dietary approaches to healthy weight gain during pregnancy focus almost exclusively on nutrition education and individual control of food intake [24]. Programs based solely on nutritional recommendations have limited success in preventing excessive gestational weight gain [25, 26], perhaps because they rarely address the root causes of the strong drive to overeat. A successful program to address excessive weight gain during pregnancy must also integrate behavioral strategies for managing appetitive drive, knowledge of the psychology of eating and behavior change, and the neuroscience of stress, appetite, and reward.

Mindfulness-based interventions are receiving increasing attention and empirical support for reducing stress and addressing stress-related medical problems and behaviors [27–29]. Mindfulness skills may be important for combating non-homeostatic eating in three ways. First, stress is a fundamental but sometimes overlooked factor that both predicts and interacts with eating behaviors to increase risk for obesity. Mindfulness skills can target the stress-eating interaction because they are effective for reducing anxiety, depression, and stress [30, 31], which should in turn help to reduce stress-eating. Second, the psychological causes of emotional eating are believed to involve poor awareness of internal physiological states and differentiation of hunger cues and emotional arousal [32, 33]. Mindfulness increases attention to and awareness of internal sensations, which may help individuals develop a heightened ability to differentiate hunger cues from emotion responses, and detect and respond to satiety cues. Consequently, the frequency of binge eating can be reduced [34–37]. Third, mindfulness practices are aimed at increasing attention to and awareness of thoughts and emotions. Emotional eating is thought to be a self-regulation process, where one's attention is shifted away from negative affect or negative self-appraisals towards an immediately available reward-stimulus such as food [38, 39]. Mindfulness allows individuals to gain awareness of, acknowledge, and tolerate their internal states without immediately responding to them, thus possibly reducing their need to shift their attention to food. At the same time, these practices may facilitate awareness of the thoughts and feelings that trigger emotional eating. In addition, mindfulness-based interventions are short-term, low-cost, and feasible to integrate into standard prenatal care [40–42].

The aim of this project was to develop a psychoeducational intervention for overweight or obese pregnant women to encourage better nutrition and healthy weight gain during pregnancy by teaching mindfulness skills for stress reduction integrated with nutritional and exercise recommendations. The overall project utilized the Obesity-Related Behavioral Intervention Trials (ORBIT) model for developing behavioral treatments to prevent and/or manage chronic disease [43]. Our specific model (see Fig. 1) was that women enter into pregnancy with a diverse array of factors influencing pre-pregnancy weight and nutrition, including life stressors and stress-resilience, food security/availability, and eating behavior patterns. We hypothesized that the Mindful Moms Training (MMT) would, through increasing mindfulness of stress, hunger, fullness, and satiety cues, reduce stress and increase resilience to stressors, improve eating behaviors, and modify to a certain extent the coupling between stress and overeating. By doing this, we hoped that the intervention would result in healthy gestational weight gain within IOM guidelines, and theoretically improve maternal outcomes, neonatal outcomes, and offspring outcomes postpartum. The area within the curved blue box illustrates the portion of the study this paper focuses on: development of the intervention and assessment of its impact on hypothesized mediators. The rectangular box indicates how our model follows the application of the ORBIT model.

In this paper we describe a) our process model for intervention development; b) the content of the intervention resulting from this process; c) attendance, feasibility and teacher fidelity to the intervention; d) the intervention's effects on proposed mechanisms of change (mindfulness, acceptance, emotion regulation); and e) whether these were related to well-being (reductions in stress, depressed mood) and non-homeostatic eating behaviors (emotional eating and external eating), focusing only on the participants who received the intervention (not including the comparison group).

Methods

The Maternal Adiposity, Metabolism, And Stress (MAMAS) study was funded by a National Institutes of Health U01 collaborative research mechanism intended to facilitate developmental approaches to translating basic research into effective behavioral interventions for chronic disease. We used the Obesity-Related Behavioral Intervention Trials (ORBIT) model of intervention development [43], which outlines clear phases for a flexible and progressive process, with clinically relevant milestones for forward movement and return to earlier stages for refinement and optimization.

The MAMAS study began with focus groups with overweight and obese pregnant women (n = 59) representative of the target population to assess interest in, and identify potential barriers to, participating in a mindfulness-based prenatal behavioral intervention for health weight gain during pregnancy [44, 45]. We found that the participants in our target population faced substantial stressors in multiple domains of financial, relationship, pregnancy-related, and weight and health-related situations. They were very interested in the idea of a stress-reduction intervention and were open to the mindfulness approach that we described. Next we conducted a proof-of-concept pilot study, which informed recruitment methods, data-driven selection of intervention content, and intervention delivery logistics. This was followed by the MAMAS intervention trial, which is the primary focus of this paper. We first describe the overview of the study and sample, then intervention development and content, and end with quantitative analyses of proposed mechanisms.

Participants and setting

Participants in the San Francisco Bay Area were recruited between 8 and 20 weeks gestation and screened for eligibility, completed clinical assessments, and began the intervention between 12 and 20 weeks gestation. Inclusion criteria were: being pregnant, age 18 to 45 years, pre-pregnancy BMI minimum = 25 and maximum = 41 or < 300 pounds, and income to poverty ratio ≤ 500% (median income to poverty ratio in the Bay Area, specific to family size). We utilized a wide array of direct and indirect recruitment strategies and found that in-person recruitment at hospital-based prenatal clinics produced the highest yield of participants. Establishing close relationships with prenatal care providers, clinic staff, social service agencies and study participants was an essential precursor to successful recruitment and retention of our study participants [45].

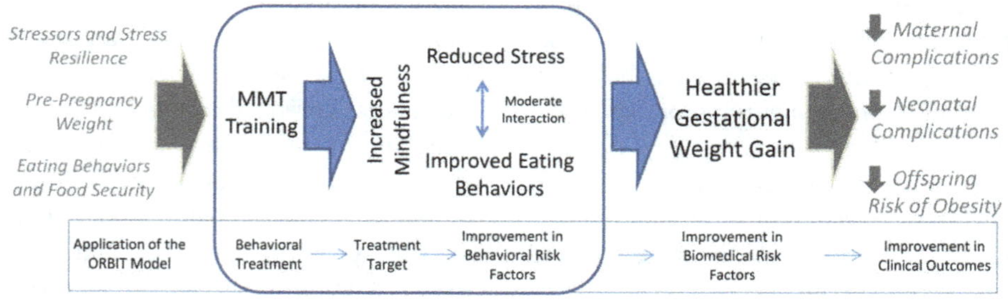

Fig. 1 Theoretical Model

Prospective participants engaged in a group or individual orientation session to learn more about the study requirements and informed consent was obtained from those who chose to participate [46]. A total of 110 pregnant women were recruited to participate in 11 waves of the intervention with 7–13 participants in each wave between 2011 and 2013. One hundred non-randomized treatment-as-usual participants were recruited as a comparison group: their data are not provided in this paper. Orientations and intervention sessions were conducted at CPMC's St. Luke's Hospital and community health centers in the San Francisco Bay Area. The clinical assessments took place at the UCSF General Clinical Research Center where hospital emergency care was immediately available.

Intervention development

Intervention development proceeded in three stages. First, we created an initial provisional intervention. Second, the intervention was refined and optimized through an iterative process over the course of eleven waves of participants (n = 110). Participants in each wave received successive versions of the intervention. Intervention facilitators were selected based on three criteria: 1) experience facilitating mindfulness-based health interventions, 2) experience working with pregnant women and new mothers matching the target population, and 3) willingness to adhere to a research protocol by a) adhering to a manualized intervention, b) providing facilitator feedback, and c) participating in intervention refinement. Two facilitators were selected for this project, one a Masters-level psychology student, and the other a certified nurse midwife (CNM) and family nurse practitioner (FNP), both with extensive experience working with diverse populations formally training in mindfulness-based interventions. Both were trained and supervised by the primary MMT intervention developers (CV and JK). Third, we assessed participants' retention, engagement and subjective response to the intervention and examined pre- to post-intervention changes in hypothesized mediators of mindfulness, mindful eating, activity levels, and acceptance-based coping.

First stage of intervention manual

The initial intervention manual was created using a problem-formulation approach [47] which calls for tailoring interventions to match the population and problem being addressed. We developed the initial content and structure of the intervention based on a theory of change, literature review, and qualitative analysis of focus group responses of 59 stressed, low-income, overweight/obese pregnant women [44]. We then selected components from existing mindfulness-based eating and stress reduction interventions that have shown promise for improving eating, stress, and mood [40, 48–52] and would be suitable to the specific sources of stress, needs and capacities of the target population. These data also informed recruitment materials, reading levels and language used to describe concepts, and incentives for participating.

We selected intervention components designed to achieve the intended outcomes (healthy gestational weight gain and reduced distress) through our theorized mechanisms of action (eating behavior, mindfulness of food choices and hunger, fullness, and taste satiety cues; acceptance-based coping, mindfulness, and improved emotion regulation through reappraisal rather than suppression of distress). Components were selected that demonstrated evidence for 1) reducing distress and improving mood in pregnant women and new mothers (the Mindful Motherhood Training [53]); 2) reducing overeating and binge eating (Mindfulness-Based Eating Awareness Training (MB-EAT) [54]) and Supporting Health by Integrating Nutrition and Exercise (SHINE) [49]). These components were modified to be appropriate for the target population, and to more directly target the stress-overeating interaction. The overall format from these mindfulness intervention derivatives were inspired by Mindfulness-Based Stress Reduction (MBSR) [55]. Like other mindfulness-based interventions that have been empirically supported, an eight-week length of intervention was determined to be suitable for delivering information in a relatively brief window that would provide enough time for participants to introduce and incorporate new concepts and behaviors, while allowing for potential short-term changes in weight gain trajectories.

Intervention manual refinement

Intervention sessions were audio-recorded and the intervention facilitators met weekly with clinical supervisors (CV and JK) by phone to review and discuss feasibility, effectiveness, and areas for improvement. Changes to the initial intervention were made through an iterative process based on: 1) weekly facilitator feedback; 2) supervisor review and assessment of audio recordings of sessions, and 3) mid-course and post-course participant evaluations. Proposed changes were made in consensus decision making sessions among the curriculum development team and were then included in the manual for the subsequent wave. Substantial changes were made during waves 1–5, such as simplifying the movement series and moving it to the beginning of each session, reducing time spent on and simplifying delivery of stress-reduction concepts, increasing focus and time spent on nutritional recommendations with more concrete examples and the "what to eat, how to eat, and how much to eat" framework, and changing exercises and metaphors to ones that were more relatable to the population (such as stress from feeling overwhelmed at work to stress from having the car break down on the freeway). More subtle refinements were made during waves 6–11, such as creating more time for question and answer periods after specific exercises, and making exercises more interactive to assure participants were engaged and following the material. The process led to several key decisions about the structure and content of the training, and changes from the provisional version to the resulting final intervention.

Final intervention

The resulting intervention, the Mindful Moms Training (MMT), is an experiential training where pregnant participants attend a two-hour group session once a week for eight weeks and are asked to engage in assigned readings and experiential practice daily between sessions (note: the terms "training" and "session" are used intentionally rather than "class" to imply an active rather than passive stance of participants). Each session begins with a period of mindful movement, such as gentle stretching and beginner level yoga (~ 15 min), followed by a verbal check-in regarding home practice and progress toward goals in the previous week (~ 15 min), discussion of a mindful stress reduction topic (~ 15 min), mindful eating and nutritional recommendations (~ 30–40 min), mindfulness practice (~ 15 min), review of home practice and goals for the coming week (~ 10 min) , and review/checkout/closing (~ 10 min).

Participants were asked to complete all 8 sessions to the best of their ability, and participants who thought they might not be able to attend more than two sessions at the scheduled times were not enrolled. Participants who missed a session were called the next day by the teaching assistant, and the content of the session and recommended homework was reviewed with them. Class sessions were held at 5:30 pm on a weekday for the most part, which was determined through focus groups to be the best time for most pregnant women since many of them worked during the day, or needed to wait until a partner or grandparent came home from work to care for other children. Participants were welcomed to bring food to the sessions since they occurred during most people's dinner time. We provided incentives for attending group sessions including free gifts such as water bottles, yoga mats, baby clothing, and other items donated by local companies. Each participant was reimbursed $25 at the end of each session for childcare and transportation costs. We did not offer childcare due to potential the liability involved.

The training focuses equally on 1) nutritional and eating behavior recommendations, 2) mindful awareness of hunger, fullness, taste satiety, and food choices, and 3) mindfulness skills for stress reduction (sitting meditation, gentle stretching, acceptance-based stress coping concepts, and informal practices in daily living) (Table 1). A strong social support component organically emerged in which women described feeling relief through sharing their experiences and hearing about the experiences of other women.

1) *Nutrition and Eating Behavior Recommendations.* The nutritional components included 1) "What to Eat" - including recommendations for choosing more fresh whole foods, and less high sugar/ processed foods, discussion of nutritional content, recipes and cooking instructions, drinking more water, replacing foods with more nutritional options, and reading or scanning labels & calories; 2) "How Much to Eat" - discussion of portion sizes and proportions of vegetables, proteins, grains, fruits, dairy, and fats, using the plate method and food pyramid as tools, and 3) "How and When to Eat" - discussion of changing unhealthy eating behaviors such as eating in front of the TV or eating chips out of the bag, and encouraging healthy eating behaviors like eating more small meals per day rather than few large ones, and using small-sized plates.
2) *Mindful eating.* The mindful eating portions of the course were adapted from the Mindfulness-Based Eating Awareness Training (MB-EAT) program [56, 57]. MB-EAT focuses on fostering mindful awareness while eating (i.e., paying attention rather than distracting or "zoning out" while eating). In particular, participants learned and practiced in class: 1) mindful awareness of hunger and fullness; 2) mindful awareness of taste satisfaction and satiety; and 3) mindful awareness of food choices. They also learned to be more aware of thoughts and feelings related to eating, including discussion of stress and emotional eating, and learning how to use mini-meditations before meals. A key element of this component of the program were in-depth experiential eating exercises using food in class, such as exploring taste satiety through mindful eating of potato chips, learning to rate level of hunger prior to eating a piece of chocolate cake, and assessing fullness while drinking a bottle of water. As in MB-EAT, we made the distinction that mindful eating entailed cultivating "inner wisdom," while adapting nutritional recommendations to personal needs was "outer wisdom," so that participants could understand the distinction between the two and utilize both in their eating behaviors and food choices.
3) *Mindfulness for stress reduction.* Content for this portion was adapted from Mindfulness-Based Stress Reduction [58], Mindfulness-Based Cognitive Therapy [52], and the Mindful Motherhood Training [40], with inspiration from Mindfulness-

Table 1 Mindful Moms Training primary intervention components

Nutritional/Eating Behavior	Mindful Eating	Mindful Stress Reduction
What to Eat	Mindful vs. Mindless Eating	Acceptance-Based Coping
How Much to Eat	Hunger and Fullness	Present Moment Awareness
How and When to Eat	Taste Satisfaction and Satiety	Awareness of Breathing
	Food Choices	Body Scan
	Stress and Emotional Eating	Observing Thoughts and Feelings
	Mini-Meditations Before Meals	Mindful Connection with Baby
		Self-Compassion

Based Childbirth and Parenting [41]. Elements of Mindful Self-Compassion training [59] were included as well, since many women reported experiencing stress from their own perceived failings. This was also designed to buffer against stress potentially caused by the intervention's focus on weight and eating, which for many women can result in shame or self-criticism. The stress reduction components of the course were delivered through interactive discussion, small group and dyad work, and experiential exercises focused on acceptance-based coping techniques.

Five types of mindfulness were taught: awareness of breathing, awareness of body sensations (both sitting and while moving), awareness of thoughts and feelings, awareness of connection with the baby, and mindful awareness in everyday life (including eating, but also extending to such activities as being mindful while showering, or while washing dishes). It also included mini-discussions on topics such as "The Observing Self," "What is Acceptance?," "Thoughts are not Facts," "Focusing on the Present Moment," "Mindfulness in Relationships," "Mindful Decision Making," and "Self-Compassion." We found it very important to make these topic discussions highly interactive rather than didactic, using Socratic methods, metaphors, and frequent real-world examples.

The overall course content was summarized for participants in what we called the "Three Commitments" represented by the slogan "Mindful Eating, Move My Body, Breathe!" (see Fig. 2). Throughout each session, the three commitments were reinforced. Participants were provided with laminated cards summarizing the primary program components (see Fig. 1). At the beginning of each session, the group discussed progress and obstacles from the previous week and troubleshooting, problem solving, and goal setting for the coming week. At the end of each session, homework for the coming week was reviewed (e.g., reading assignments, mindful eating, nutrition and exercise recommendations, and recorded guidance for mindful awareness practice). A brief practice of compassion/self-compassion meditation closed each session.

Measures

An array of measures was administered as part of the larger MAMAS study and are reported elsewhere (Epel E, Laraia B, Coleman-Phox K, Leung C, Vieten C, Mellin L, Kristeller J, Thomas M, Stotland N, Bush N et al: Effects of a mindfulness-based intervention on distress, weight gain, and glucose control in pregnant low-income women: a controlled trial, in preparation, [60]) (see Additional file 1 – MAMAS Study Demographics Questionnaire in supplementary materials online). Measures specific to the intervention development portion of the project are reported here:

1) *Participant Retention/Attendance.* Participants were asked to report how many hours they practiced homework per week, and attendance at sessions was tracked by facilitators.
2) *Instructor Fidelity Assessment.* All session were audio-recorded, and between 2 and 5 sessions from each wave were randomly selected to be assessed by trained graduate psychology students, using a checklist for the extent to which facilitators delivered the primary components of the intervention as outlined in the manual (see Additional file 2 – MAMAS Study Fidelity Assessments in the supplementary materials online). A total of 32 sessions were reviewed.
3) *Participant Response.* A Final Evaluation Questionnaire was given to participants in Waves 1–11 at the end of the final class for each wave or was mailed to participants who did not attend the last class (see Additional file 3 – MAMAS Study Final Evaluation in supplementary materials online).

   Fifty-eight questionnaires were returned, of 110 total participants. The questionnaire included structured and open-ended questions about the program including convenience of class location and time, reasons for enrolling, teacher attention, satisfaction with the program, likes and dislikes, usefulness and frequency of use of program components (Mindful Awareness of Breathing,

MINDFUL MOMS DAILY COMMITMENTS

1. Mindful Eating

Inner Wisdom	Outer Knowledge
Hunger and Fullness	Tips for Healthy Eating
Taste Satisfaction	Eat More, Eat Less
Food Choices	Plate Method

2. Move My Body

1) Mindful Stretching
2) Mindful Walking

3. Breathe Awareness of Breathing, Baby, Body Sensations, Feelings & Thoughts

MINDFUL EATING, MOVE MY BODY, BREATHE

Fig. 2 Mindful Moms Three Daily Commitments

Mindful Movement, Mindful Eating), comprehension of mindfulness and acceptance, use of mindfulness skills outside of program, and amount of time outside of program spent using new skills each week.

4) *Self-Report Questionnaires.* Participants were asked to complete baseline measures upon enrollment and post-intervention measures nine weeks later, including:

The *Five Facet Mindfulness Questionnaire (FFMQ)* [61] assesses the general tendency to be mindful in daily life with subscales to assess respondents' ability to act with awareness (α = .86), observe experiences (α = .78), describe feelings (α = .91), non-judging (α = .86), and non-reactivity (α = .73) [62]. The FFMQ has been shown to have convergent and discriminant validity in relation to other psychological constructs in meditating and non-meditating samples. The intervention was designed to increase mindfulness generally, and thus all subscales were included.

To assess the potential mechanism of mindful eating, we utilized two scales from the *Mindful Eating Questionnaire (MEQ)* [63]: mindful awareness of eating, such as noticing flavors, sweetness, colors, and smells of food) (α = .74), and eating in response to external cues (e.g. eating because the food is there, such as eating popcorn in a movie theater or candy from a dish) instead of in response to hunger, (α = .70).

The *Acceptance and Action Questionnaire (AAQ)* [64] is a ten-item questionnaire that measures psychological flexibility, or the ability tolerate negative thoughts and feelings (acceptance) in the pursuit of goals or, depending upon the situation, change behavior to accomplish goals (action) (α = .84). The intervention was designed to increase psychological flexibility/acceptance and decrease experiential avoidance.

The *Emotion Regulation Questionnaire (ERQ)* [65] is a 10-item questionnaire that assesses positive reappraisal (the ability to reframe or look at situations in a positive light) (α = .79), and emotional suppression (the tendency to suppress and avoid negative emotional responses) (α = .73).

The *Perceived Stress Scale (PSS)* [66] was used to measure the degree to which situations in one's life are appraised as stressful, or how unpredictable, uncontrollable, and overloaded respondents find their lives (α = .91). The *Patient Health Questionnaire (PHQ-9)* [67] was used to measure depressive symptoms (α = .86–.89) [68].

To assess eating behavior outcomes, we utilized two scales of the *Dutch Eating Behavior Questionnaire* [69]: emotional eating (α = .93), or overeating in response to emotions, and external eating (α = .80), or eating in response to food-related stimuli, regardless of the internal states of hunger and satiety.

Statistical analyses

We compiled descriptive results (means, standard deviations, or frequencies) for teacher fidelity to the critical domains of the intervention, class attendance and adherence. To assess change in presumed mechanisms, we used paired *t*-tests comparing baseline and endpoint scores. Pearson correlation coefficients were calculated to evaluate changes in general mindfulness, acceptance, mindful eating correlated with perceived stress score changes. All analyses were conducted using SAS software [70].

Results

Demographics

As shown in Table 2, participants in the intervention were an average of 28 years old, predominantly low

Table 2 Demographics

	MMT ($n = 110$)
Age (years), mean (SD)	27.8 (5.7)
	N (%)
Race/ethnicity	
White	14 (12.8)
African American	39 (35.8)
Latino	35 (32.1)
Other/ Multiracial	21 (19.2)
Education	
< 12 years	10 (9.1)
High school graduate/GED	30 (27.3)
Any college or vocational training	56 (50.9)
College graduate or higher	14 (12.7)
Marital status	
Married or in committed relationship	74 (67.3)
Single, separated or divorced	36 (32.7)
Household income, mean (SD)	$24,723 ($22,459)
Number of previous children, mean (SD)	0.8 (1.0)
Pre-pregnancy weight status	
Normal or overweight	58 (55.2)
Class I obese	30 (28.6)
Class II obese	17 (16.2)
Food-Insecure	44 (41.9)
Smoking status	
Current smoker	5 (4.8)
Former smoker	44 (42.3)
Never smoker	55 (52.9)
Leisure-time physical activity	
Inactive or light activity	58 (56.9)
Moderate or vigorously around 3 times/week	21 (20.6)
Moderate or vigorously on most days	23 (22.6)

income, women of color, 78.2% had a high school diploma and/or some college or vocational training, and 13% had a college degree. Thirty-three percent were single, separated, or divorced. There was a notable amount of food insecurity (42%) [71]. Around 45% were obese, and 55% were overweight. Women started the intervention at a mean of 15.9 (SD = 3.8) weeks gestation and completed it at a mean of 24 (SD = 3.0) weeks gestation.

Participant retention/attendance

Of the 114 women enrolled in the intervention, eight women did not complete the baseline questionnaires and thus their quantitative data are not reported here. Four women miscarried and 7 were lost to follow up (1 moved, 1 unable to attend classes, and 5 unable to contact). Participants attended a mean of 5.73 (*SD* 2.31) sessions out of 8 with a median of 7 (see Table 3 for number of participants and percent of total sessions attended by wave). Overall, the mean number of classes attended was 0.79 (SD .06) On average, women reported spending 4.1 h (range 0.16–17.5) outside of class practicing the new skills they learned each week.

Table 3 Participant percentage of total sessions attended by wave

Wave	% of total sessions attended	SD	N
W1	0.83	0.29	8
W2	0.71	0.26	12
W3	0.84	0.23	12
W4	0.84	0.32	7
W5	0.69	0.28	10
W6	0.78	0.23	8
W7	0.83	0.15	9
W8	0.88	0.19	6
W9	0.75	0.26	13
W10	0.84	0.28	9
W11	0.75	0.36	12
Total	0.79	0.06	106

Facilitator Fidelity

Intervention fidelity was good. In 93% of the sessions reviewed, the intervention facilitators "mostly" or "completely" implemented the "Move My Body" gentle stretching aspect of the intervention. In 88% of the sessions the facilitators "mostly" or "completely" provided the "Mindful Eating" portion of the intervention. In 69.2% of the sessions facilitators "mostly" or "completely" delivered the "Breathe" mindfulness-stress reduction component. Facilitators "completely" reviewed the three commitments at the end of each session 88.5% of the time, and 73% of sessions ended in the compassion meditation as indicated in the manual.

Participant response

Fifty-eight women (53%) completed a Final Evaluation Questionnaire. The lower response was due to the questionnaire being sent after the completion of the post-intervention research assessment. We strongly recommend in future studies that program evaluation questionnaires be completed in class or at assessment visits to improve response rates. Among those who responded, most reported that the class location was either "very convenient" (60%) or "somewhat convenient" (29%), as was the day and time of the class ("very convenient"

55%; "somewhat convenient" 41%). Almost all participants felt they had enough opportunities to ask any questions they had of the teachers during or after class (95%; 3% did not have any questions to ask). Most participants were "very satisfied" 71% or "satisfied" 29% overall. No one endorsed being "dissatisfied" or "very dissatisfied". All participants reported understanding of the idea of acceptance ("understood it very well" 65%; "understood it somewhat" 35%).

Participants reported finding the three major program components useful, and most participants practiced at least one mindfulness skill at least a few times over the past week (Table 4). The eating and movement advice for outside of class (the three basic commitments and tips for eating healthy and movement) was also found to be useful ("very useful" 46%; "useful" 49%; "not very useful" 4%; and "not at all useful" 2%). Ninety-five percent of the participants used one or more of the skills or concepts learned in the program outside of class. Mindful breathing was most endorsed (48%), followed by mindful eating (36%), and mindful movement (33%).

Changes in aspects of mindfulness and emotion regulation

We assessed changes in mindfulness in several domains (mindful eating, psychological flexibility/acceptance, the five facets of mindfulness captured by the FFMQ, and emotion regulation), from pre-intervention to post-intervention, within subjects. There were significant increases in mindful eating (awareness of eating, $p < .01$), and non-significant reductions in external eating ($p = .09$). There were improvements in three of the five mindfulness subscales of the FFMQ: observe ($p < .0001$), non-judging ($p = .03$), and non-reactivity ($p = .002$) with a non-significant trend toward improvement in the "act with awareness" subscale ($p = .08$). There were also increases in AAQ psychological flexibility/acceptance (which can also be described as reductions in experiential avoidance) ($p < .0001$), and in adaptive emotion regulation in the tendency toward reappraisal ($p = .002$), with no change in tendency for emotional suppression (see Table 5). There were significant improvements in PSS perceived stress ($p < .0001$) and PHQ depression ($p < .0001$) from pre-intervention to post-intervention.

Correlations between changes in targets and outcomes

As shown in Table 6, as hypothesized, there was a pattern showing that increases in measures of mindfulness were associated with decreases in distress (stress and depression) and self-reported eating behavior. Specifically, increases in psychological flexibility (acceptance) were significantly correlated with decreases in stress, depression and emotional eating (but not external eating). Similarly, improvements in all five of the mindfulness (FFMQ) subscales were correlated with decreases in either stress or depression or both. Increases in the mindfulness subscales measuring "acting with awareness" and "non-judging" were correlated with a decrease in emotional eating and external eating. Finally, increases in the reappraisal form of emotion regulation were correlated with decreased stress and emotional eating, whereas increases in emotion suppression were correlated with increased stress, depression, and a non-significant increase in emotional eating. There were no associations between the mindful eating subscales of "awareness" and "external eating" with stress, depression, or eating behaviors.

Discussion

In this study, we developed and tested an eight-week mindfulness-based intervention directed toward reducing stress and overeating in pregnancy. We have described both the content of the intervention, and the iterative process of intervention development required to adequately tailor and optimize the intervention for a high-risk sample. We utilized the ORBIT model, which recognizes that interventions must be customized to meet the needs of special vulnerable populations, and intervention development must be strongly informed by iterative feasibility testing with the target population.

The resulting Mindful Moms Training (MMT) is a mindfulness-based psychosocial intervention for low- to middle-income overweight/obese pregnant women that was designed to foster healthy weight gain during pregnancy and reduction of transmission of obesity to infants by targeting 1) reductions in stress and negative mood, through acceptance-based coping, and 2) improved nutrition and healthy eating behavior during pregnancy

Table 4 Participant reported usefulness and frequency of use of intervention components ($n = 58$)

Program Components	How useful?				How often used over past week?			
	Not at all useful	Not very useful	Useful	Very useful	Did not use	A few times	1×/day most days	Several times most days
Mindful Awareness of Breathing	0%	3%	41%	55%	2%	31%	40%	27%
Mindful Movement	0%	7%	44%	53%	7%	32%	30%	32%
Mindful Eating	0%	7%	40%	53%	11%	39%	30%	20%
Three Basic Commitments	2%	4%	49%	46%	N/A	N/A	N/A	N/A

Table 5 Changes in mindfulness and emotion regulation from pre- to post- intervention

	Pre	Post	Change in Intervention Group[a]
	Mean (SD)	Mean (SD)	P
Mindful Eating – Awareness (MEQ) $N = 79$	2.55 (0.6)	2.73 (0.7)	**0.01**
Mindful Eating – External (MEQ) $N = 77$	2.31 (0.6)	2.43 (0.8)	0.09
Psychological Flexibility (AAQ) $N = 80$	49.92 (10.1)	53.67 (8.9)	**< 0.0001**
Mindfulness – Observe (FFMQ) $N = 81$	25.64 (6.2)	28.61 (6.1)	**< 0.0001**
Mindfulness - Describe (FFMQ) $N = 81$	29.05 (5.6)	29.67 (5.2)	0.19
Mindfulness - Act w/Awareness (FFMQ) $N = 80$	28.40 (6.0)	29.28 (5.0)	0.08
Mindfulness - Nonjudge (FFMQ) $N = 80$	27.48 (5.9)	28.76 (5.6)	**0.03**
Mindfulness - Nonreact (FFMQ) $N = 80$	19.60 (4.7)	21.27 (4.0)	**0.002**
Emotion Regulation - Reappraisal (ERQ) $N = 78$	28.29 (6.5)	30.46 (6.5)	**0.002**
Emotion Regulation - Suppression (ERQ) $N = 80$	12.51 (5.0)	12.88 (4.8)	0.51
Perceived Stress (PSS) $N = 82$	18.62 (6.1)	15.77 (5.7)	**< 0.0001**
Depression (PHQ9) $N = 82$	7.12 (5.6)	4.57 (3.8)	**< 0.0001**

[a]Paired *t*-tests

through mindful eating practices, stress reduction, and increased activity.

We were able to obtain excellent retention, attendance, and reporting of home practice outside of the class setting. Attendance was similar across waves. Participants reported high satisfaction with the program, in terms of content and logistics. We also found strong facilitator fidelity to the intervention.

Partial support was found for the hypothesized mechanisms of change: general mindfulness, mindful eating, acceptance, and emotion regulation. We found improvement in awareness of eating, and three facets of mindfulness - the ability to observe inner experiences (e.g., distressing thoughts, sensations, or emotions), non-judgment, and non-reactivity to those experiences. In addition, we found increases in psychological flexibility, which is defined by greater acceptance of experiences (i.e., reductions in experiential avoidance), as well as the ability to regulate emotions by reappraising situations. Further, we found evidence that improvements in mindfulness were correlated with decreases in stress, depression, and emotional and external eating (i.e., eating to soothe distress or in response to environmental cues instead of hunger or caloric need).

Table 6 Pearson correlations between change in mindfulness measures and changes in distress and eating behavior

Changes in Mindfulness Variables	n	Change in Perceived Stress (PSS)	Change in Depression (PHQ-9)	Change in Emotional Eating (DEBQ)	Change in External eating (DEBQ)
Mindful Eating Questionnaire					
Mindful Eating - Awareness (MEQ)	58–79	−0.10	−0.02	−0.18	−0.02
Mindful Eating - External (MEQ)	56–77	−0.00	−0.08	−0.06	0.04
Acceptance and Action Questionnaire					
Psychological Flexibility (AAQ)	59–80	− 0.26*	− 0.40***	− 0.22*	− 0.02
Five Factor Mindfulness Questionnaire					
Mindfulness - Observe (FFMQ)	59–81	− 0.33**	− 0.06	− 0.17	0.00
Mindfulness - Describe (FFMQ)	59–81	− 0.36***	− 0.42***	− 0.13	− 0.12
Mindfulness - Act With Awareness (FFMQ)	59–80	− 0.18	− 0.46***	−0.25*	− 0.32**
Mindfulness - Nonjudge (FFMQ)	59–80	−0.14	− 0.26*	−0.28*	− 0.33**
Mindfulness - NonReact (FFMQ)	58–80	−0.36**	− 0.13	−0.16	− 0.05
Emotion Regulation Questionnaire					
Emotion Regulation - Reappraisal (ERQ)	58–78	−0.28*	−0.03	− 0.25*	−0.19+
Emotion Regulation - Suppression (ERQ)	59–80	0.22*	0.26*	0.18	0.13

*** = $p < .001$, ** = $p < .01$, * = $p < .05$, + = $p < .10$

The sample size (n) varies, ranging from 56 to 80, as shown, due to missing data

These results support the presumed mechanisms of mindfulness practices in reducing distress and improving eating behavior in pregnant women. The primary outcomes from the nonrandomized trial that utilized this intervention (reported elsewhere (Epel E, Laraia B, Coleman-Phox K, Leung C, Vieten C, Mellin L, Kristeller J, Thomas M, Stotland N, Bush N et al: Effects of a mindfulness-based intervention on distress, weight gain, and glucose control in pregnant low-income women: a controlled trial, in preparation)) showed that women who were enrolled in MMT, compared to a non-randomized comparison group of women receiving treatment as usual, had significant reductions in perceived stress, depressive symptoms, and glucose levels after an oral glucose tolerance test (glucose regulation), but no differences in whether they met Institute of Medicine (IOM) criteria for recommended weight gain. Although there were no detectable effects on the primary outcome of weight, the positive effects on mothers' mental health are important. Those in MMT had lower depression, not just post-intervention but throughout the postpartum period [72]. Additionally, their offspring had fewer medical visits [73]. We are currently following this sample to examine developmental effects on offspring.

Our results should be interpreted while bearing in mind the study's limitations. We had a substantial rate of missing final participant evaluations of the intervention that may have led to biased results, and could not compare those who completed the final evaluations with those who did not because we collected them anonymously (to help participants feel completely free to be critical in light of the power differential). Also, because the intervention was developed through an iterative process over the course of the study, each wave of participants provided data based on slightly different intervention designs. While statistically significant, changes in mindful eating (awareness) and mindfulness (observe, nonjudge, and nonreact) subscales were small (< 12%). Since there are not yet norms established for clinically meaningful improvements, it is possible that these improvements are clinically negligible. It is also possible that even minor improvements in these variables can make a difference in the outcomes of interest. Reductions in perceived stress and depression were 15 and 36% respectively, which are more noticeable clinically. Reported relationships between increased mindfulness/acceptance and reduced stress, depression, emotional eating and external eating were based on correlations, and thus, we cannot infer causal relationships. Power was not adequate to conduct a more thorough analysis of the relationships between these change scores while controlling for potentially confounding variables.

Another limitation of this project was that pregnant women began the intervention in the second trimester, which is potentially late for addressing eating behaviors and weight gain. It is difficult to recruit subjects and implement a group intervention during the first trimester since many women do not realize that they are pregnant, or trust in the viability of the pregnancy, until the end of the first trimester. Future studies could focus on pre-pregnancy women, or provide a drop-in style group format immediately upon confirmation of pregnancy.

While the brief and nonpharmacological nature of this intervention makes it a promising candidate for widespread use in supporting well-being in pregnancy, a longer, more intensive intervention may be more effective in limiting excessive weight gain. When a sample has high food insecurity, as this sample did, providing healthy food directly or easier access to healthy food may improve efficacy. We are pilot testing further curriculum development to augment MMT by providing both cooking skills (hands on kitchen training) and fresh grocery bags each week, and preliminary feedback from participants has been favorable. In their evaluations, participants suggested that the MMT program could also expand mindfulness meditation and sharing time, and meet every other week until later in the pregnancy.

Recruitment and retention were difficult, requiring tremendous staff effort and devotion of study resources, which has implications for scaling to a community setting. The narrow window of eligibility for enrolling women in a group intervention during the 2nd trimester of pregnancy presents unique obstacles. Logistical issues particularly common in low-income samples, such as inflexible work schedules, lack of transportation/reliance on public transit, and need for childcare also created barriers. In order to optimize recruitment and retention efficiency for future interventions, it may be useful to more fully integrate the program with existing support programs or organizations/communities for low-income pregnant mothers.

Conclusions

Pregnancy is a critical period for both maternal and offspring health, and there is need to reduce distress and unhealthy eating during pregnancy, particularly for women at greatest risk for high stress and excessive gestational weight gain. Through an iterative process of intervention development, we have developed a mindfulness-based program designed to reduce stress and encourage healthy weight gain that we have demonstrated is feasible to utilize with a high-stress diverse pregnant population. Partial support was found for effects of the intervention on hypothesized mechanisms of change: general mindfulness, mindful eating, acceptance, and emotion regulation. Improvements in mindfulness were correlated with decreases in stress, depression, and self-reported emotional and external eating.

By sharing our process of intervention development and initial findings regarding the mechanisms of MMT effects, we hope to make future studies in this area easier to implement. Our intervention manual is available upon request to be tailored for other populations. These findings should encourage practitioners and policy-makers that even in very high risk samples, pregnancy is a window of opportunity for behavior change that can improve metabolic and mood trajectories both for women and their offspring.

Abbreviations

AAQ: Acceptance and action questionnaire; BMI: Body mass index; CNM: Certified Nurse Midwife; CPMC: California Pacific Medical Center; CRC: Clinical Research Center; DEBQ: Dutch eating behavior questionnaire; ERQ: Emotion Regulation Questionnaire; FFMQ: Five factor mindfulness questionnaire; FNP: Family Nurse Practitioner; IOM: Institute of Medicine; MAMAS: Maternal adiposity, metabolism, and stress; MBCT: Mindfulness-based cognitive therapy; MB-EAT: Mindfulness-Based Eating Awareness Training; MBSR: Mindfulness-based stress reduction; MEQ: Mindful eating questionnaire; MMT: Mindful moms training; ORBIT: Obesity-Related Behavioral Intervention Trials; PANAS: Positive and negative affective scale; PSS: Perceived stress scale; SHINE: Supporting Health by Integrating Nutrition and Exercise; UCSF: University of California, San Francisco

Acknowledgments

We thank Holly Wing, Gwen Valencia-Moscoso, Nina Fry, Ingrid Ammondson, Amber Benson, Samantha Schilf, Vanessa Tearnan, for their assistance with participant recruitment and data collection; Cy de Groat, Michael Coccia, and Alan Pierce for assistance with data management and statistical analysis; the California Pacific Medical Center (CPMC) Research Institute Clinical Research Team, the University of California, San Francisco (UCSF) Clinical Research Center (CRC); and the CPMC, San Francisco General Hospital, UCSF, and community women's health facilities. We also thank Hokhmah Joyallen, Shahara Godfrey, Karen Sharifa Krongold for leading the mindfulness groups; and our study participants.

Funding

Support for this work was provided by The National Institutes of Health (NHLBI U01 HL097973-02; NCCIH K01 AT005270); the Aetna Foundation, the Bella Vista Foundation, the Mental Insight Foundation, and the Lisa and John Pritzker Foundation. Funding agencies had no role in the design of the study and collection, analysis, and interpretation of data and in writing the manuscript.

Authors' contributions

CV was primarily responsible for intervention development, in collaboration with JK and the team. EE, BL, and NA were principal investigators responsible for the overall study design and implementation. KC-P was responsible for overall project management. NB designed and implemented the follow-up of participants and their infants, LD contributed to intervention content, HW assisted with data analysis and creation of tables, CV, HW & EE drafted the manuscript, and all authors contributed to manuscript editing and read and approved the final manuscript.

Competing interests

The authors declare that they have no competing interests.

Author details

[1]California Pacific Medical Center Research Institute, 475 Brannan Street, San Francisco, CA 94120, USA. [2]Institute of Noetic Sciences, 625 Second Street, # 200, Petaluma, CA 94952, USA. [3]Center for Health and Community, University of California, San Francisco, 3333 California St., Suite 465, Box 0844, San Francisco, CA 94143-0844, USA. [4]School of Public Health, University of California, Berkeley, 207-B University Hall, Berkeley, CA 94720-7360, USA. [5]Department of Psychology, Indiana State University, Terre Haute, Indiana 47809, USA. [6]Department of Pediatrics, University of California, San Francisco, 550 16th Street, San Francisco, CA 94158, USA. [7]School of Human Ecology, University of Wisconsin-Madison, 1300 Linden Drive, Madison, WI 53706, USA.

References

1. Ogden CL, Carroll MD, Lawman HG, Fryar CD, Kruszon-Moran D, Kit BK, Flegal KM. Trends in obesity prevalence among children and adolescents in the United States, 1988-1994 through 2013-2014. JAMA. 2016;315(21):2292–9.
2. Flegal KM, Kruszon-Moran D, Carroll MD, Fryar CD, Ogden CL. Trends in obesity among adults in the United States, 2005 to 2014. JAMA. 2016; 315(21):2284–91.
3. Institute of Medicine. Weight gain during pregnancy: reexamining the guidelines. Washington DC: National Academies Press; 2009.
4. Catalano P, Ehrenberg H. The short-and long-term implications of maternal obesity on the mother and her offspring. BJOG. 2006;113(10):1126–33.
5. Hedderson MM, Weiss NS, Sacks DA, Pettitt DJ, Selby JV, Quesenberry CP, Ferrara A. Pregnancy weight gain and risk of neonatal complications: macrosomia, hypoglycemia, and hyperbilirubinemia. Obstet Gynecol. 2006; 108(5):1153–61.
6. Li C, Liu Y, Zhang W. Joint and independent associations of gestational weight gain and pre-pregnancy body mass index with outcomes of pregnancy in Chinese women: a retrospective cohort study. PLoS One. 2015;10(8):e0136850.
7. Oken E, Rifas-Shiman SL, Field AE, Frazier AL, Gillman MW. Maternal gestational weight gain and offspring weight in adolescence. Obstet Gynecol. 2008;112(5):999.
8. Kiel DW, Dodson EA, Artal R, Boehmer TK, Leet TL. Gestational weight gain and pregnancy outcomes in obese women: how much is enough? Obstet Gynecol. 2007;110(4):752–8.
9. Bray GA, Champagne CM. Beyond energy balance: there is more to obesity than kilocalories. J Am Diet Assoc. 2005;105(5 Suppl 1):S17–23.
10. Adam TC, Epel ES. Stress, eating and the reward system. Physiol Behav. 2007;91(4):449–58.
11. Garg N, Wansink B, Inman JJ. The influence of incidental affect on consumers' food intake. J Mark. 2007;71(1):194–206.
12. Rutters F, Nieuwenhuizen AG, Lemmens SG, Born JM, Westerterp-Plantenga MS. Acute stress-related changes in eating in the absence of hunger. Obesity. 2009;17(1):72–7.
13. Rolls BJ, Roe LS, Meengs JS, Wall DE. Increasing the portion size of a sandwich increases energy intake. J Am Diet Assoc. 2004;104(3):367–72.
14. Wansink B, Kim J. Bad popcorn in big buckets: portion size can influence intake as much as taste. J Nutr Educ Behav. 2005;37(5):242–5.
15. Wansink B, Van Ittersum K, Painter JE. Ice cream illusions: bowls, spoons, and self-served portion sizes. Am J Prev Med. 2006;31(3):240–3.
16. Yeomans MR, Gray RW. Opioid peptides and the control of human ingestive behaviour. Neurosci Biobehav Rev. 2002;26(6):713–28.
17. Dallman MF. Stress-induced obesity and the emotional nervous system. Trends Endocrinol Metab. 2010;21(3):159–65.
18. Boggiano MM, Chandler PC, Viana JB, Oswald KD, Maldonado CR, Wauford PK. Combined dieting and stress evoke exaggerated responses to opioids in binge-eating rats. Behav Neurosci. 2005;119(5):1207.
19. Artiga A, Viana J, Maldonado C, Chandler-Laney P, Oswald K, Boggiano M. Body composition and endocrine status of long-term stress-induced binge-eating rats. Physiol Behav. 2007;91(4):424–31.
20. Eisenmann JC. Insight into the causes of the recent secular trend in pediatric obesity: common sense does not always prevail for complex, multi-factorial phenotypes. Prev Med. 2006;42(5):329–35.

21. Stotland NE, Cheng YW, Hopkins LM, Caughey AB. Gestational weight gain and adverse neonatal outcome among term infants. Obstet Gynecol. 2006; 108(3, Part 1):635–43.
22. Jain NJ, Denk CE, Kruse LK, Dandolu V. Maternal obesity: can pregnancy weight gain modify risk of selected adverse pregnancy outcomes? Am J Perinatol. 2007;24(5):291–8.
23. Koza RA, Nikonova L, Hogan J, Rim J-S, Mendoza T, Faulk C, Skaf J, Kozak LP. Changes in gene expression foreshadow diet-induced obesity in genetically identical mice. PLoS Genet. 2006;2(5):e81.
24. Garmendia ML, Corvalan C, Araya M, Casanello P, Kusanovic JP, Uauy R. Effectiveness of a normative nutrition intervention (diet, physical activity and breastfeeding) on maternal nutrition and offspring growth: the Chilean maternal and infant nutrition cohort study (CHiMINCs). BMC Pregnancy Childbirth. 2015;15:175.
25. Tanentsapf I, Heitmann BL, Adegboye AR. Systematic review of clinical trials on dietary interventions to prevent excessive weight gain during pregnancy among normal weight, overweight and obese women. BMC Pregnancy Childbirth. 2011;11:81.
26. Dodd JM, Grivell RM, Crowther CA, Robinson JS. Antenatal interventions for overweight or obese pregnant women: a systematic review of randomised trials. BJOG. 2010;117(11):1316–26.
27. Hartmann M, Kopf S, Kircher C, Faude-Lang V, Djuric Z, Augstein F, Friederich H-C, Kieser M, Bierhaus A, Humpert PM. Sustained effects of a mindfulness-based stress-reduction intervention in type 2 diabetic patients design and first results of a randomized controlled trial (the Heidelberger diabetes and stress-study). Diabetes Care. 2012;35(5):945–7.
28. Hoffman CJ, Ersser SJ, Hopkinson JB, Nicholls PG, Harrington JE, Thomas PW. Effectiveness of mindfulness-based stress reduction in mood, breast-and endocrine-related quality of life, and well-being in stage 0 to III breast cancer: a randomized, controlled trial. J Clin Oncol. 2012;30(12):1335–42.
29. Hou RJ, Wong S-S, Yip B-K, Hung AT, Lo H-M, Chan PH, Lo CS, Kwok T-Y, Tang WK, Mak WW. The effects of mindfulness-based stress reduction program on the mental health of family caregivers: a randomized controlled trial. Psychother Psychosom. 2013;83(1):45–53.
30. Brown K, Ryan R, Creswell JD. Mindfulness: theoretical foundations and evidence for its salutary effects. Psychol Inq. 2007;18(4):211–37.
31. Goyal M, Singh S, Sibinga EM, Gould NF, Rowland-Seymour A, Sharma R, Berger Z, Sleicher D, Maron DD, Shihab HM, et al. Meditation programs for psychological stress and well-being: a systematic review and meta-analysis. JAMA Intern Med. 2014;174(3):357–68.
32. van Strien T. Ice-cream consumption, tendency toward overeating, and personality. Int J Eat Disord. 2000;28(4):460–4.
33. van Strien T, Ouwens MA. Counterregulation in female obese emotional eaters: Schachter, Goldman, and Gordon's (1968) test of psychosomatic theory revisited. Eat Behav. 2003;3(4):329–40.
34. Guardino CM, Dunkel Schetter C, Bower JE, Lu MC, Smalley SL. Randomised controlled pilot trial of mindfulness training for stress reduction during pregnancy. Psychol Health. 2014;29(3):334–49.
35. Katterman SN, Kleinman BM, Hood MM, Nackers LM, Corsica JA. Mindfulness meditation as an intervention for binge eating, emotional eating, and weight loss: a systematic review. Eat Behav. 2014;15(2):197–204.
36. Kristeller JL, Hallett B. An exploratory study of a meditation-based intervention for binge eating disorder. J Health Psychol. 1999;4(3):357–63.
37. Kristeller J, Wolever RQ, Sheets V. Mindfulness-based eating awareness training (MB-EAT) for binge eating: a randomized clinical trial. Mindfulness. 2014;5(3):282–97.
38. Heatherton T, Jenn R. Stress and the disinhibition of behavior. Mind Body Med. 1995;1:72–81.
39. Wallis DJ, Hetherington MM. Stress and eating: the effects of ego-threat and cognitive demand on food intake in restrained and emotional eaters. Appetite. 2004;43(1):39–46.
40. Vieten C, Astin J. Effects of a mindfulness-based intervention during pregnancy on prenatal stress and mood: results of a pilot study. Arch Womens Ment Health. 2008;11(1):67–74.
41. Duncan LG, Bardacke N. Mindfulness-based childbirth and parenting education: promoting family mindfulness during the perinatal period. J Child Fam Stud. 2010;19(2):190–202.
42. Dunn C, Hanieh E, Roberts R, Powrie R. Mindful pregnancy and childbirth: effects of a mindfulness-based intervention on women's psychological distress and well-being in the perinatal period. Arch Womens Ment Health. 2012;15(2):139–43.
43. Czajkowski SM, Powell LH, Adler N, Naar-King S, Reynolds KD, Hunter CM, Laraia B, Olster DH, Perna FM, Peterson JC, et al. From ideas to efficacy: the ORBIT model for developing behavioral treatments for chronic diseases. Health Psychol. 2015;34(10):971–82.
44. Thomas M, Vieten C, Adler N, Ammondson I, Coleman-Phox K, Epel E, Laraia B. Potential for a stress reduction intervention to promote healthy gestational weight gain: focus groups with low-income pregnant women. Womens Health Issues. 2014;24(3):e305–11.
45. Coleman-Phox K, Laraia BA, Adler N, Vieten C, Thomas M, Epel E. Recruitment and retention of pregnant women for a behavioral intervention: lessons from the maternal adiposity, metabolism, and stress (MAMAS) study. Prev Chronic Dis. 2013;10 https://doi.org/10.5888/pcd10.120096.
46. Goldberg JH, Kiernan M. Innovative techniques to address retention in a behavioral weight-loss trial. Health Educ Res. 2005;20(4):439–47.
47. Teasdale JD, Segal Z, Williams M. Mindfulness training and problem formulation. Clin Psychol. 2003;10(2):157–60.
48. Miller JJ, Fletcher K, Kabat-Zinn J. Three-year follow-up and clinical implications of a mindfulness meditation-based stress reduction intervention in the treatment of anxiety disorders. Gen Hosp Psychiatry. 1995;17(3):192–200.
49. Mason AE, Daubenmier J, Moran PJ, Kristeller J, Dallman M, Lustig RH, Acree M, Bacchetti P, Laraia B, Epel ES. Increases in mindful eating predict reductions in consumption of sweets and desserts: data from the supporting health by integrating nutrition and exercise (SHINE) clinical trial. J Altern Complement Med. 2014;20(5):A17.
50. Kristeller JL, Baer RA, Quillian-Wolever R. Mindfulness-based approaches to eating disorders, Mindfulness-based treatment approaches: Clinician's guide to evidence base and applications; 2006. p. 75–91.
51. Hayes SC, Hayes SC, Strosahl KD, Wilson KG. Acceptance and commitment therapy. New York: Guilford Press; 2012.
52. Segal ZV, Williams JMG, Teasdale JD. Mindfulness-based cognitive therapy for depression. New York: Guilford Publications; 2018.
53. Vieten C. Mindful Motherhood: Practical Tools for Staying Sane During Pregnancy and Your Child's First Year. Oakland: New Harbinger Publications; 2009.
54. Kristeller JL, Wolever RQ. Mindfulness-based eating awareness training: treatment of overeating and obesity, Mindfulness-based treatment approaches: Clinician's guide to evidence base and applications, vol. 119; 2014.
55. Kabat-Zinn J. An outpatient program in behavioral medicine for chronic pain patients based on the practice of mindfulness meditation: theoretical considerations and preliminary results. Gen Hosp Psychiatry. 1982;4(1):33–47.
56. Kristeller JL, Wolever RQ. Mindfulness-based eating awareness training for treating binge eating disorder: the conceptual foundation. Eat Disord. 2010; 19(1):49–61.
57. Kristeller J, Bowman A. The joy of half a cookie: using mindfulness to lose weight and end the struggle with food: TarcherPerigee; 2015.
58. Kabat-Zinn J. Full catastrophe living: using the wisdom of your body and mind to face stress, pain, and illness. New York: Delta; 2009.
59. Neff KD, Germer CK. A pilot study and randomized controlled trial of the mindful self-compassion program. J Clin Psychol. 2013;69(1):28–44.
60. Hayes SC, Hayes SC, Strosahl KD, Wilson KG. Acceptance and therapy. New York: Guilford Press; 2012.
61. Baer RA, Smith GT, Hopkins J, Krietemeyer J, Toney L. Using self-report assessment methods to explore facets of mindfulness. Assessment. 2006; 13(1):27–45.
62. Bohlmeijer E, ten Klooster PM, Fledderus M, Veehof M, Baer R. Psychometric properties of the five facet mindfulness questionnaire in depressed adults and development of a short form. Assessment. 2011;18(3):308–20.
63. Framson C, Kristal AR, Schenk JM, Littman AJ, Zeliadt S, Benitez D. Development and validation of the mindful eating questionnaire. J Am Diet Assoc. 2009;109(8): 1439.
64. Bond FW, Hayes SC, Baer RA, Carpenter KM, Guenole N, Orcutt HK, Waltz T, Zettle RD. Preliminary psychometric properties of the acceptance and action questionnaire-II: a revised measure of psychological inflexibility and experiential avoidance. Behav Ther. 2011;42(4):676–88.
65. Gross JJ, John OP. Individual differences in two emotion regulation

processes: implications for affect, relationships, and well-being. J Pers Soc Psychol. 2003;85(2):348–62.
66. Cohen S, Janicki-Deverts D. Who's stressed? Distributions of psychological stress in the United States in probability samples from 1983, 2006, and 20091. J Appl Soc Psychol. 2012;42(6):1320–34.
67. Spitzer RL, Kroenke K, Williams JB, Group PHQPCS. Validation and utility of a self-report version of PRIME-MD: the PHQ primary care study. JAMA. 1999; 282(18):1737–44.
68. Kroenke K, Spitzer RL, Williams JB, Löwe B. The patient health questionnaire somatic, anxiety, and depressive symptom scales: a systematic review. Gen Hosp Psychiatry. 2010;32(4):345–59.
69. Van Strien T, Frijters JE, Bergers G, Defares PB. The Dutch eating behavior questionnaire (DEBQ) for assessment of restrained, emotional, and external eating behavior. Int J Eat Disord. 1986;5(2):295–315.
70. SAS Institute Inc. SAS/AF® 9.4 procedure guide, second edition. Cary: SAS Institute Inc.; 2013.
71. Bickel G, Nord M, Price C, Hamilton W, Cook J: Guide to measuring household food security. US Department of Agriculture, Food and Nutrition Service, Office of Analysis, nutrition, and evaluation 2000 http://www.fns.usda.gov/fsec/FILES/Guide%20to%20Measuring%20Household%20Food%20Security(3-23-00).pdf.
72. Felder JN, Roubinov D, Bush N, et al. Effect of prenatal mindfulness training on depressive symptom severity through 18-months postpartum: A latent profile analysis. J Clin Psychol. 2018;1–9. https://doi.org/10.1002/jclp.22592.
73. Roubinov DS, Felder JN, Vieten C, Coleman-Phox K, Laraia B, Adler N, Wilson L, Epel E, Bush NR. Maternal depressive symptoms and infant healthcare utilization: The moderating role of prenatal mindfulness. General Hospital Psychiatry. 2018.

8

The effectiveness of an online intervention in preventing excessive gestational weight gain

Christine M. Olson[1*], Susan W. Groth[2], Meredith L. Graham[3], Jennifer E. Reschke[4], Myla S. Strawderman[3] and Isabel Diana Fernandez[4]

Abstract

Background: Excessive gestational weight gain (GWG) is common and contributes to the development of obesity in women and their offspring. Electronic or e-health interventions have the potential to reach large groups of women and prevent excessive GWG, but their effectiveness has not been demonstrated. The purpose of this study was to evaluate, in a real-world setting, the effectiveness of a self-directed, integrated online and mobile phone behavioral intervention in preventing excessive GWG.

Methods: This effectiveness trial was a double-blind, three-arm trial with a parallel group design. Two arms received the same e-health intervention during pregnancy with the third arm serving as the placebo control. The intervention was based on a previously efficacious non-digital intervention that was adapted to electronic format. It included three behavior change tools: a weight gain tracker, and separate diet and physical activity goal-setting and self-monitoring tools. Both treatment conditions received access to informational tools, event reminders, and a blogging feature. Healthy pregnant women age 18-35 years with body mass indexes (BMI) ≥18.5 and < 35, at ≤20 weeks gestation, and an e-mail address were eligible. The proportion of women with excessive total GWG, as defined by the Institute of Medicine (IOM), was the primary outcome. 1689 randomized women were analyzed in the intent-to-treat (ITT) analysis. The study was designed to have 87% power to detect a 10 percentage point reduction from a control rate of 55% with a sample of 1641 ($p = 0.0167$, two-sided).

Results: In the ITT sample, 48.1% (SD = 2.0%) gained excessively in the intervention group as did 46.2% (SD = 2.4%) in the placebo control group. These proportions were not significantly different (RR 1.09; 95% CI 0.98, 1.20, $p = 0.12$). The results were not altered in several sensitivity analyses.

Conclusion: The addition of three behavior change tools to an informational placebo control did not result in a difference in the proportion of women with excessive total GWG compared to the placebo control in this effectiveness trial of an online, self-directed intervention. The similarity of intervention and control treatments and low usage of the behavior change tools in the intervention group are possible explanations.

Keywords: Gestational weight gain, Behavior change, Online intervention, Pregnancy, Randomized controlled trial

* Correspondence: cmo3@cornell.edu
[1]Division of Nutritional Sciences, 406 Savage Hall, Cornell University, Ithaca, NY 14853, USA
Full list of author information is available at the end of the article

Background

Excessive gestational weight gain (GWG) is a risk factor for postpartum weight retention that contributes to long-term weight gain in women [1–3]. It is also related to increased risk of obesity in offspring [2, 4]. In the US in 2015, about 39% of normal weight, 61% of overweight, and 55% of obese women, gained more than the recommended amount of weight during pregnancy [5]. Obesity experts have called for obesity prevention to begin during pregnancy and early infancy [6].

A recent Cochrane review found diet and/or exercise interventions during pregnancy reduced the risk of excessive GWG by 20% [7]. The estimate was robust and supported by high-quality evidence. Electronic communication technologies have the potential to reach large numbers of women during pregnancy with behavioral interventions to prevent excessive weight gain. However, there is currently a paucity of data on their effectiveness for this purpose [8, 9]. There is a growing body of evidence that electronic communication interventions, often called e- and m-health interventions, are efficacious in several different domains of health behavior change including weight loss and weight gain prevention among non-pregnant individuals [10, 11].

The aim of this study was to evaluate the effectiveness of a self-directed, integrated mobile phone and online behavior change intervention in preventing excessive GWG in a real-world setting.

Methods

Overview and design

The overall goal of the project of which this study is a part was to expand the understanding of how to slow the accumulation of weight in childbearing women. This paper reports on the pregnancy portion of a longer study that followed women until 12 months postpartum in order to evaluate the effectiveness of pregnancy intervention and combined pregnancy and postpartum intervention on weight retention at 12 months postpartum. Thus during pregnancy, two arms received the same intervention (one of these arms becomes a control postpartum) and the third arm was the placebo control (Fig. 1). The primary hypothesis for the pregnancy portion of the study was that the intervention would lead to a 10 percentage point reduction in the proportion of women with excessive total GWG in the intervention arms (45%) compared to the placebo control arm (55%).

This trial was a double-blind, three-arm randomized trial with a parallel group design with the individual as the unit of randomization and analysis [12]. Pregnant women were screened by research staff in prenatal clinics, private obstetric practices, ultra-sound offices, and over the phone and online in a large Northeastern US city from May 2011 through July 2012. Inclusion criteria were age 18-35 years and gestational age $\leq$ 20 weeks at time of enrollment. Exclusion criteria included body mass index (BMI) < 18.5 and ≥ 35 kg/m^2, multiple gestation, weight-affecting medical or psychiatric conditions, and no e-mail address [12]. The age limits were set by the Early Adult Reduction of Weight through LifestYle interventions (EARLY) consortium of weight management studies of which this trial was a part [13]. Eligible women provided written informed consent and signed a form for release of their medical records. Upon consent, participants were electronically randomized via computer to 2 intervention arms and 1 control arm within 4 income (with low income defined by Medicaid eligibility) and BMI (normal BMI and overweight plus obese class 1 BMI) strata in blocks of six: strata 1 - normal BMI low income; strata 2 - normal BMI high income; strata 3 - overweight plus obese class 1 low income; and strata 4 - overweight plus obese class 1 high income. The study protocol was approved by the University of Rochester Research Subject Review Board and the Cornell University Institutional Review Board.

Intervention

Participants assigned to the intervention arms received access to the intervention website and those assigned to the placebo control condition received access to the control website, both of which were password protected. A more detailed description of the theory, development and implementation of the pregnancy intervention is available [14, 15]. Briefly, the self-directed, integrated online and mobile phone behavioral intervention was designed using the Integrative Model of Behavior Prediction [16] and the Behavior Model for Persuasive Design [17] in addition to formative research with the target population [14]. It was based on a non-electronic pregnancy lifestyle intervention that was demonstrated to be efficacious in low-income women [18]. Women in the intervention arms received access to three behavior change tools including a weight gain tracker, a diet and a physical activity goal-setting and self-monitoring tool, as well as, health information including tips, articles, frequently asked questions; a description of pregnancy and parenting-related resources available in the local community; a blogging tool; and an event and appointment reminder. Fig. 2 shows these tools, their behavioral targets and leverage points from the theoretical model [17]. Fig. 3 shows the dashboard available to participants in the intervention group. The placebo control arm received access to all the features above except the weight gain tracker and the diet and physical activity goal-setting and self-monitoring tools since the latter were hypothesized to be the active ingredients of the intervention. Reminders and informational content, that differed by arm, were distributed weekly via e-mail messages to all participants. In

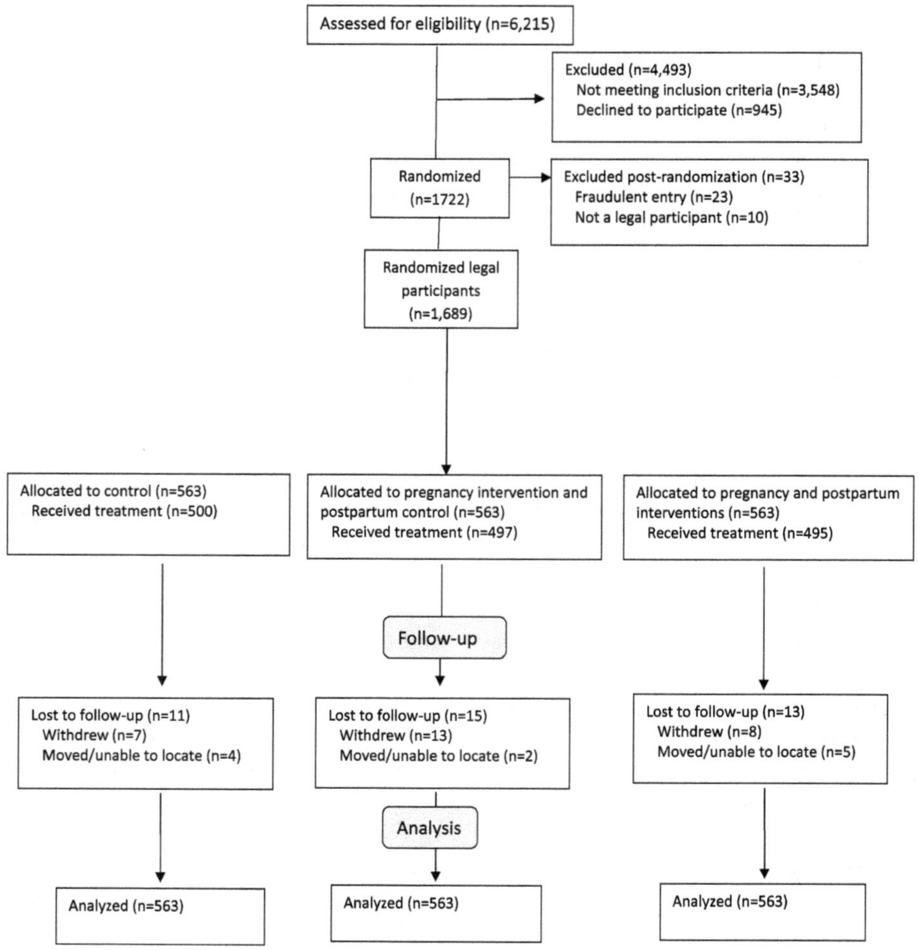

Fig. 1 Participant flow diagram. [a] Fraudulent entries were multiple entries from women who were seeking to enter the study multiple times for monetary purposes. [b] Illegal participants were females who were too young to give informed consent or women whose signed consent forms were missing

summary, two different suites of tools were made available to trial participants on a password protected study website and mobile phone platform. Women were reminded weekly to login, and they decided what, when, and how much they would use the tools made available to them. All women in the trial received standard prenatal care from their self-selected health care provider.

Measures and data collection

Data were collected at screening by research staff, with two online surveys completed by participants during pregnancy (one before 28 weeks gestation and one from 32 weeks until delivery), and through an audit of the women's prenatal, labor and delivery, and 6 week postpartum medical records by research staff. Sociodemographic, behavioral, psychosocial and adverse event data were collected through online surveys [12]. Health and weight data were abstracted from the medical record [12]. Participants received financial incentives for enrolling in the study and for each of the online questionnaires they completed. They could earn up to $45 for completing all data collection activities during pregnancy. They were not paid for engaging with intervention or control treatments. An online satisfaction survey using EARLY questions and for which no financial incentive was provided was made available to participants to complete at 6 weeks postpartum [13].

The pre-specified primary outcome for evaluating the effectiveness of the intervention was the proportion of women with total GWG above the upper limit of the range for total GWG defined by the Institute of Medicine (IOM) for each BMI group [1]. Total GWG was calculated as the difference between the first weight at < 14 weeks gestation and the last weight at ≥37 weeks in pregnancy. The binary outcome, the proportion of women with excessive total GWG, was determined by comparing the difference for each woman to the IOM upper limit for GWG range for each BMI group: normal BMI - > 16 kg; overweight BMI - > 11.5 kg; and obese

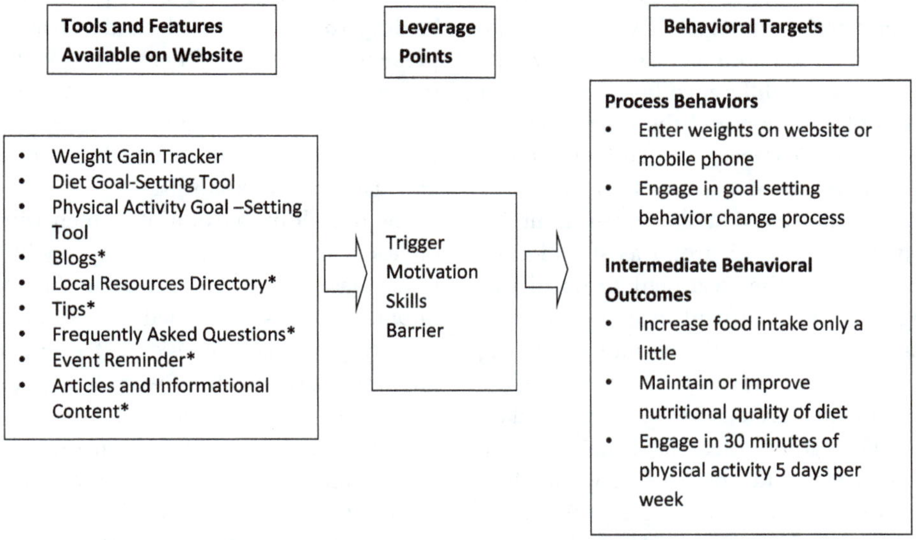

Features with an * were available to participants in the intervention and placebo control conditions.

Fig. 2 Website features, leverage points and behavioral targets for intervention

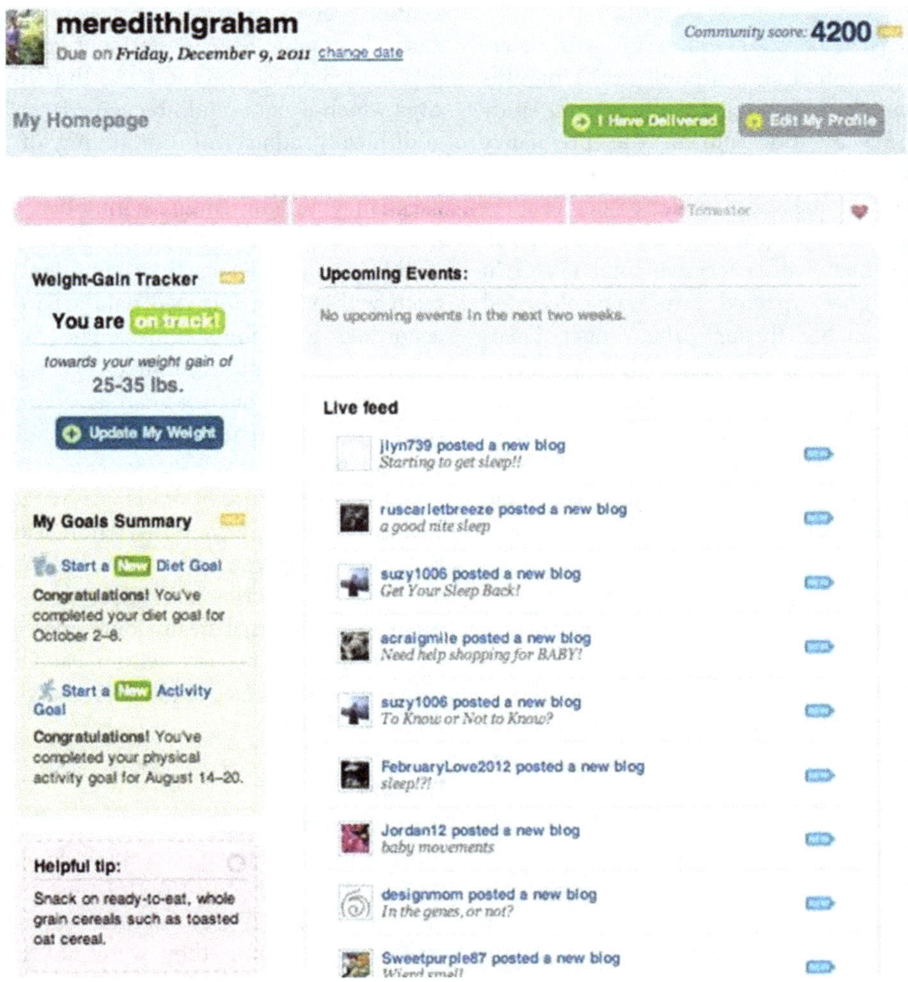

Fig. 3 Dashboard for women on intervention arm

class 1 BMI - > 9 kg [1]. Excessive average weekly GWG in the last half of pregnancy and total GWG in kg were pre-specified secondary outcomes. Average weekly GWG was calculated as the difference between the last weight at ≥37 weeks of gestation and the weight nearest to 20 weeks gestation (+/− 2 weeks) divided by the number of weeks between the two weights. This value was defined as excessive if it exceeded the upper limit for weekly weight gain for each BMI group as specified by the IOM [1]. Adherence to the treatment protocol was defined as logging into the treatment arm specific project website at least once in each 45 day interval during pregnancy. This time interval was based on the schedule of prenatal care visits which are on average every 30 days during pregnancy. Formative research showed that a large proportion of women did not have scales in their homes and thus in order to use the weight gain tracker they needed to use the weights measured at their prenatal care visits [14]. This level of adherence was considered as providing a minimal possibly effective dose of exposure to treatment.

Sample size

The target sample size of 1641 (547/arm) was determined by the weight retention endpoint at 12 months postpartum, the ending time point for the overall study [12]. Assuming 15% attrition during the pregnancy period, yielding 465 controls and 930 intervention subjects, we estimated 87% statistical power to detect a reduction of 10 percentage points from the overall expected 55% of women with excessive total GWG in the control group. The expected rate was calculated from data made available through the Finger Lakes Perinatal Data System which aggregates birth certificate information from hospitals in the region. (See Additional file 1: Table S1.) The study was not powered to examine intervention effects within strata. A Bonferroni-corrected significance level of 1.67% (2-sided), reflecting the three primary comparisons in the entire study, was applied to the primary analysis of excessive total GWG. Otherwise, no multiple comparison procedures were applied and a significance level of 5% was used.

Statistical analysis

Missing data were handled using multiple imputation to address issues of bias which may result from analyzing only complete cases [19]. Sufficient weight information for the calculation of the primary outcome required having a measured weight at both < 14 weeks and ≥ 37 weeks of gestation. If weight information was insufficient, the first, 20 week, and/or last weights were imputed using Statistical Analysis System (SAS) Proc MI. A previous evaluation of the non-electronic version of the intervention indicated that both income and BMI affected GWG outcomes, leading to the stratified randomization design for the present study [18]. Therefore, to allow for a potential interaction between income, BMI, and intervention within the imputed data, 60 imputed data sets were created within each income and BMI group and used in the analysis.

The overall proportion of women with excessive GWG on each arm was estimated by pooling across the imputed data sets, accounting for the variability between imputations, as described by Ratitch, Lipkovich and O'Kelly [20]. Relative risk (RR) estimates for the binary outcomes (proportion of women with excessive total and weekly GWG) were obtained from log-binomial regression models. In two of the sensitivity analyses, some of the log-binomial models did not converge in a few of the 60 imputed data sets. The COPY method was then applied to address the computational issues [21] and was successful in addressing convergence issues in all cases. Mean differences in total GWG (kg) were similarly estimated from least-squares regression models. All multivariable model estimates for the overall effect of intervention versus control arms were adjusted for strata, early pregnancy BMI, gestational age at delivery (to adjust for length of gestation and thus the amount of time over which weight could be gained), and two variables to additionally adjust for the timing of weight measurements: the number of weeks between the first and last pregnancy weight, and the number of weeks between the last pregnancy weight and delivery. SAS Proc MIANALYZE was then used to combine the model results from within each imputed data set in the standard way according to Rubin's Rules. The interaction between treatment arm and the four category strata variable was assessed as a secondary analysis. Several sensitivity analyses were conducted with various subsamples of study participants.

Descriptive information is presented on engagement within treatment arm. Satisfaction with study participation was compared by treatment arm using chi-square analysis. To describe the safety of the intervention, 10 infant and maternal health outcomes and complications were compared by arm within each of the four strata using Fisher's Exact Test. Birthweight was compared using the T-Test.

Results

Description of sample

Of the 6215 women screened, 945 (15.2%) declined participation and 3548 (57.1%) were not eligible (Fig. 1). Of the 1722 (27.7%) women randomized, 23 were fraudulent meaning they were not individual women. They were multiple entries from women who eluded checkpoints and entered the study multiple times for monetary purposes. In addition, 10 women misreported their ages and were too young to give informed consent or their signed consent forms were missing. A sample of 1689 pregnant women was included in the intention-to-treat (ITT) analysis (Fig. 1).

Participants' socio-demographic characteristics were similar between randomized arms (Table 1). Overall, the sample was about 43% low income which means they qualified to received Medicaid (government subsidized prenatal care) during pregnancy and had household incomes < 185% of the Federal poverty threshold. In each treatment group, 53.4% of women had a BMI in the normal range and 46.6% were overweight or class 1 obese. The sample was about 64% non-Hispanic white with African Americans making up 21.1% of the control group and 23.5% of the intervention group. The sample recruited into the study had a higher rate of overweight and obese low income women compared to the population who met study eligibility criteria and delivered infants at the four participating hospitals in the study area (22.3% vs. 15.3%) and had a lower rate of normal BMI high income women compared to the population (32.3% vs. 40.6%). Otherwise, the sample was similar to the population (Additional file 1: Table S1).

Table 1 Baseline characteristics of sample by treatment arm ($n = 1689$)

Characteristic[a]	Placebo control $n = 563$	Intervention $n = 1126$
BMI Income Strata	*n* (%)	n (%)
Normal Low Income	115 (20.4)	242 (21.5)
Normal Not-Low Income	186 (33.0)	359 (31.9)
Overweight + Obese Low Income	125 (22.2)	252 (22.4)
Overweight + Obese Not-Low Income	137 (24.3)	273 (24.3)
Initial BMI (kg/m^2)		
Median (25th, 75th percentile)	24.7 (21.9, 28.3)	24.7 (22.0, 28.6)
Age at entry		
18 to 24.99 y	167 (29.7)	358 (31.8)
25 to 29.99 y	205 (36.4)	366 (32.5)
30 to 34.99 y	191 (33.9)	402 (35.7)
Race and ethnicity		
Non-Hispanic white	340 (64.8)	667 (63.8)
Non-Hispanic African American	111 (21.1)	246 (23.5)
Hispanic/Latina	27 (5.1)	73 (7.0)
Other	47 (9.0)	60 (5.7)
Missing (*n*)	38	80
Parity		
Nulliparous	264 (47.1)	511(45.4)
Primiparous	172 (30.7)	378 (33.6)
Multiparous	125 (22.3)	236 (21.0)
Missing (*n*)	2	1
Education		
High school or less	91 (20.2)	200 (22.5)
Some college	133 (29.6)	258 (29.0)
College graduate	113 (25.1)	213 (23.9)
Graduate or professional degree	113 (25.1)	219 (24.6)
Missing (*n*)	113	236
Smoked in pregnancy		
Yes	66 (12.6)	114 (11.0)
No	457 (87.4)	923 (89.0)
Missing (*n*)	40	89
Home internet use		
Most days/week	335 (71.7)	665 (72.0)
A few times or less	132 (28.3)	259 (28.0)
Missing (*n*)	96	202

[a]Table entries are shown as frequency and percent of known values, n (%), unless specified differently. Subjects with missing values are shown in the missing row for each characteristic

Engagement with treatment

Participants engaged with their treatment arm specific website beginning at a median of 12 weeks of gestation and 34.6% of the placebo control and 46.1% of the intervention arms logged into the website at least once in each 45-day interval of participation and thus were defined as adherent to treatment (Table 2). Control and intervention women had access to the study website a median of 199 and 196 days, respectively, and they logged in a median of 3.2% and 5.6% of those days. The median number of logins and web page views for the placebo control and intervention women were 6 and 10 for logins and 15 and 24 for page views, respectively, with 6 of the page views for behavior change tools in the intervention group.

Additional file 2 Table S2 displays the exposure to and engagement with the information and social content (the placebo content) by treatment arm. The two arms were sent an equal number of weekly e-mail messages, at a median of 28. Overall, the two arms were very similar in their exposure to the placebo content.

Overall, 1169 women (69.2%) submitted a satisfaction survey with no difference in the completion rate by arm. Of these women, 930 (80%) completed the two satisfaction questions reported here. On the 0 to 10 point scale, the majority of participants (53.6%) in both arms scored a 9 or 10 on the item related to recommending the website to other pregnant women (Additional file 3: Table S3). A significantly greater proportion of women in the intervention group scored 9 or 10 on the item asking about enjoying participation in the trial compared to the placebo control group (45.5% vs 37.6%; $p = 0.02$).

Table 2 Engagement with treatment assignment ($n = 1689$)

Indicator of engagement[a]	Placebo control $n = 563$	Intervention $n = 1126$
Logged into study web site at least once, n (%)	473 (84.0)	946 (84.0)
Week of pregnancy of first login	11.8 (8.9, 15.4)	12.0 (8.6, 16.0)
Logged-in each 45 days of participation (adherent), n (%)	195 (34.6)	519 (46.1)
Number of days with access to website	199 (166, 220)	196 (161, 220)
Percent of access days with a login	3.2 (0.9, 6.7)	5.6 (0.2, 11.7)
Number of logins for treatment[b]	6 (2, 14)	10 (2, 24)
Number of web page views	15 (2, 48)	24 (3,62)
Number of web page views of control content	15 (2, 48)	17 (3, 48)
Number of web page views of behavior change tool content	0 (0, 0)	6 (0, 14)

[a]Table entries are median (25th percentile, 75th percentile) unless otherwise noted
[b]This excludes logins for questionnaire completion and other study administrative tasks

Gestational weight gain (GWG) outcomes

Forty-eight and one-tenth percent of women in the intervention arm gained excessively as did 46.2% of women in the placebo control arm (Table 3). In the adjusted analysis, no differences between treatment arms were found in the ITT sample for the primary and secondary outcomes: proportion with excessive total GWG, proportion with excessive weekly GWG, and total GWG in kg (RR 1.09; 95% CI 0.98, 1.20; $p = 0.12$; RR 1.00; 95% CI 0.94, 1.07; $p = 0.90$; mean difference 0.10 kg; 95% CI -0.58, 0.77; $p = 0.78$), respectively. The interaction of treatment with the four-category strata variable (strata 1 - normal BMI low income; strata 2 - normal BMI high income; strata 3 - overweight plus obese class 1 low income; and strata 4 - overweight plus obese class 1 high income) was not significant for any outcome ($p = 0.19$, $p = 0.22$, and $p = 0.16$, respectively). The sensitivity analyses are shown in Table 4 for both excessive total GWG and excessive weekly GWG. Since the results between the two outcomes do not differ, only those for the primary outcome, excessive total GWG, are described in the text. The eligible and participating (treated) sample ($n = 1335$) showed results that were similar to those in the ITT sample: RR 1.10; 95% CI 0.98, 1.22; $p = 0.09$. Additional analyses with the complete case sample ($n = 1337$) for whom no weights were imputed and the per-protocol sample ($n = 714$) that only included women who were defined as adherent by logging in at least once in each 45 day interval of participation, also showed no significant difference between treatment arms. A sensitivity analysis that used self-reported pre-pregnancy weight rather than first measured weight at < 14 weeks gestation for the calculation of gestational weight gain showed no intervention effect, nor did an analysis that included only those who had not gained excessively at the time they started treatment (Table 4).

Safety and clinical outcomes

Two of the 40 maternal and neonatal outcomes and complications compared by treatment arm within strata differed in the eligible and participating sample: the proportion of cesarean deliveries that were repeat cesarean deliveries was significantly greater in the intervention than the control arm (92.3% vs. 66.7%; $p \leq 0.05$) in strata 4 (overweight plus obese class 1 high income) and macrosomia (birthweight > 4000 g) was significantly less common in the intervention than control arm (6.8% vs. 14.0%; $p \leq 0.05$) in strata 2 (normal BMI high income) (Additional file 4: Table S4). Thus, there is little evidence indicating the intervention harmed women or infants.

Table 3 Primary and secondary gestational weight gain (GWG) outcomes in the ITT sample

	Intervention[a] $n = 1126$	Placebo control[a] $n = 563$	Adjusted estimate[b] (95% CI)	P-value
Primary outcome - % exceeding the upper limit of guidelines for total GWG				
Intervention effect	48.1% (2.0%)	46.2% (2.4%)	1.09 (0.98, 1.20)	0.12
Intervention x Strata interaction (3df)				0.19
Secondary outcome - % exceeding the upper limit of weekly GWG rate (kg/week)				
Intervention effect	66.4% (2.0%)	67.9% (2.3%)	1.00 (0.94, 1.07)	0.90
Intervention x Strata interaction (3df)				0.22
Secondary outcome analysis- total GWG (kg)				
Intervention effect	13.73 (0.46)	13.73 (0.45)	0.10 (−0.58, 0.77)	0.78
Intervention x Strata interaction (3df)				0.16

[a]Results are pooled across imputed data sets and are unadjusted for other factors ($n = 1689$)
[b]Relative Risk (RR) estimates of excessive total and weekly GWG from log-binomial model for intervention vs placebo adjusted for strata, gestational age at delivery, continuous BMI, and two timing of weight measurement variables. For total GWG, the mean difference (kg) between intervention and placebo from least squares regression model was adjusted for strata, gestational age at delivery, continuous BMI, and two timing of weight measurement variables. The COPY method was used if any of the 60 log-binomial models did not converge [20]

Table 4 Sensitivity analyses for excessive total gestational weight gain (GWG) and excessive weekly GWG

Sensitivity Sample	Outcome	Intervention[a]	Placebo control[a]	Adjusted estimate[b] (95% CI)	*P*-value
Eligible and participating sample[c]	Excessive total GWG	47.6% (1.7%)	45.9% (2.4%)	1.10 (0.98, 1.22)	0.09
	Excessive weekly GWG	66.8% (1.6%)	68.9% (2.3%)	0.99 (0.93, 1.07)	0.85
Complete case sample[d]	Excessive total GWG	47.0%	45.1%	1.11 (1.00, 1.24)	0.06
	Excessive weekly GWG	67.0%	68.4%	1.01 (0.94, 1.08)	0.85
Per-protocol sample[e]	Excessive total GWG	45.5% (2.3%)	41.6% (3.6%)	1.14 (0.96, 1.37)	0.14
	Excessive weekly GWG	64.2% (2.2%)	62.2% (3.7%)	1.07 (0.95, 1.20)	0.28
As treated sample[f]	Excessive total GWG	47.4% (1.8%)	46.6% (2.2%)	1.08 (0.97, 1.2)	0.15
	Excessive weekly GWG	66.6% (1.7%)	68.8% (2.0%)	1.00 (0.93, 1.07)	0.89
Self-reported pre-pregnancy weight[g]	Excessive total GWG	53.9% (1.9%)	53.1% (2.4%)	1.05 (0.96, 1.15)	0.26
	Excessive weekly GWG	Not applicable	Not applicable	Not applicable	Not applicable
Not excessive GWG at start of treatment[h]	Excessive total GWG	42.8% (2.0%)	39.3% (2.7%)	1.12 (0.96, 1.30)	0.15
	Excessive weekly GWG	65.6% (2.0%)	66.3% (2.6%)	1.02 (0.93, 1.11)	0.68

[a]Results are pooled across imputed data sets (except for the complete case sample) and are not adjusted for other factors, [Mean % (SD)]
[b]Relative Risk (RR) estimates of excessive GWG from log-binomial model for intervention vs placebo adjusted for strata, gestational age at delivery, continuous BMI, and two timing of weight measurements variables. The COPY method was used if any of the 60 log-binomial models did not converge
[c]Eligible and participating sample: $N = 1335$; Intervention arm ($n = 898$), Placebo control arm ($n = 437$)
[d]Complete case sample for excessive total GWG: $N = 1337$; Intervention arm ($n = 891$), Placebo control arm ($n = 446$). Complete case sample for excessive weekly GWG rate: $N = 1364$; Intervention arm ($n = 912$), Placebo control arm ($n = 452$)
[e]Per protocol sample comprised of subjects who logged into website within each 45 day interval of participation: $N = 714$; Intervention arm ($n = 519$), Placebo control arm ($n = 195$)
[f]The as treated sample moves all those in the intervention arm who did not login or when they logged in, did not view the behavior change tools to the placebo control condition: $N = 1335$; Intervention arm ($n = 788$), Placebo control arm ($n = 547$)
[g]ITT sample with excessive GWG determined using self-reported pre-pregnancy weight rather than first measured weight ≤ 14 weeks gestation
[h]ITT sample not excessive GWG by first login to website (nearest weight within 6 weeks): $N = 1055$; Intervention arm ($n = 709$), Placebo control arm ($n = 346$)

Discussion

A socio-economically and racially diverse sample of women that was similar in terms of income and BMI to the population from which it was recruited entered into the study. The integrated online and mobile phone intervention that included 3 behavior change tools had no significant effect beyond the informational placebo control on any of the primary or secondary GWG outcomes. The result was robust to several sensitivity analyses.

In effectiveness trials with self-directed, online interventions focused on preventing excessive GWG, the level of engagement required to achieve a successful outcome is not known. In this trial, the level of engagement with the treatment arm specific website, also called adherence, was determined by research participants. In the intervention arm women, adherence at a level considered to be a minimum possibly effective dose was 46.1% (Table 2), despite the weekly e-mail reminders to login and view new content on the website that was also listed in the message.

Currently five relatively small pilot or feasibility efficacy trials in the literature used mobile and web-based communication technologies to address excessive GWG [22–26]. Among those with positive results, engagement with behavior change interventions was higher than for this study, ranging from 61 to 86%. These findings suggest that the low prevalence of adherence in the intervention arm may have contributed to the null findings of this effectiveness trial with its self-directed, online intervention.

While the placebo control and intervention participants had a similar number of web page views of informational content (the majority of page views), the intervention arm members had only 6 page views of the behavioral change tools. In addition, 135 of the 1126 women in the intervention group (12%) only viewed placebo control content, essentially self-assigning themselves to the control group. The weight gain tracker was the most widely used behavior change tool with 70% of intervention arm women using the tool at least once [14] and 27.3% using it consistently across pregnancy [27]. In an analysis of usage of intervention website features, using the weight gain tracker consistently across pregnancy was associated with a reduction in the proportion of women with excessive total and weekly GWG and mean total GWG among not-low income women [27, 28]. These results support the supposition that the low prevalence of consistent engagement with a key behavior change tool, the weight gain tracker, was not sufficient to produce a difference in weight outcomes between treatment arms and demonstrate the challenge of implementing the IOM guidelines in public health contexts.

Pregnancy has been described as a teachable moment when women are highly motivated to engage in healthy behaviors [29]. For motivated women in the placebo control arm, the information and blogging tools may have been sufficient for preventing excessive GWG. Another RCT with a health coaching intervention to prevent excessive GWG that had an education only control condition also saw no difference in weight gain outcomes between treatment groups [30]. However, no associations were found in this trial between the amount of use of the website and weight outcomes in the placebo control arm decreasing the likelihood of this explanation for the null findings [28].

In this study, personal contact with study staff was limited and similar across treatment arms. A recent review of mobile phone interventions for weight management has shown that the amount of personal contact was significantly ($p = 0.05$) related to differences in weight outcomes [31].

This study has several limitations related to the measurement of weight outcomes and the design of the intervention. This study used a weight < 14 weeks gestation from women's medical records for calculating total GWG. These medical records came from 29 different practices and clinics likely leading to measurement error and inflating the variability in GWG. However, the sensitivity analyses showed that using self-reported pre-pregnancy weights for calculating GWG, as is done in most studies of this topic, did not alter trial outcomes, indicating that the lack of an intervention effect is not highly sensitive to measurement error.

The study relied on self-reported weight and height for calculating BMI for strata assignment and identifying the upper limit for GWG for the weight gain tracker. If women under-reported their pre-pregnancy weight, which was likely, that would lead to a lower BMI and potential misclassification by BMI group. The results would be that under-reporting women would have been told by the study website to gain too much weight during pregnancy. This would decrease the likelihood that the intervention would have a positive effect compared to no weight advice given to the placebo control condition. In future trials, women should be weighed at entry in early pregnancy by research staff in order to correctly identify the upper limit of GWG and avoid giving incorrect advice on appropriate GWG.

Another limitation of the study was that the intervention was self-directed. This was done to meet the very diverse needs of the population of women [32] and to mimic real-world conditions for this translational research trial. The goal was to provide an intervention that was similar to what women could find on their own in the online environment. This may have been an unwise decision. A recent review of the literature on e-behavioral nutrition interventions showed that structured, tailored interventions were more likely to be successful in achieving dietary change [33].

A major strength of this study that supports the importance of publishing this null findings paper is that it is the first large RCT to test a self-directed, integrated e- and m-health intervention to prevent excessive GWG in a real-world setting, much like what any woman could access on her own in an online environment. A related strength is that the trial included a socio-economically, racially, and ethnically diverse sample and used a theory-based suite of behavior change intervention features.

Conclusion

This trial failed to show a positive effect of a self-directed, integrated online and mobile phone behavior change intervention on the proportion of the sample with excessive total GWG compared to an information only placebo control condition. The lack of effect was robust to several sensitivity analyses. There are likely multiple explanations for this result. Our view is that in the overall sample, the behavior change features in the intervention were used too little by too few women to produce a difference from the information only placebo control condition. The behavior change features, particularly the weight gain tracker, could possibly have had an effect if they had been more widely and consistently used across pregnancy. Finally, obtaining an accurate measured body weight very early in pregnancy is essential for giving the correct advice on GWG and for the calculation of the GWG outcome.

Several large trials are currently underway to evaluate the efficacy of various intervention approaches to preventing excessive GWG in overweight and obese women [34]. The results of these trials plus the results of this trial have the potential to enhance the understanding of how to utilize e-and m-health interventions in population-wide obesity prevention programs during pregnancy.

Additional files

Additional file 1: Table S1. Description of population and intent-to-treat (ITT) sample by strata; text

Additional file 2: Table S2. Engagement with informational content by treatment arm; text

Additional file 3: Table S3. Proportion of participants with very high satisfaction scores (9 or 10) by treatment arm; text

Additional file 4: Table S4. Infant and maternal health outcomes and complications; text

Abbreviations

BMI: Body mass index,; CI: Confidence interval; EARLY: Early Adult Reduction of Weight through LifestYle; GWG: Gestational weight gain; IOM: Institute of Medicine; ITT: Intention to treat; kg: kilograms; m: meters; RR: Relative risk; SAS: Statistical Analysis System; SD: Standard deviation; US: United States; y: years

Acknowledgements

The authors would like to thank professors Geri Gay and Jeff Niederdeppe from the Department of Communication at Cornell University for their work on developing the pregnancy intervention and Christian Schimke, Joe Tunis, and Jeremy Larkin of Form Collective for the design, development, and maintenance of the participant website. The authors are grateful to Eva Pressman, Chair of Obstetrics and Gynecology at the University of Rochester School of Medicine and Dentistry and Patrick Stover, Director of the Division of Nutritional Sciences at Cornell University for their administrative leadership that allowed completion of this project.

Funding

National Heart, Lung and Blood Institute and the Eunice Kennedy Shriver National Institute of Child Health and Human Development, Grant No. U01HL096760. The content of this article is solely the responsibility of the authors and does not necessarily represent the official views of the National Institutes of Health.

Authors' contributions

CMO, SWG, MLG, MSS, and IDF designed the research; SWG, MLG, JER, MSS conducted research with JER serving as the study coordinator; MSS analyzed the data; CMO, IDF, SWG, MSS, JER, MLG interpreted the data; CMO and MSS wrote the initial draft of the paper, and SWG, MLG, JER and IDF provided critical reviews and comments. All authors (CMO, SWG, MLG, JER, MSS and IDF) have read and approved the final manuscript.

Competing interests

The authors declare that they have no competing interests.

Author details

[1]Division of Nutritional Sciences, 406 Savage Hall, Cornell University, Ithaca, NY 14853, USA. [2]School of Nursing, University of Rochester, Box SON, 601 Elmwood Ave., Rochester, NY 14642, USA. [3]Division of Nutritional Sciences, 352 MVR Hall, Cornell University, Ithaca, NY 14853, USA. [4]Department of Public Health Sciences, University of Rochester School of Medicine and Dentistry, 265 Crittenden Blvd, CU420644, Rochester, NY 14642, USA.

References

1. Institute of Medicine, National Research Council. Weight gain during pregnancy: reexamining the guidelines. Washington, DC: National Academy of Sciences; 2009.
2. Zilko C, Rehkopf D, Abrams B. Association of maternal gestational weight gain with short- and long-term maternal and child health outcomes. Am J Obstet Gynecol. 2010;202:574. e1-8
3. Linne Y, Dye L, Barkeling B, Rossner S. Weight development over time in parous women—the SPAWN study—15 years follow-up. Int J Obes. 2003;27:1516–22.
4. Sridhar SB, Darbinian J, Ehrlich SF, et al. Maternal gestational weight gain and offspring risk for childhood overweight or obesity. Am J Obstet Gynecol. 2014;211:259. e1-8
5. Branum AM, Sharma AJ, Deputy NP. Gestational weight gain among women with full term, singleton births compared with recommendations–48 states and the District of Columbia, 2015. Morb Mortal Wkly Rep. 2016;65:1121.
6. Gillman M, Ludwig D. How early should obesity prevention start? N Engl J Med. 2013;369(23):2173–5.
7. Muktabhant B, Lawrie TA, Lumbiganon P, Laopaiboon M. Diet or exercise, or both, for preventing excessive weight gain in pregnancy. Cochrane Database of Syst Rev. 2015;(Issue 6, Art. No:CD007145). https://doi.org/10.1002/14651858.CD007145.pub3.
8. O'Brien OA, McCarthy M, Gibney ER, McAuliffe FM. Technology-supported dietary and lifestyle interventions in healthy pregnant women: a systematic review. Eur J Clin Nutr. 2014;68(7):760–6.
9. Sherifali D, Nerenberg KA, Wilson S, Semeniuk K, Ali MU, Redman LM, Adamo KB. The effectiveness of ehealth technologies on weight management in pregnant and postpartum women: systematic review and meta-analysis. J Med Internet Res. 2017;19(10):e337.
10. Tang J, Abraham C, Greaves C, Yates T. Self-directed interventions to promote weight loss: A systematic review of reviews. J Med Internet Res. 2014;16(2):e58.
11. Wantland D, Portillo C, Holzemer W, Slaughter R, McGhee E. The effectiveness of web-based vs. non-web-based interventions: a meta-analysis of behavioral change outcomes. J Med Internet Res. 2004;6(4):e40.
12. Fernandez I, Groth S, Reschke J, Graham M, Strawderman M, Olson C. Electronically-mediated weight interventions for pregnant and postpartum women. Study design and baseline characteristics. Contemp Clin Trials. 2015;43:63–74.
13. Lytle LA, Svetkey LP, Patrick K, Belle SH, Fernandez ID, Jakicic JM, Johnson KC, Olson CM, Tate DF, Wing R, Loria CM. The EARLY trials: a consortium of studies targeting weight control in young adults. Transl Behav Med. 2014; 4(3):304–13.
14. Graham ML, Uesugi KP, Niederdeppe J, Gay GK, Olson CM. The theory, development, and implementation of an online intervention to prevent excessive gestational weight gain: eMoms roc. Telemed J E Health. 2014; 20(12):1–8.
15. Demment M, Graham M, Olson C. How an online intervention to prevent excessive gestational weight gain is used and by whom: a randomized controlled process evaluation. J Med Internet Res. 2014;16(8):e194.
16. Fishbein M, Yzer MC. Using theory to design effective health behavior interventions. Communication Theory. 2003;13:164–83.
17. Fogg B. Persuasive technology. Using computers to change what we think and do. San Francisco: Morgan Kaufmann; 2002.
18. Olson CM, Strawderman MS, Reed RG. Efficacy of an intervention to prevent excessive gestational weight gain. Am J Obstet Gynecol. 2004;191(2):530–6.
19. Graham J. Missing data analysis: making it work in the real world. Ann Rev Psychol. 2009;60:549–76.
20. Ratitch B, Lipkovich I, O'Kelly M. Combining analysis results from mutiply imputed catagorical data. In: PharmaSUG 2013. Conference proceedings. 2013; https://www.pharmasug.org/2013-proceedings.html. Accessed 15 May 2017
21. Deddens JA, Petersen MR. Approaches for estimating prevalence ratios. Occup Environ Med. 2008;65:501–6.
22. Herring SJ, Cruice JF, Bennett GG, Rose MZ, Davey A, Foster GD. Preventing excessive gestational weight gain among African American women: a randomized clinical trial. Obesity (Silver Spring). 2016;24(1):30–6.
23. Pollak KI, Alexander SC, Bennett G, Lyna P, Coffman CJ, Bilheimer A, Farrell D, Bodner ME, Swamy GK, Ostbye T. Weight-related SMS texts promoting appropriate pregnancy weight gain: a pilot study. Patient Educ and Couns. 2014;97:256–60.
24. Soltani H, Duxbury AMS, Arden MA, Dearden A, Furness PJ, Garland C. Maternal obesity management using mobile technology: a feasibility study to evaluate text messaging-based complex intervention during pregnancy. J Obesity. 2015;2015:814830.

25. Willcox JC, Wilkinson SA, Lappas M, Ball K, Crawford D, McCarthy EA, Fjeldsoe B, Whittaker R, Maddison R, Campbell KH. A mobile health intervention promoting healthy gestational weight gain form women entering pregnancy at a high body mass index: the txt4two pilot randomised controlled trial. BJOG. 2017; https://doi.org/10.1111/1471-0528.14552.
26. Redman LM, Gilmore LA, Breaux J, Thomas DM, Elkind-Hirsch K, Stewart T, Hsia DS, Burton J, Apolzan JW, Cain LE, Altazan AD, Ragusa S, Brady H, Davis A, Tilford JM, Sutton EF, Martin CK. Effectiveness of SmartMoms, a novel ehealth intervention for management of gestational weight gain: randomized controlled pilot trial. JMIR Mhealth and Uhealth. 2017;5(9):e133.
27. Olson CM, Strawderman MS, Graham ML. Association between consistent weight gain tracking and gestational weight gain: Secondary analysis of a randomized trial. Obesity (Sliver Spring). 2017;25:1217–27.
28. Graham ML, Strawderman MS, Demment M, Olson CM. Does usage of an ehealth intervention reduce the risk of excessive gestational weight gain? Secondary analysis from a randomized controlled trial. J Med Internet Res. 2017;19(1):e6.
29. Phelan S. Pregnancy: a "teachable moment" for weight control and obesity prevention. Am J Obstet Gynecol. 2010;202:135. e1-8
30. Skouteris H, McPhie S, Hill B, McCabe M, Milgrom J, Kent B, Bruce L, Herring S, Gale J, Mihalopoulos C, et al. Health coaching to prevent excessive gestational weight gain: a randomized-controlled trial. Br J Health Psychol. 2016;21(1):31–51.
31. Schippers M, Adam PCG, Smolenski DJ, Wong HTH, de Wit JBF. A meta-analysis of overall effects of weight loss interventions delivered via mobile phones and effect size differences according to delivery mode, personal contact, and intervention intensity and duration. Obes Rev. 2017;18:450–9.
32. Paul KH, Graham ML, Olson CM. The web of risk factors for excessive gestational weight gain in low income women. Matern Child Health J. 2013;17:344–51.
33. Olson CM. Behavioral nutrition interventions using e- and m-health communication technologies: a narrative review. Annu Rev Nutr. 2016;36:647–64.
34. The LIFE-Moms Research Group. Design of lifestyle intervention trials to prevent excessive gestational weight gain in women with overweight or obesity. Obesity (Silver Spring). 2016;24:305–13.

9

The characterisation of overweight and obese women who are under reporting energy intake during pregnancy

L. J. Moran[1,2*], S. A. McNaughton[3], Z. Sui[1], C. Cramp[1], A. R. Deussen[1], R. M. Grivell[1,4] and J. M. Dodd[1,4]

Abstract

Background: Misreporting of energy intake is common and can contribute to biased estimates of the relationship between diet and disease. Energy intake misreporting is poorly understood in pregnancy and there is limited research assessing characteristics of women who misreport energy intake or changes in misreporting of energy intake across pregnancy.

Methods: An observational study in $n = 945$ overweight or obese pregnant women receiving standard antenatal care who participated in the LIMIT randomised trial. Diet, physical activity, psychological factors, body image satisfaction and dieting behaviour were assessed at trial entry (10–20 weeks gestation) and 36 weeks gestation. Energy misreporting status was assessed through the ratio of daily energy intake over basal metabolic rate. Logistic regression analyses were conducted with the dependent variable of under reporting of energy intake at study entry or 36 weeks in separate analysis.

Results: At study entry and 36 weeks, women were classified as under reporters (38 vs 49.4%), adequate reporters (59.7 vs 49.8%) or over reporters of energy intake (2.3 vs 0.8%) respectively. The prevalence of under reporting energy intake at 36 weeks was higher than at study entry (early pregnancy). Body mass index (BMI) at study entry and 36 weeks and socioeconomic status, dieting behaviour and risk of depression at 36 weeks were independent predictors of under reporting of energy intake.

Conclusions: Under reporting of energy intake was present in over a third of overweight and obese pregnant women and was higher in late compared to early pregnancy. Characteristics such as BMI, socioeconomic status, past dieting behaviour and risk of depression may aid in identifying women who either require support in accurate recording of food intake or attention for improving diet quality. Results were unable to distinguish whether under reporting reflects misreporting or a true restriction of dietary intake.

Keywords: Under reporting of energy, Diet, Pregnancy, Obesity, Overweight

Background

There are recognised limitations to the measurement of dietary intake in clinical or epidemiological research. Commonly used tools including food frequency questionnaires (FFQ), 24-h dietary recalls and dietary records can result in misreporting (low or high reporting) of dietary intake in comparison with gold-standard measures such as doubly labelled water and 24-h urinary nitrogen excretion [1]. The prevalence of misreporting varies but is estimated at ~ 30% for under reporting of energy intake and ~ 10% for over reporting of energy intake in the general adult population [2]. Misreporting also varies depending on the dietary assessment tool used with a lower level of low energy reporting for multiple 24-h recalls compared with a FFQ [3]. Misreporting is related to characteristics including adiposity, socioeconomic status

* Correspondence: lisa.moran@monash.edu
[1]The Robinson Research Institute, Discipline of Obstetrics and Gynaecology, School of Paediatrics and Reproductive Health, The University of Adelaide, Adelaide, VIC 3168, Australia
[2]Monash Centre for Health Research Implementation, School of Public Health and Preventive Medicine, Monash University, Clayton, Australia
Full list of author information is available at the end of the article

and education, age, gender, psychological status such as depression or poor body image, or health-related activities such as smoking or dieting [2, 4]. Misreporting of energy intake could reflect intentional under recording which can be related to social desirability bias. In particular, low energy reporting may result from biasing of reported intake towards foods deemed more appropriate [4, 5] with a lower intake of unhealthier foods high in fat and sugar or unhealthy eating habits resulting in an overall lower diet quality [4]. It may also be related to failure to record accurate food intake due to recall bias or memory lapses, poor awareness of quantities or types of foods eaten [2], the inconvenience of reporting, or reporting an incomplete or simplified version of what is consumed secondary to inaccurate portion size estimation [6].

The misreporting of dietary intake, particularly if systematic and non-random, can result in incorrect assessments of the relationships between dietary components and clinical outcomes. The common under reporting of energy intake or specific dietary components in obesity may also result in a specific bias in studies investigating the relationship between the aetiology and consequences of obesity. Stronger associations between diet, obesity or obesity-associated health conditions or biomarkers of diet or obesity-related health have been previously reported in adequate compared to under reporters of energy intake [7, 8].

Ensuring adequate dietary intake during pregnancy is crucial for optimising maternal, fetal, and infant outcomes [9, 10]. This is important with regards to ensuring micronutrient adequacy and preventing excess energy and macronutrient intake. The identification of women who misreport energy intake in pregnancy is important in identifying any associations between maternal antenatal diet and subsequent health outcomes. This is also relevant in overweight and obese pregnant women as they are more likely to have a higher prevalence of under reporting of energy intake [11], and an increased risk of adverse pregnancy and birth complications. [12] Furthermore, children born to women who are overweight or obese have a higher prevalence of childhood and adult obesity, and obesity-related conditions [13, 14]. However, there is limited literature examining the characteristics of pregnant women who misreport energy intake. While psychological characteristics are associated with under-reporting in the general population [4, 15], there is minimal examination of depression [16] and no examination of the contribution of anxiety, body image status or dieting behaviour to misreporting in pregnancy. There is also limited and contradictory literature examining changes in misreporting status across pregnancy [17, 18], it being unclear if there is a true reduction in energy intake related dietary restriction or to a higher level of energy misreporting.

The aim of this study was to perform a comprehensive assessment of energy misreporting status across two time-points in pregnancy (early and late pregnancy) in a large population of overweight and obese women. Specifically, we aimed to assess the demographic, behavioural and psychological characteristics of overweight and obese pregnant women who misreported energy intake or who had changes in energy misreporting status across pregnancy.

Methods

Study design and population

This study involved women who participated in the LIMIT randomised controlled trial, and who were randomised to receive Standard Antenatal Care. The detailed methodology and primary trial findings have been reported [19]. Briefly, $n = 2122$ women with a body mass index (BMI) ≥25 kg/m^2, with a singleton pregnancy between 10 and 20 weeks gestation (defined as trial entry) and no current diagnosis of diabetes were recruited from the three main maternity hospitals in metropolitan Adelaide, South Australia. The ethics committee at each collaborating hospital independently approved the study protocol (Women's and Children's Hospital (Adelaide, South Australia); Flinders Medical Centre (Adelaide, South Australia); Lyell McEwin Health Service (Adelaide, South Australia); The Queen Elizabeth Hospital (Adelaide, South Australia), and eligible women provided written informed consent. At the time of study entry, women were stratified according to the following domains; parity (0 versus 1 or more), BMI at antenatal booking visit (25.1–29.9 kg/m^2 versus > 30 kg/m^2) and collaborating centre. The LIMIT trial was registered at the Australian and New Zealand Clinical Trials Registry (ACTRN12607000161426).

Outcomes

Demographics and maternal and obstetric outcomes

Baseline demographic details were collected including parity, age, ethnicity, smoking, and past obstetric, medical and family history. Socioeconomic index for area of disadvantage score (SEIFA) [20] was calculated from postcode of residence, with quintile 1 indicating the most disadvantaged women. Women had their weight and height measured by research staff at their first trimester antenatal visit (median 14 weeks gestation) [19] using calibrated scales and stadiometer and weight measured again at 36 weeks gestation. BMI was calculated as their weight divided by the square of their height. Gestational weight gain was calculated as the change in their weight between measurements. BMI was categorised as overweight (25 to 29.9 kg/m^2), obese class I (30–34.99 kg/m^2), class II (35–39.99 kg/m^2) or class III (≥40 kg/m^2) according to World Health Organization guidelines [21] and gestational weight gain was classified as below (inadequate), within (adequate) or above (excessive) according to the Institute of Medicine guidelines [22] of 7–11.5 kg for overweight and 5–9 kg for obese women for total weight gain.

Risk of depression, anxiety symptoms and body image

At study entry and 36 weeks gestation, women were asked to complete questionnaires assessing risk of depression and anxiety as previously reported [23], in addition to questionnaires assessing weight and shape satisfaction. Risk of depression was measured using the Edinburgh Postnatal Depression Scale (EPDS), with increased risk of depression defined as a score of ≥12 [24]. Maternal anxiety symptoms were assessed using the Spielberger State-Trait Inventory Self Evaluation Questionnaire (STAI), comprising of 6 questions, with scores below 15 considered to be within the normal range [25, 26].

At study entry women were asked to complete questionnaires relating to their visual perception of body image in which standard silhouettes were presented corresponding to different BMI categories (Stunkard Figure Rating Scale) [27]. Women were asked to indicate the silhouette that most closely resembled how they usually look (prior to pregnancy), and that which represented how they would like to look. This produced a measure of current size, desired size and a discrepancy score (desired-measured) as a measure of body dissatisfaction. In addition, women were asked to indicate the number of times in the previous year they had attempted to limit the amount of food eaten in order to lose weight (responses never, 1 to 10 times or more than 10 times) and their satisfaction with their weight and body shape (classified as satisfied if they indicated markedly satisfied, moderately satisfied or slightly satisfied versus not at all satisfied) as previously described [28].

Dietary intake, physical activity and energy reporting status

At trial entry and 36 weeks, dietary intake was assessed with the Harvard Semi-quantitative FFQ (The Willett Questionnaire). The reference period for the FFQ was the past 12 months (for trial entry questionnaires) and for the time period from week 28–36 (for the 36 week questionnaire due to the administration of an additional FFQ at 28 weeks). The Willett questionnaire was developed in 1985 in the USA to measure the daily intake of nutrients from 126 food items, with an indication of standard portion size, divided into seven food groups [29], and has been validated for use during pregnancy [30], and in an Australian pregnancy setting [31]. Questions were asked about the relative frequency of consumption of specific food items, use of supplements, cooking methods used and addition of sugar to foods. An open-ended question allowed record of consumption of other foods, which were then categorised by the study investigators. Daily energy, macronutrient and micronutrient intakes were estimated by multiplying frequency responses by the nutrient compositions of the specified portion size of each food item according to Australian food composition tables [32], reflecting standard food fortification with both folate and iodine, utilising the Food Works Nutrient Analysis Software Package (FoodWorks, v.7 Professional; Xyris Software 2012; Australia). Glycemic index values for each food using glucose as the reference standard were obtained from published international [33] and online (http://www.glycemicindex.com/) glycemic index tables according to a prior published protocol [34]. Dietary glycaemic index was determined as the sum of the glycaemic index for all carbohydrates consumed in the diet, with a proportional weighting to account for the relative contribution of each food. Dietary glycemic load was calculated by multiplying the glycemic index of each food with the amount of carbohydrate per serve (from Australian food composition tables [32]) with the overall glycemic load summed from all foods. Diet quality was assessed through the 2005 Healthy Eating Index (HEI) as previously described calculated on an energy-adjusted density [35]. The maximum score is 100 with a HEI score above 80 considered good, a score between 50 and 80 needing improvement and scores below 50 considered poor. If missing data exceeded 25% the questionnaire was excluded from the analysis. At trial entry and 36 weeks total, work, housework, commuting and leisure-time physical activity in metabolic equivalents (MET)/minute/week were assessed with the Short Questionnaire to Assess Health-enhancing physical activity (SQUASH) as previously described [35].

Adequate reporting of energy intake was determined by Goldberg's method using the ratio of daily energy intake to estimated basal metabolic rate (BMR). BMR was calculated for each woman using Schofield equations using age, gender and weight [36] as previously reported in pregnancy [37, 38]. The extra energy requirement for different trimesters was then added to BMR according to National Health and Medical Council reference values (1.4 MJ/day for the 2nd and 1.9 MJ/day for the 3rd trimester) [39]. Under reporters of energy intake, adequate reporters and over reporters of energy intake were classified as an energy intake of < 0.9, 0.9 to 2.1 and > 2.1 BMR respectively as this has been previously used to assess misreporting in pregnant populations [37, 38, 40, 41].

Statistical analysis

Two-tailed statistical analyses were performed using Stata (Stata/IC 13.1 for Windows 2014) with statistical significance set at a P value of < 0.05. Data are presented as mean ± standard deviation (SD) except where indicated.

Data transformations were not used to correct for any departures from normality, since the sample size was sufficient for the central limit theorem to apply [42]. Cross-sectional data were assessed using t test or chi square test and comparisons between time points were assessed using Wilcoxon test for non-parametric and paired t test for parametric data with energy reporting status as the between subject factor. Logistic regression analyses were conducted with the dependent variable of under reporting of energy intake at study entry or 36 weeks in separate analysis. Independent variables were selected based on hypothesis testing and association with under reporting of energy intake on univariate analysis ($p < 0.2$) with the final model constructed with simultaneous entry of preselected predictors. Regression models were constructed to avoid collinearity and assessed for standard assumptions.

Results

Participant characteristics

This study comprises $n = 945$ women randomised to the routine care group of LIMIT (age 29.6 ± 5.4 years; weight 87.7 ± 17.1 kg and BMI 32.3 ± 5.8 kg/m^2). Of these women, data were available at 36 weeks for $n = 508$ women. For the total sample, women were classified as under reporters of energy intake [359/945 (38.0%) at study entry; and 251/508 (49.4%) at 36 weeks respectively], adequate reporters of energy intake [564/945 (59.7%) and 253/508 (49.8%)] or over reporters of energy intake [22/945 (2.3%) and 4/508 (0.8%)]. These proportions were numerically similar when assessing the completers analyses only (Table 1). As there were only a small number of women who over reported their energy intake at each time point, further statistical analysis with this subgroup was not possible and they were excluded from all further analyses.

Table 1 reports participant characteristics according to energy reporting status for the total sample and the completers analysis. In the total sample, women who under reported energy intake were younger, had lower physical activity, higher weight and higher BMI at study entry and 36 weeks, and a higher prevalence of smoking at 36 weeks, when compared with women who adequately reported their energy intake. Under reporting of energy intake was more likely among obese women compared with overweight women at both study entry (66.9% vs 33.1%, $p < 0.001$) and 36 weeks gestation (51.4% vs 35.8%, $p = 0.032$). Women who under reported energy intake had poorer diet quality at study entry (Table 1), specifically in relation to consumption of whole fruit, total vegetables, total grains, wholegrains or milk (Additional file1: Table S1). Women who under reported energy intake also had a lower intake of energy (Table 1), macronutrients, fibre, glycaemic load and all micronutrients both at study entry and 36 weeks. These relationships were maintained in the completers analysis for all variables with the exception of physical activity and diet quality (total and wholegrains) at study entry. On completers analysis women who under reported also had lower diet quality in relation to consumption of total fruit (Additional file 1: Table S1).

For the completers analysis, the prevalence of under reporting of energy intake was significantly higher at 36 weeks gestation in comparison to early pregnancy ($p < 0.001$). There was also a pattern of women changing their energy reporting status from early to late pregnancy. 30.1% of women were considered under reporters of energy intake at both time points, 41.4% adequate energy reporters at both time points. 7.9% considered under reporters of energy intake at study entry but adequate energy reporters at 36 weeks and 20.6% were adequate energy reporters at study entry but under reporters of energy intake at 36 weeks. The women who changed from adequate to under reporters of energy intake were older than women who were under reporters of energy intake at both time points (30.6 ± 5.1 vs 28.6 ± 5.1 years, $p = 0.012$), and of higher weight (87.0 ± 16.1 vs 81.5 ± 13.4 kg, $p = 0.026$) and BMI (32.6 ± 5.6 vs 30.0 ± 4.4 kg/m^2, $p = 0.001$) than those who were adequate energy reporters at both time points.

Gestational weight gain by energy misreporting status

For the completers analysis, the mean gestational weight gain was 9.8 ± 5.7 kg. 44.3% of women gained above, 21.2% gained below and 34.5% gained within the Institute of Medicine gestational weight gain recommendations. There was no association between under reporting of energy intake and gestational weight gain ($p = 0.536$), or the proportion of women achieving weight gain within the Institute of Medicine recommendations ($p = 0.444$). However, there was a significant time-by-energy reporter status interaction for the change in energy intake across pregnancy ($p < 0.001$). Women who under reported energy intake had a reduction (− 1087.2 ± 2271.9 kJ, $p < 0.001$) and adequate reporters had an increase (649.3 ± 3209.9 kJ, $p < 0.001$) in energy intake from trial entry to 36 weeks.

Characteristics of women who under reported energy intake

For the completers analysis there were no differences in the risk of depression or anxiety symptoms, dieting behaviour or BMI estimation at either study entry or 36 weeks for women who did or did not under report energy intake (Table 2). While energy reporting status was not associated with body image discrepancy score at study entry, women who under reported energy intake

Table 1 Participant characteristics according to energy reporting status

Outcomes		10–20 weeks (total sample, $n = 923$)			10–20 weeks (completers, $n = 497$)			36 weeks ($n = 504$)		
		UR $N = 359$ (38.9%)	AR $N = 564$ (61.1%)	P	UR $N = 188$ 37.8%)	AR $N = 309$ (62.2%)	P	UR $N = 251$ (49.8%)	AR $N = 253$ (50.2%)	P
EI/BMR	mean ± SD	0.71 ± 0.15	1.25 ± 0.26	< 0.001	0.72 ± 0.13	1.25 ± 0.27	< 0.001	0.68 ± 0.14	1.21 ± 0.26	< 0.001
Physical activity (MET/min/wk)	mean ± SD	6838.3 ± 4309.1	7661.5 ± 198.1	0.008	6877.8 ± 4073.6	7555.7 ± 4099.4	0.074	5489.0 ± 3889.7	5568.3 ± 3680.9	0.816
Energy intake (kJ)	mean ± SD	5707.5 ± 1215.0	9726.3 ± 2082.2	< 0.001	5776.8 ± 1142.9	9673.7 ± 2101.0	< 0.001	5986.5 ± 1258.9	10,400.8 ± 2202.9	< 0.001
HEI total	mean ± SD	71.5 ± 7.8	73.0 ± 7.0	0.002	72.2 ± 7.7	73.4 ± 6.9	0.085	70.8 ± 7.9	71.5 ± 7.5	0.319
Age (years)	mean ± SD	28.5 ± 5.5	30.2 ± 5.2	< 0.001	28.9 ± 5.1	30.4 ± 29.9	0.001	29.4 ± 5.2	30.4 ± 5.0	0.029
	< 20 years	16 (4.5%)	10 (1.8%)	0.002	4 (2.1%)	5 (1.6%)	0.241	5 (2.0%)	4 (1.6%)	0.505
	20- < 30 years	193 (53.8%)	255 (45.2%)		96 (51.1%)	134 (43.4%)		123 (49.0%)	109 (43.1%)	
	30- < 40 years	141 (39.3%)	276 (48.9%)		85 (45.2%)	159 (51.5%)		117 (46.6%)	131 (51.8%)	
	≥40 years	9 (2.5%)	23 (4.1%)		3 (1.6%)	11 (3.6%)		6 (2.4%)	9 (3.6%)	
Weight (kg)	mean ± SD	92.7 ± 18.0	84.7 ± 15.8	< 0.001	91.7 ± 17.6	83.3 ± 14.5	< 0.001	99.4 ± 17.4	93.4 ± 13.3	< 0.001
BMI (kg/m^2)	mean ± SD	33.9 ± 6.1	31.3 ± 5.4	< 0.001	33.5 ± 6.2	30.8 ± 5.0	< 0.001	36.7 ± 5.8	34.3 ± 4.6	< 0.001
	Overweight	119 (33.1%)	287 (50.9%)	< 0.001	65 (34.6%)	162 (52.4%)	< 0.001	20 (8.0%)	34 (13.4%)	< 0.001
	Obese class I	98 (27.3%)	163 (28.9%)		56 (29.8%)	96 (31.1%)		97 (38.6%)	129 (51.0%)	
	Obese class II	81 (22.6%)	70 (12.4%)		38 (20.2%)	34 (11.0%)		72 (28.7%)	63 (24.9%)	
	Obese class III	61 (17.0%)	44 (7.8%)		29 (15.4%)	17 (5.5%)		62 (24.7%)	27 (10.7%)	
Parity	0	155 (43.2%)	219 (38.8%)	0.190	84 (44.7%)	130 (42.1%)	0.569	115 (45.8%)	102 (40.3%)	0.212
	≥1	204 (56.8%)	345 (61.2%)		104 (55.3%)	179 (57.9%)		136 (54.2%)	151 (59.7%)	
Smoking	No	308 (88.0%)	498 (90.5%)	0.224	165 (89.7%)	286 (94.4%)	0.054	25 (89.8%)	11 (95.6%)	0.014
	Yes	42 (12.0%)	52 (9.5%)		19 (10.3%)	17 (5.6%)		221 (10.2%)	237 (4.4%)	
SEIFA	Quintile 1	105 (29.3%)	164 (29.1%)	0.194	48 (25.5%)	72 (23.3%)	0.382	70 (27.9%)	50 (19.8%)	0.056
	Quintile 2	102 (28.5%)	124 (22.0%)		58 (30.9%)	75 (24.3%)		73 (29.1%)	64 (25.3%)	
	Quintile 3	48 (13.4%)	92 (16.3%)		29 (15.4%)	54 (17.5%)		41 (16.3%)	43 (17.0%)	
	Quintile 4	51 (14.2%)	93 (16.5%)		28 (14.9%)	54 (17.5%)		35 (13.9%)	48 (19.0%)	
	Quintile 5	52 (14.5%)	91 (16.1%)		25 (13.3%)	54 (17.5%)		32 (12.7%)	48 (19.0%)	
Ethnicity	Caucasian	330 (91.9%)	515 (91.3%)	0.745	176 (93.6%)	288 (93.2%)	0.858	233 (92.8%)	236 (93.3%)	0.157
	Non-Caucasian	29 (9.1%)	49 (8.7%)		12 (6.4%)	21 (6.8%)		18 (7.2%)	17 (6.7%)	

Data are presented as mean ± SD or proportions and were analysed by independent t test or chi squared tests
Over reporters were excluded from analysis
AR Adequate reporter, *ATSI* Aboriginal or Torres Strait Islander, *EI/BMR* energy intake: basal metabolic rate, *GDM* gestational diabetes mellitus; *HEI* Healthy Eating Index, *MET* Metabolic equivalent, *SD* Standard deviation, *SEIFA* Socioeconomic indices for areas disadvantage score South Asian: Indian/Pakistan/Sri Lankan, *UR* under reporter

Table 2 Risk of depression, anxiety symptoms, dieting behaviour and weight and shape satisfaction according to energy reporting status

Outcomes		10–20 weeks (completers, $n = 497$)			36 weeks ($n = 504$)		
		UR	AR	*P*	UR	AR	*P*
Risk of depression	mean ± SD	5.4 ± 4.5	5.6 ± 4.2	0.554	5.2 ± 4.6	5.8 ± 4.7	0.175
	Yes	15 (8.6%)	21 (7.3%)	0.613	16 (6.4%)	28 (11.1%)	0.064
	No	159 (91.4%)	266 (92.7%)		234 (93.6%)	225 (88.9%)	
Anxiety symptoms	mean ± SD	10.2 ± 3.4	10.4 ± 3.8	0.530	10.0 ± 3.4	10.5 ± 3.6	0.164
	Yes	24 (12..8%)	40 (13.0%)	0.856	28 (11.2%)	32 (12.7%)	0.593
	No	163 (87.2%)	268 (87.0%)		223 (88.8%)	220 (87.3%)	
Dieting behaviour (times in previous year)	Never	10 (17.9%)	32 (31.7%)	0.164	13 (16.5%)	30 (36.1%)	0.013
	1–10 times	40 (71.4%)	61 (59.8%)		56 (70.9%)	47 (56.6%)	
	> 10 times	6 (10.7%)	9 (8.8%)		10 (12.7%)	6 (7.2%)	
BMI estimate	Underestimate	24 (42.9%)	47 (45.6%)	0.931	38 (48.1%)	40 (47.6%)	0.579
	Correctly estimate	27 (48.2%)	48 (46.6%)		33 (41.8%)	39 (46.4%)	
	Overestimate	5 (8.9%)	8 (7.8%)		8 (10.1%)	5 (6.0%)	
Discrepancy score	mean ± SD	4.1 ± 0.7	3.9 ± 0.6	0. 115	4.1 ± 0.7	3.8 ± 0.6	0.034
Weight satisfaction	Not satisfied	25 (44.6%)	69 (67.0%)	0.006	39 (49.4%)	57 (67.9%)	0.016
	Satisfied	31 (55.4%)	34 (33.0%)		40 (50.6%)	27 (32.1%)	
Shape satisfaction	Not satisfied	25 (44.6%)	71 (68.9%)	0.003	41 (51.9%)	58 (69.0%)	0.025
	Satisfied	31 (55.4%)	32 (31.1%)		38 (48.1%)	26 (31.0%)	

Data are presented as mean ± SD or proportions and were analysed by independent t test or chi squared tests
Over reporters were excluded from analysis
AR Adequate reporter, *BMI* Body mass index, *SD* Standard deviation, *UR* Under reporter

were more likely to report greater dissatisfaction at 36 weeks gestation. Women who under reported their energy intake at 36 weeks were also more likely to report a history of multiple dieting attempts in the previous 12 months, when compared with women who reported an adequate energy intake. Women who under reported their energy intake were less likely to also report dissatisfaction with their weight and shape at both study entry and 36 weeks when compared with women who adequately reported their energy intake.

The independent contribution of demographic, anthropometric and psychosocial factors to under reporting of energy intake at study entry or 36 weeks is reported in Table 3 for the completers analysis. At study entry, higher social disadvantage and BMI were the only significant independent predictors of under reporting of energy intake. At 36 weeks, higher social disadvantage, higher BMI and greater dieting behaviour were all significantly predictive of under reporting of energy intake (Table 3). Women identified to be at a higher risk of depression were less likely to under report energy intake.

Discussion

We report for the first time the association of behavioural and psychological factors with energy misreporting status in a large population of overweight or obese women across pregnancy. At 10–36 weeks gestation under reporting of energy intake was present in up to 50% of women and was independently related to BMI, SEIFA, prior dieting behaviour and depression. The level of under reporting was higher in late pregnancy in comparison to early pregnancy. Diet quality was lower among women who under reported energy intake. We reported a low prevalence of women who over reported intake (0.2–2.3%), in contrast to other reports of up to 12% during pregnancy [11, 16].

As previously reported, under reporting of energy intake was present in a third of overweight or obese women at study entry [16, 37]. As not all overweight and obese women misreport energy intake it is important to identify characteristics that may be predictive of misreporting status. Under reporting of energy intake was more common among obese women compared with overweight women [11, 16, 37] consistent with general population data [2]. The association of low socioeconomic status or education with under reporting of energy intake in the general population or in pregnancy has also been previously reported, and may reflect poor literacy skills [2, 37]. Alternatively, a positive association has also been reported between education and under reporting [43] which may reflect those with a greater knowledge about healthy eating being more prone to selective misreporting. Women may also experience pressure and guilt in relation to achieving an optimal

Table 3 Logistic regression of under reporter status at trial entry or 36 weeks

Outcomes		10–20 weeks			36 weeks		
		OR	95% CI	*P*	OR	95% CI	*P*
SEIFA	1	1	–	–	1	–	–
	2	0.56	0.20, 1.55	0.262	0.19	0.06, 0.60	0.003
	3	0.45	0.13, 1.59	0.215	0.15	0.04, 0.56	0.005
	4	0.25	0.07, 0.87	0.029	0.16	0.05, 0.58	0.005
	5	0.34	0.09, 1.29	0.113	0.15	0.04, 0.59	0.007
BMI (kg/m^2)	25–29.99	1	–	–	1	–	–
	30–34.99	1.09	0.43, 2.78	0.850	2.07	0.58, 7.46	0.265
	35–39.99	1.61	0.52, 4.96	0.405	2.60	0.58, 11.66	0.212
	≤40	23.10	2.44, 218.6	0.006	10.27	1.75, 60.30	0.010
Age (years)		1.01	0.93, 1.09	0.786			
Smoking	No	1	–	–			
	Yes	1.57	0.21, 11.7	0.659			
Weight satisfaction	Satisfied	1	–	–	1		
	Not satisfied	0.49	0.16, 1.48	0.207	0.38	0.11, 1.21	0.101
Shape satisfaction	Satisfied	1	–	–	1		
	Not satisfied	0.87	0.29, 2.58	0.806	1.35	0.42, 4.33	0.611
BMI estimate	Correctly estimate	1	–	–			
	Under estimate	0.80	0.36, 1.77	0.576			
	Over estimate	0.68	0.16, 2.82	0.595			
Dieting behaviour	Never				1	–	–
	1–10 times				2.38	1.00, 5.65	0.051
	> 10 times				4.52	1.11, 18.29	0.035
Discrepancy score					1.06	0.55, 2.03	0.864
Risk of depression	No				1	–	–
	Yes				0.20	0.04, 0.93	0.040

Data were analysed by logistic regression
Over reporters were excluded from analysis
BMI Body mass index, *CI* Confidence interval, *OR* Odds ratio, *SEIFA* Socioeconomic indices for areas disadvantage score

diet during pregnancy [44] which increases as pregnancy progresses and may be compounded by socioeconomic status reflecting poorer health literacy and differences in knowledge and attitudes towards nutrition [45].

We report a range of behavioural or psychological factors that are independently associated with under reporting of energy intake during pregnancy. Specifically, we have identified an independent association between risk of depression and a lower prevalence of under reporting of energy intake in late pregnancy. This is in contrast to prior reports, in which there was no association between risk of depression and low energy reporting, but positive associations with high energy reporting in the second trimester of pregnancy [16]. We found no association between symptoms of anxiety and energy misreporting, which is in contrast to reports from the general population [46]. Increased dieting behaviour prior to pregnancy, greater body dissatisfaction and less dissatisfaction with weight or shape were all associated with a higher level of under reporting of energy intake, in keeping with general population data [4, 47]. However, weight and shape satisfaction associations were attenuated in the logistic regression models indicating a likely indirect relationship between body image and to energy reporting through its relationship with BMI.

There is limited and conflicting literature assessing changes in energy reporting status across pregnancy. A lower level of under reporting of energy intake later in pregnancy assessed by 24-h recall was reported in $n = 490$ pregnant Indonesian women [17]. However, others have reported a higher level of under reporting of energy intake later in pregnancy in 12 women, in the only study utilising the gold-standard assessment of energy expenditure of doubly labelled water [18] consistent with our results presented here. The reason for the higher under reporting occurring at week 36 in our current study is unclear. It was not possible to identify characteristics of women who modified their energy reporting status across pregnancy due to the small event number with the exception of age and BMI. It may be related to factors such as increased time pressures or the effect of weight increasing as pregnancy progresses. We have also previously reported a reduction in depression across pregnancy in this cohort [23]. Given that we reported higher depression was related to lower under reporting on logistic regression analysis, the higher under reporting may be a reflection of this previously observed lower level of depression. While under reporting of energy intake commonly reflects inadequate reporting of dietary intake, it may also reflect an actual restriction in food intake. This may be particularly relevant in overweight or obese women during pregnancy as an attempt to prevent excess weight gain [48]. However, while women who under reported their energy intake at 36 weeks were more likely to report a history of multiple dieting attempts in the previous 12 months, we did not assess if women perceived themselves to be under any dietary restraint during pregnancy itself. In early pregnancy, under reporting of energy intake may also reflect dietary intake secondary to nausea or food aversions. We didnot specifically measure these issues as many women attended the trial entry visit in the second trimester where some of these symptoms may have abated. As these symptoms may affect a large proportion of women (up to 72% in a Norwegian cohort study of $n = 51{,}675$ women) [49], it is crucial to report this in future research assessing dietary misreporting during pregnancy.

We also identified that women who under report energy intake have a subtly poorer diet quality, largely reflecting reduced core food group intake, as has previously been reported [37]. This is in contrast to data from the general population where under reporters of energy intake have improved diet quality [4], more optimal dietary intake by dietary pattern analysis, [50] or micronutrient densities [2, 7], a lower proportional intake of fat, [4] and lower consumption of non-core foods [4]. Our study comprised only women who were overweight or obese and it is possible that this precluded an accurate assessment of changes in dietary intake across all energy reporting groups. Alternatively, if low energy reporting in pregnancy reflects an actual reduction in food intake then a subset of overweight and obese pregnant women are limiting their dietary intake, which in turn potentially impacts their diet quality.

Our study has focused on women who were overweight and obese, which limits therefore the generalisability of our results. We note that the self-reporting of dietary intake data is associated with a degree of inherent measurement errors [51]. In particular, the use of FFQ is associated with a higher level of under energy reporting of intake, when compared with other tools of dietary assessment, such as multiple 24-h recalls. [3]. This may reflect a number of underlying factors including measurement error relating to recall bias, categorisation of portion size and food items lists that may not reflect a changing and diverse food supply [52]. However, the use of the FFQ is more practical and feasible for use in a large scale clinical trial such as ours, and for ranking individuals in large epidemiological or clinical trials. We note the different recall periods used for the FFQ (12 months versus 8 weeks). This may result in capturing a combination of pre-pregnancy and pregnancy dietary intake for the trial entry FFQ in comparison to only pregnancy dietary intake for the 36 week questionnaire which may introduce bias into our dietary information. SEIFA is also an estimate of socioeconomic status that may not accurately reflect individual or familial disadvantage. [20] The influence of family income, education or occupation on energy misreporting in pregnancy should be considered in future studies. The strengths of this study include the large sample size, a comprehensive assessment of women's psychological wellbeing and assessment at two time points across pregnancy.

Our detailed assessment of demographic, behavioural and psychological characteristics has identified factors independently associated with energy misreporting across pregnancy. It is important to identify women who are at high risk of energy intake under reporting across pregnancy, who may be suitable for a more intensive and tailored intervention during pregnancy. Furthermore, if under reporting of energy intake in pregnancy reflects a true reduction in food intake, this also highlights a proportion of overweight and obese pregnant women who may have suboptimal dietary intake, and who warrant specific attention for improving their diet quality and nutrient adequacy.

Conclusion

Under reporting of energy intake was present in over a third of overweight and obese pregnant women and was higher in late compared to early pregnancy. Characteristics such as BMI, socioeconomic status, past dieting behaviour and risk of depression may aid in identifying women who either require support in accurate recording of food intake or attention for improving diet quality.

Additional file

Additional file 1: Table S1. Dietary intake at trial entry and 36 weeks according to energy reporting status. Supplemental Table describing differences in dietary at trial entry and 36 weeks comparing women who were under reporters or adequate reporters of energy.

Abbreviatons

BMR: Basal metabolic rate; BMI: Body mass index; EPDS: Edinburgh Postnatal Depression Scale; FFQ: Food frequency questionnaires; GI: Glycaemic index; GL: Glycaemic load; HEI: Healthy Eating Index; SEIFA: Socioeconomic index for area of disadvantage score; SQUASH: Short Questionnaire to Assess Health-enhancing physical activity; STAI: Spielberger State-Trait Inventory Self Evaluation Questionnaire

Acknowledgements

The following individuals and institutions (except where indicated, in Adelaide, South Australia) participated in the LIMIT Trial:
Steering Group: JM Dodd (Chair), D Turnbull, A McPhee, RM Grivell, C Crowther, M Gillman (Obesity Prevention Program, and Harvard University, Boston, Massachusetts, USA), G Wittert, JA Owens, JS Robinson.
Co-ordinating Team: JM Dodd, A Deussen, RM Grivell, L Yelland, L Moran, C Cramp, A Newman, L Kannieappian, S Hendrijanto, M Kelsey, J Beaumont, C Danz, J Koch, A Webber, C Holst, K Robinson, S Zhang, V Ball, K Ball, H Deussen, N Salehi, R Bartley, R Stafford-Green, S Ophel, M Cooney, M Szmeja, A Short, A Melrose, S Han, I Mohamad, L Chapple.
Statistical Analyses: L Yelland.
Serious Adverse Events Committee: RM Grivell, J Svigos, V Bhatia, N Manton.
Writing Group: JM Dodd, D Turnbull, A McPhee, A Deussen, RM Grivell, L Yelland, C Crowther, G Wittert, JA Owens, JS Robinson.
Collaborating Hospitals (total number of women recruited from each site in parentheses). *Indicates named associate investigator for the NHMRC grant.
• Flinders Medical Centre (South Australia) (669): J McGavigan*, R Bryce, S Coppi, C Fanning, G Hannah, M Ignacio, H Pollard, F Schmidt, Y Shinners.
• Lyell McEwin Hospital (South Australia) (505): G Dekker*, S Kennedy-Andrews, R Beaven, J Niven, S Burgen, J Dalton, N Dewhurst, L Forst, V Mugg, C Will, H Stone.
• Women's and Children's Hospital (South Australia) (1,038): JM Dodd, JS Robinson, A Deussen, C Crowther*, C Wilkinson*, H Purcell, J Wood, D Press, K Ralph, S Donleavy, S Seager, F Gately, A Jolly, L Lahnstein, S Harding, K Daw, M Hedges, R Fraser-Trumble.
We are indebted to the 2,212 women who participated in this randomised trial.

Funding

The LIMIT Randomised Trial was funded by a four-year project grant from the National Health and Medical Research Council, Australia (ID 519240). Ancillary studies to The LIMIT Randomised Trial are supported by a National Institute of Health Program Grant (ID: 5R01HL94235-4). JM Dodd is supported through a National Health and Medical Research Council Practitioner Fellowship (ID 627005). RG is supported by a National Health and Medical Research Council Early Career Research Fellowship (ID 1073514). LM is supported by a SACVRDP Fellowship; a program collaboratively funded by the NHF, the South Australian Department of Health and the South Australian Health and Medical Research Institute. The funders had no role in the design, analysis or writing of this article.

Authors' contributions

All authors were involved equally in the development, design and conduct of the LIMIT trial. Conception and design or acquisition of data: LM, SM, ZS, CC, AD, RG, JD. Analysis and interpretation of data: LM, SM, ZS, CC. Drafting the article or revising it critically for important intellectual content: LM, SM, ZS, CC, AD, RG, JD. Final approval of the version to be published: LM, SM, ZS, CC, AD, RG, JD.

Competing interests

The authors declare that they have no competing interests.

Author details

[1]The Robinson Research Institute, Discipline of Obstetrics and Gynaecology, School of Paediatrics and Reproductive Health, The University of Adelaide, Adelaide, VIC 3168, Australia. [2]Monash Centre for Health Research Implementation, School of Public Health and Preventive Medicine, Monash University, Clayton, Australia. [3]Institute for Physical Activity and Nutrition (IPAN), Deakin University, Geelong, VIC, Australia. [4]Department of Perinatal Medicine, Women's & Babies Division, Women's and Children's Hospital, North Adelaide, Adelaide, Australia.

References

1. Black AE, Cole TJ. Biased over- or under-reporting is characteristic of individuals whether over time or by different assessment methods. J Am Diet Assoc. 2001;101(1):70–80.
2. Poslusna K, Ruprich J, de Vries JH, Jakubikova M, van't Veer P. Misreporting of energy and micronutrient intake estimated by food records and 24 hour recalls, control and adjustment methods in practice. Br J Nutr. 2009; 101(Suppl 2):S73–85.
3. Freedman LS, Commins JM, Moler JE, Arab L, Baer DJ, Kipnis V, Midthune D, Moshfegh AJ, Neuhouser ML, Prentice RL, et al. Pooled results from 5 validation studies of dietary self-report instruments using recovery biomarkers for energy and protein intake. Am J Epidemiol. 2014;180(2):172–88.
4. Lutomski JE, van den Broeck J, Harrington J, Shiely F, Perry IJ. Sociodemographic, lifestyle, mental health and dietary factors associated with direction of misreporting of energy intake. Public Health Nutr. 2011;14(3):532–41.
5. Scagliusi FB, Polacow VO, Artioli GG, Benatti FB, Lancha AH, Jr.: Selective underreporting of energy intake in women: magnitude, determinants, and effect of training. J Am Diet Assoc 2003, 103(10):1306-1313.
6. Mela DJ, Aaron JI. Honest but invalid: what subjects say about recording their food intake. J Am Diet Assoc. 1997;97(7):791–3.
7. Rosell MS, Hellenius ML, de Faire UH, Johansson GK. Associations between diet and the metabolic syndrome vary with the validity of dietary intake data. Am J Clin Nutr. 2003;78(1):84–90.
8. Mendez MA, Wynter S, Wilks R, Forrester T. Under- and overreporting of energy is related to obesity, lifestyle factors and food group intakes in Jamaican adults. Public Health Nutr. 2004;7(1):9–19.
9. Dyer JS, Rosenfield CR. Metabolic imprinting by prenatal, perinatal, and Postnatal Overnutrition. Semin Reprod Endocrinol. 2011;29(3):266–76.
10. Kind KL, Moore VM, Davies MJ. Diet around conception and during pregnancy–effects on fetal and neonatal outcomes. Reprod BioMed Online. 2006;12(5):532–41.
11. Mullaney L, O'Higgins AC, Cawley S, Doolan A, McCartney D, Turner MJ. An estimation of periconceptional under-reporting of dietary energy intake. Journal of public health. 2014;37(8):728–36.
12. Dodd JM, Grivell RM, Ngyuen MA, Chan A, Robinson JS. Maternal and perinatal health outcomes by maternal body mass index category. ANZJOG. 2011;51(2):136–40.
13. Catalano PM, Farrell K, Thomas A, Huston-Presley L, Mencin P, de Mouzon SH, Amini SB. Perinatal risk factors for childhood obesity and metabolic dysregulation. Am J Clin Nutr. 2009;90(5):1303–13.
14. Hochner H, Friedlander Y, Calderon-Margalit R, Meiner V, Sagy Y, Avgil-Tsadok M, Burger A, Savitsky B, Siscovick DS, Manor O. Associations of maternal prepregnancy body mass index and gestational weight gain with adult offspring cardiometabolic risk factors: the Jerusalem perinatal family follow-up study. Circulation. 2012;125(11):1381–9.
15. Kretsch MJ, Fong AK, Green MW. Behavioral and body size correlates of energy intake underreporting by obese and normal-weight women. J Am Diet Assoc. 1999;99(3):300–6.
16. Nowicki E, Siega-Riz AM, Herring A, He K, Stuebe A, Olshan A. Predictors of measurement error in energy intake during pregnancy. Am J Epidemiol. 2011;173(5):560–8.
17. Winkvist A, Persson V, Hartini TN. Underreporting of energy intake is less common among pregnant women in Indonesia. Public Health Nutr. 2002;5(4):523–9.

18. Goldberg GR, Prentice AM, Coward WA, Davies HL, Murgatroyd PR, Wensing C, Black AE, Harding M, Sawyer M. Longitudinal assessment of energy expenditure in pregnancy by the doubly labeled water method. Am J Clin Nutr. 1993;57(4):494–505.
19. Dodd JM, Turnbull D, McPhee AJ, Deussen AR, Grivell RM, Yelland LN, Crowther CA, Wittert G, Owens JA, Robinson JS, et al. Antenatal lifestyle advice for women who are overweight or obese: LIMIT randomised trial. BMJ. 2014;348:g1285.
20. Australian Bureau of Statistics. Socio-Economic Indexes for Areas (SEIFA) - Technical Paper 2006, vol. 2008. Canberra: Australian Bureau of Statistics.
21. WHO Obesity and overweight fact sheet (number 311; March 2011): WHO; http://www.who.int/mediacentre/factsheets/fs311/en/index.html.
22. National Research Council Institute of Medicine. In: Rasmussen KM, Yaktine AL, editors. Weight gain during pregnancy: reexamining the guidelines. Washington D.C; 2009.
23. Dodd JM, Newman A, Moran LJ, Deussen AR, Grivell RM, Yelland LN, Crowther CA, McPhee AJ, Wittert G, Owens JA, et al. The effect of antenatal dietary and lifestyle advice for women who are overweight or obese on emotional well-being: the LIMIT randomized trial. Acta Obstet Gynecol Scand. 2016;95(3):309–18.
24. Cox JL, Holden JM, Sagovsky R. Detection of postnatal depression - development of the 10 item Edinburgh postnatal depression scale (EDPS). Brit J Psych. 1987;154:782–6.
25. Marteau TM, Bekker H. The development of a six item form of the state scale of the Spielberger state trait anxiety inventory (STAI). Br J Clin Psychol. 1992;31:301–6.
26. Spielberger CD. The state-trait anxiety inventory: consulting psychologists press, Inc; 1970.
27. Bulik CM, Wade TD, Heath AC, Martin NG, Stunkard AJ, Eaves LJ. Relating body mass index to figural stimuli: population-based normative data for Caucasians. Int J Obes Relat Metab Disord. 2001;25(10):1517–24.
28. Sui Z, Turnbull D, Dodd J. Effect of body image on gestational weight gain in overweight and obese women. Women and birth : journal of the Australian College of Midwives. 2013;26(4):267–72.
29. Willett WC, Reynolds RD, Cottrell-Hoehner S, Sampson L, Browne ML. Validation of a semi-quantitative food frequency questionnaire: comparison with a 1-year diet record. J Am Diet Assoc. 1987;87(1):43–7.
30. Fawzi WW, Rifas-Shiman SL, Rich-Edwards JW, Willett WC, Gillman MW. Calibration of a semi-quantitative food frequency questionnaire in early pregnancy. Ann Epidemiol. 2004;14(10):754–62.
31. Rumbold AR, Crowther CA, Haslam RR, Dekker GA, Robinson JS, Group AS. Vitamins C and E and the risks of preeclampsia and perinatal complications. N Engl J Med. 2006;354(17):1796–806.
32. NUTTAB. Australian food composition tables. Canberra: Zealand FSAN; 2010.
33. Atkinson FS, Foster-Powell K, Brand-Miller JC. International tables of glycemic index and glycemic load values: 2008. Diabetes Care. 2008;31(12):2281–3.
34. Louie JC, Flood V, Turner N, Everingham C, Gwynn J. Methodology for adding glycemic index values to 24-hour recalls. Nutrition. 2011;27(1):59–64.
35. Dodd JM, Cramp C, Sui Z, Yelland LN, Deussen AR, Grivell RM, Moran LJ, Crowther CA, Turnbull D, McPhee AJ, et al. The effects of antenatal dietary and lifestyle advice for women who are overweight or obese on maternal diet and physical activity: the LIMIT randomised trial. BMC Med. 2014;12(1):161.
36. Schofield WN. Predicting basal metabolic rate, new standards and review of previous work. Human nutrition Clinical nutrition. 1985;39(Suppl 1):5–41.
37. McGowan CA, McAuliffe FM. Maternal nutrient intakes and levels of energy underreporting during early pregnancy. Eur J Clin Nutr. 2012;66(8):906–13.
38. Horan MK, McGowan CA, Gibney ER, Byrne J, Donnelly JM, McAuliffe FM. Maternal nutrition and Glycaemic index during pregnancy impacts on offspring adiposity at 6 months of age–analysis from the ROLO randomised controlled trial. Nutrients. 2016;8(1)
39. NHMRC. Nutrient reference values for Australia and New Zealand. In: Canberra: Australian government publishing service; 2005.
40. Lindsay KL, Heneghan C, McNulty B, Brennan L, McAuliffe FM. Lifestyle and dietary habits of an obese pregnant cohort. Matern Child Health J. 2015;19(1):25–32.
41. Goldberg GR, Black AE, Jebb SA, Cole TJ, Murgatroyd PR, Coward WA, Prentice AM. Critical evaluation of energy intake data using fundamental principles of energy physiology: 1. Derivation of cut-off limits to identify under-recording. Eur J Clin Nutr. 1991;45(12):569–81.
42. Lumley T, Diehr P, Emerson S, Chen L. The importance of the normality assumption in large public health data sets. Annu Rev Public Health. 2002;23:151–69.
43. Yannakoulia M, Panagiotakos DB, Pitsavos C, Bathrellou E, Chrysohoou C, Skoumas Y, Stefanadis C. Low energy reporting related to lifestyle, clinical, and psychosocial factors in a randomly selected population sample of Greek adults: the ATTICA study. J Am Coll Nutr. 2007;26(4):327–33.
44. Wennberg AL, Lundqvist A, Hogberg U, Sandstrom H, Hamberg K. Women's experiences of dietary advice and dietary changes during pregnancy. Midwifery. 2013;29(9):1027–34.
45. Inglis V, Ball K, Crawford D. Why do women of low socioeconomic status have poorer dietary behaviours than women of higher socioeconomic status? A qualitative exploration. Appetite. 2005;45(3):334–43.
46. Taren DL, Tobar M, Hill A, Howell W, Shisslak C, Bell I, Ritenbaugh C. The association of energy intake bias with psychological scores of women. Eur J Clin Nutr. 1999;53(7):570–8.
47. Rennie KL, Siervo M, Jebb SA. Can self-reported dieting and dietary restraint identify underreporters of energy intake in dietary surveys? J Am Diet Assoc. 2006;106(10):1667–72.
48. Storti KL, Arena VC, Barmada MM, Bunker CH, Hanson RL, Laston SL, Yeh JL, Zmuda JM, Howard BV, Kriska AM. Physical activity levels in American-Indian adults: the Strong Heart Family Study. Am J Prev Med. 2009;37(6):481–7.
49. Chortatos A, Haugen M, Iversen PO, Vikanes A, Magnus P, Veierod MB. Nausea and vomiting in pregnancy: associations with maternal gestational diet and lifestyle factors in the Norwegian mother and child cohort study. BJOG. 2013;120(13):1642–53.
50. Scagliusi FB, Ferriolli E, Pfrimer K, Laureano C, Cunha CS, Gualano B, Lourenco B, Lancha AH. Under-reporting of energy intake is more prevalent in a healthy dietary pattern cluster. Br J Nutr. 2008;100(5):1060–8.
51. Subar AF, Freedman LS, Tooze JA, Kirkpatrick SI, Boushey C, Neuhouser ML, Thompson FE, Potischman N, Guenther PM, Tarasuk V, et al. Addressing current criticism regarding the value of self-report dietary data. J Nutr. 2015;145(12):2639–45.
52. Prentice RL, Mossavar-Rahmani Y, Huang Y, Van Horn L, Beresford SA, Caan B, Tinker L, Schoeller D, Bingham S, Eaton CB, et al. Evaluation and comparison of food records, recalls, and frequencies for energy and protein assessment by using recovery biomarkers. Am J Epidemiol. 2011;174(5):591–603.

10

Is birth weight the major confounding factor in the study of gestational weight gain?

Amy C. O'Higgins*, Anne Doolan, Thomas McCartan, Laura Mullaney, Clare O'Connor and Michael J. Turner

Abstract

Background: Much interest has been focussed on both maternal obesity and gestational weight gain (GWG), particularly on their role in influencing birth weight (BW). Several large reviews have reported that excessive GWG is associated with an increase in BW· However recent large, well-designed, randomized controlled trials studying interventions aimed at reducing GWG have all consistently failed to show a reduction in BW despite achieving a reduction in GWG. The aim of this longitudinal prospective study was to examine the relationship between GWG and birth weight in women where GWG and Body Mass Index (BMI) were measured accurately in a strictly standardized way.

Methods: Women were enrolled at their convenience before 18 weeks gestation. Height and weight were measured accurately at the first antenatal visit and BMI calculated. Maternal weight was measured again after 37 weeks gestation. The weight of the baby was measured at birth. Relationships were tested using linear regression analysis, chi-squared tests and t-tests as appropriate.

Results: Of the 522 women studied, the mean BMI was 25.3 kg/m^2 and 15.7% were obese. The mean BW at term was 3576 g (2160–5120) and 2.7% ($n = 14$) weighed ≥4500 g. The mean GWG overall was 12.3 kg (4.6 to 28.4) and GWG decreased as BMI increased. The mean GWG was less in obese women, at 8.7 kg (− 4.6 to 23.4), compared to non-obese,13.0 kg (0.6–28.4) ($p < 0.001$). Mean BW in obese women was 3630 g vs 3565 g in non-obese ($p = 0.27$). The total GWG correlated positively with BW ($p < 0.001$). When BW was subtracted from total GWG, GWG no longer correlated with BW ($p = 0.12$).

Conclusions: The positive correlation between GWG in pregnancy and BW can be accounted for by the contribution of fetal weight to GWG antenatally without a contribution from increased maternal adiposity. There was a wide range of BW irrespective of the degree of GWG and obese women had a lower GWG than non-obese women. These findings help explain why Randomized Controlled Trials (RCTs) designed to reduce GWG have failed to decrease BW and suggest there is no causative link between excessive GWG and increased BW.

Keywords: Gestational weight gain, Maternal obesity, Birth weight

* Correspondence: amyohiggins@rcsi.ie
UCD Centre for Human Reproduction, Coombe Women and Infants University Hospital, Dublin 8, Ireland

Background

Obesity is now a major health problem and is now associated with more deaths globally than malnutrition [1]. There are multiple, complex factors driving the increase in rates of both adult and childhood obesity [1]. Recently much interest has focussed on both maternal obesity and gestational weight gain (GWG), particularly on their role in influencing birth weight (BW). Several large reviews have reported that excessive GWG is associated with an increase in BW [2–5].

However, we are concerned that there are limitations to previous studies that have not been adequately addressed [6]. In particular, these studies are large epidemiological studies where maternal height and weight is self-reported and not measured, leading to the miscategorization of baseline BMI, the under-estimation of obesity rates and the over-estimation of the *impact* of obesity of *clinical* outcomes [7, 8]. Since the publication of revised guidelines on GWG by the Institute of Medicine (IOM) in the United States in 2009 [2], many studies of GWG have reported their outcomes in relation to 'excessive', 'adequate' or 'inadequate' GWG as defined by the IOM [9–12]. The IOM guidelines give different ranges of recommended GWG depending on a woman's baseline BMI. *Underweight women have a recommended GWG of 12.5–18.0 kg, women of normal BMI have a recommened GWG of 11.5–16.0 kg, overweight women have a recommended GWG of 7.0–11.5 kg and obese women a recommended GWG of 5.0–9.0 kg. This terminology is a source of bias in the current literature since a GWG of 10 kg is considered 'inadequate' for women of a normal BMI and 'excessive' for obese women.* It prevents correlation of maternal and fetal outcomes with absolute GWG and makes it difficult to understand the basic physiological correlations between GWG and clincial outcomes including BW.

Recently several large, well-designed, randomised controlled trials studying interventions aimed at reducing gestational weight gain have all consistenly failed to show a reduction in BW despite achieving a reduction in GWG with their intervention [13–17]. We believe these results raise doubt as to a causal relationship between GWG and BW.

We examined the relationship between absolute GWG and BW at term in a well-characterised cohort of women where the calculation of Body Mass Index (BMI) and GWG was accurately assesed in a strictly standardized way.

Methods

The study was undertaken between July 2012 and July 2014 at, *the Coombe Women and Infants Univeristy Hospital*, a large university teaching hospital with over 8500 deliveries per annum. The Hospital cares for women from rural and urban regions and from all socio-economic groups. The study was confined to white European women with a singleton pregnancy *to reduce confounding variables associated with differences in fat mass between women of differing ethnicities of the same BMI* [18]. Women with pre-existing diabetes mellitus were excluded.

Women were recruited at their first antenatal visit *which takes place in the Hospital.* An information leaflet was given and written informed consent obtained. The study was approved by the Hospital's Research Ethics Committee. At recruitment all women had their pregnancy dated by ultrasound and only women < 18 weeks gestation were included. We have previously reported in a cross-sectional study that there is no significant change in mean maternal weight or body composition before this gestation [6, 19]. Maternal sociodemographic and clinical details were recorded and computerized.

Maternal height was measured at recruitment to the nearest 0.1 cm using a digital wall-mounted stadiometer (Seca, Birmingham, United Kingdom) with the woman standing in her bare feet. *Weight was measured using a digital weighing scales* (Tanita MC-180MA, Tokyo, Japan). Women were asked to empty their bladder prior to measurement *which* was performed in light clothing and bare feet [19]. BMI was categorized according to the World Health Organization [20]. Term was defined as the period after *36* completed weeks of gestation. Maternal weight measurement was measured again at a routine antenatal visit at term.

Women with a risk factor for the development of gestational diabetes mellitus (GDM) according to the national guidelines underwent screening with a 75 g oral glucose tolerance test (GTT) between 24 and 28 weeks gestation [21, 22]. The women received their clinical care from their own obstetric teams and not from the research team.

Infants were weighed within an hour of birth using a digital scales wearing only their identification band and umbilical cord clip. We defined total GWG as the measured maternal weight from 37 weeks gestation minus the measured maternal weight at the first antenatal visit. Total GWG includes both a maternal component as well as the weight of the fetus, placenta and *amniotic fluid.* We approximated the maternal component of GWG, which we called net GWG as total GWG minus BW.

Analysis was performed using Microsoft Excel (version 14.2, Microsoft, Redmond, United States of America (USA)) and SPSS (version 20.0, IBM Corp., Armok, New York, USA). *Data were tested for normality using a Shapiro-Wilk test and a normality was taken as a significance value > 0.05.* Differences between proportions were tested using chi-squared analysis, differences between means using independent samples t-test *for normally distributed data and a Mann-Whitney U test for non-normally distributed data.* Differences between continuous variables were tested using linear regression analysis *and Pearson coefficients for normally distributed data.* A p value < 0.05 was considered statistically significant.

Results

Of the 1061 women initially recruited, four women had pre-existing diabetes mellitus, 15 miscarried, three women experienced preterm stillbirth, 31 delivered elsewhere, 46 had preterm live births and 440 did not return to the research centre to have a weight measurement performed after 37 weeks gestation. There were 522 women included in the final analysis. There were no differences in baseline characteristics between the 522 women included in the final analysis and those not included (Table 1). The mean gestation of the baseline weight measurement was 12.3 weeks (6.0 to 17.7, *SD 1.7*) and the mean gestation of the term weight measurement was 38.0 weeks (37.0 to 41.7, *SD 0.8*). *Of the cohort, 88% (n = 456) had the first weight measurement before 14 completed weeks of gestation and 12% (n = 66) had the first weight measurement between 14 and 18 weeks gestation.* The mean GWG was 12.3 kg (− 4.6 to 28.4, *SD 5.0*). The mean infant BW was 3576 g (2160 to 5120, *SD 448*). The range of GWG and BW at each level of maternal BMI was wide (Table 2).

Maternal total GWG, net GWG and BW were all normally distributed (Shapiro-Wilk $p = 0.11$, 0.11, 0.40 respectively). Total GWG correlated with infant BW assessed with the Pearson coefficient ($p < 0.001$, $r = 0.16$) and on linear regression analysis ($p < 0.001$, r^2 0.025) (Fig. 1*), however when infant BW was subtracted from the total GWG, the remaining net maternal weight gain no longer correlated with infant BW assessed by Pearson coefficient ($p = 0.12$, $r = 0.07$) and by linear regression analysis ($p = 0.12$, r^2 0.005)* (Fig. 2). *When booking BMI category was controlled for in the regression model the same relationship was found.* The range of BW seen at each quintile of net maternal weight gain was large. There was no difference in BW for infants born to mothers in the highest or lowest quintiles of net maternal weight gain (Table 3).

Discussion

In this prospective longitudinal study we found that the positive correlation between GWG in pregnancy and BW can be accounted for by the contribution of fetal weight to GWG antenatally without any contribution from increased maternal weight. Thus, epidemiological studies linking excessive GWG with increased BW or macrosomia may be statistically self-fulfilling. There was also a wide range of BW irrespective of the degree of GWG and, in the absence of any interventions, obese women had a lower GWG than non-obese women. Even when controlling for baseline BMI we found a strong relationship between total GWG and BW and no relationship between net GWG and BW. This suggests that irrespective of baseline BMI, *net* GWG does not contribute to BW. These findings help explain why RCTs designed to reduce GWG in obese women have failed to decrease BW and suggest there is no causative link between excessive GWG and increased BW.

Our study has strengths. The study population was well characterized, and both BMI and GWG were calculated using standard methodology by a single researcher. Since gestational age at delivery is one of the strongest determinants of BW our early pregnancy confirmation of gestational age by ultrasound is important. The calculation of BMI was based on the measurement of weight and height before 18 weeks gestation. We have previously directly measured maternal weight and body composition in early pregnancy and have shown that this does not alter before 18 weeks gestation [6, 19]. The calculation of GWG was also standardized.

Table 1 Characteristics of the study population compared with women who did not participate after consenting ($n = 1061$)

Characteristic	Final cohort ($n = 522$)	Women excluded ($n = 539$)	p
Mean maternal age (years)	30.2 (18.1–44.2)	29.9 (18.0–45.1)	0.79
Mean maternal BMI (kg/m^2)	25.3 (16.6–48.3)	25.5 (15.5–52.4)	0.40
Nulliparas (%)	42.3 (221)	40.8 (220/539)	0.62
Obesity (%)	15.7 (82)	15.8 (85/539)	0.98
Smoking (%)	10.7 (56)	13.9 (75/539)	0.11
GDM (%)	6.5 (34)	5.6 (27/486)	0.64
Mean GWG (kg)	12. 3 (−4.6–28.4)	n/a	
Mean birth gestation (weeks)	40. 2 (37.3–42.0)	39.7 (27.0–42.4)	0.06
Mean birth weight (g)	3576 (2160–5120)	3475 (950–5120)	0.06
Macrosomia ≥4.5 kg (%)	2.7 (14)	2.1 (10/486)	0.65
Male infants (%)	49.0 (256)	50.2 (244/486)	0.71

Table 2 Gestational weight gain and birth weight by baseline BMI category ($n = 522$)

Baseline BMI	Mean total GWG (kg)	Mean BW (g)	Mean net GWG (kg)
Underweight ($n = 15$)	12.5 (8.3–19.4)	3266 (2670–3680)	9.2 (5.5–15.7)
Normal ($n = 284$)	13.2 (3.7–26.9)	3555 (2425–4860)	9.6 (0.6–24.1)
Overweight ($n = 141$)	12.6 (0.6–28.4)	3617 (2166–4720)	8.9 (− 2.8–24.8)
Obese I ($n = 48$)	10.3 (− 4.6–21.7)	3707 (2160–5120)	6.6 (− 7.7–18.0)
Obese II & III ($n = 34$)	6.6 (− 3.3–23.4)	3523 (2880–4580)	3.1 (−6.8–19.9)

A potential weakness of our study is that the findings may not be applicable to other populations as it was confined to white European women and the study was limited to singleton pregnancies. *Our data do not allow us to assess why such large variations in GWG were seen across all levels of maternal baseline BMI, nor what factors influence GWG. Since antenatal care was not directed by the research team, factors that may have impacted on GWG such as verbal advice given during the pregnancy were not recorded.* As this was a longitudinal study requiring repeat measurement by a single researcher over the course of pregnancy, for practical reasons, recruitment was convenient rather than consecutive.

Previous reviews, including the IOM guideline review, have acknowledged the limitations of the current evidence about GWG [2, 4, 23]. There is no standardization of definitions for GWG or fetal macrosomia. The findings are not consistent, particularly across BMI categories, and GWG is usually not corrected for BW.

Since the publication of the revised IOM guidelines, studies have reported an association between higher BW and GWG exceeding the recommendations [24–26]. Again, the measurements of gestational age, BMI and GWG were not standardized and were of variable quality. The IOM designation of "excessive" GWG is stricter for obese women, both in absolute terms and as a proportion of body weight. Therefore, comparisons between BMI groups may not be biologically valid since "excessive GWG" is defined differently at each level of BMI.

We found that even in the absence of pregnancy interventions, obese women have lower GWG than non-obese women [2, 27]. At a population level, large increases in the rates of maternal obesity have not been associated with an increase in babies born weighing > 4.5 kg or > 5.0 kg and there has not been an increase in mean BW [28, 29]. Pregnancy interventions designed to modify GWG have not been shown to change BW [12–16, 30, 31]. Furthermore, our research group has shown that offspring BW is associated with maternal fat-free mass and not maternal fat mass [32]. Thus, attempts to restrict GWG by decreasing maternal adiposity are unlikely to prevent high BW and may potentially do harm by restricting fetal nutrition.

If a woman standing on a weighing scales is given her newborn baby to hold, we would expect statistically, if powered strongly, that there would be a positive association

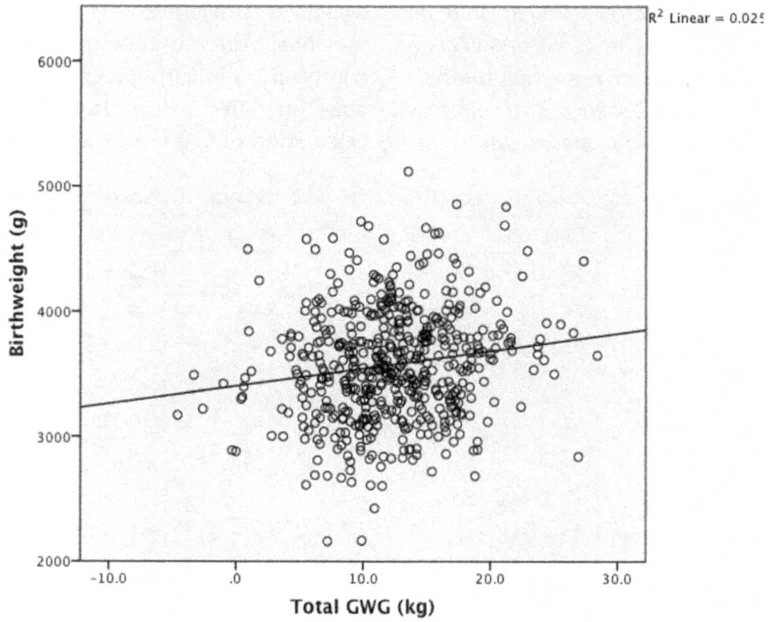

Fig. 1 Birth weight by total gestational weight gain (n=522) p<0.001, r^2 0.025

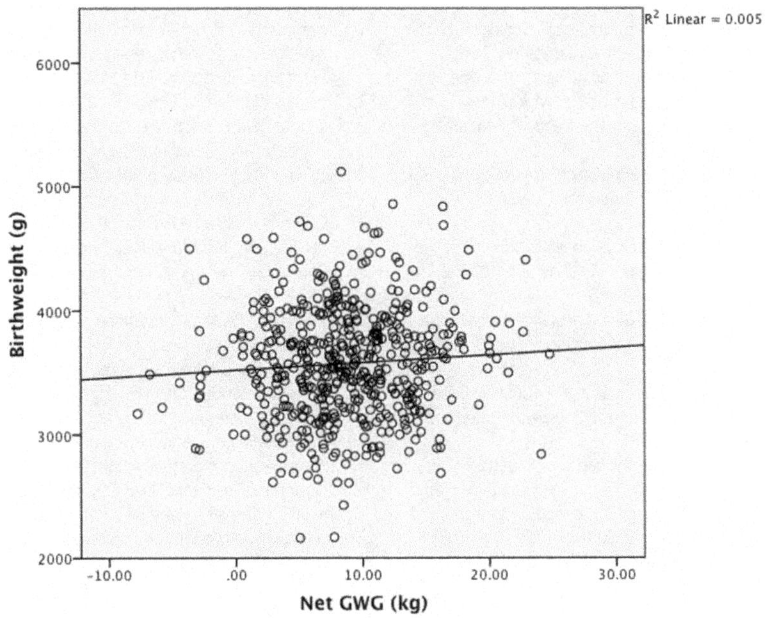

Fig. 2 Birth weight by net gestational weight gain (*n*=522) *p*=0.12, r^2 0.005

between their combined weight and the weight of the baby she is holding. It is hardly surprising therefore, that there is a positive association between total GWG antenatally and BW at term, particularly in large epidemiological studies, since total GWG includes the weight of the baby. It would also be expected that any positive association is stronger if maternal component of GWG in lower, as is generally the case in obese women.

Conclusions

Our findings show that BW varies widely for the same total GWG and that GWG does not correlate with BW once the weight of the baby is subtracted, do not support a causal relationship between GWG and BW. This absence of a causal relationship has also been supported by the results of the recent trials, all of which have failed to show a modification in BW despite modifying GWG [13–17].

We believe these results are important to all those involved in the care of pregnant women and their babies. This has important implications for those giving advice to pregnant women. Modification of GWG in obese women is unlikely to influence the growth of the baby. Focussing on dietary restriction, particularly in obese women who are at increased risk of micronutrient deficiency, has the potential to deprive the fetus of essential nutrients. We believe that the focus should be on helping women achieve a varied, well-balanced diet rather than on restricting weight gain. Future research on GWG needs to standardize the measurement of GWG and maternal adiposity.

Table 3 Mean birth weight (g) by maternal quintile of net GWG (*n* = 522)

	Birth weight	Significance of BW difference compared to quintile 3, t-test (*p*)
Quintile 1 GWG − 7.8 to 5.0 kg (*n* = 104)	3548 (2160 to 4590)	0.45
Quintile 2 GWG 5.1 to 7.6 kg (*n* = 105)	3529 (2635 to 4720)	0.28
Quintile 3 GWG 7.7 to 9.7 kg (*n* = 104)	3596 (2166 to 5120)	n/a
Quintile 4 GWG 9.8 to 12.9 kg (*n* = 105)	3591 (2720 to 4860)	0.93
Quintile 5 GWG 13.0 to 24.8 kg (*n* = 104)	3606 (2685 to 4860)	0.88

Abbreviations

BMI: Body mass index; BW: Birth weight; GDM: Gestational diabetes mellitus; GWG: Gestaional weight gain; IOM: Institute of Medicine; RCT: Randomized controlled trial

Authors' contributions

The maternal measurements were performed by AOH and the infant measurements by AD. The data collection and analysis was performed by AOH, AD, TMcC, LM and COC. The study was designed and supervised by MJT. All authors were involved in the preparation of the manuscript. All authors read and approved the final manuscript.

Competing interests

The authors declare that they have no competing interests.

References

1. World Health Organization. Division of Non-communicable diseases Obesity and Overweight: Fact Sheet. Geneva: World Health Organization; 2016.
2. Institute of Medicine and National Research Council of National Academy of Sciences. Weight gain during pregnancy. In: Rasmussen KM, Yaktine AL, editors. Reexamining the guidelines. Washington: The National Academies Press; 2009.
3. Rodrigues PL, Oliveira LC, Ados SB, Kac G. Determinant factors of insufficient and excessive gestational weight gain and maternal-child adverse outcomes. Nutrition. 2010;26:617–23.
4. Gaudet L, Ferraro ZW, Wen SW, Walker M. Maternal obesity and occurrence of fetal macrosomia: a systematic review and meta-analysis. Biomed Res Int. 2014;2014:64021.
5. Savitz DA, Stein CR, Siega-Riz AM, Herring AH. Gestational weight gain and birth outcome in relation to prepregnancy body mass index and ethnicity. Ann Epidemiol. 2011;21:78–85.
6. O'Higgins AC, Doolan A, Mullaney L, Daly N, McCartney D, Turner MJ. The relationship between gestational weight gain and fetal growth: time to take stock? J Perinat Med. 2014;42:409–15.
7. Turner MJ. The measurement of maternal obesity: can we do better? Clin Obes. 2011;1:127–9.
8. Sheilds M, Connor Gorber S, Tremblay MS. Estimates of obesity based on self-report versus direct measures. Health Rep. 2008;19:16–76.
9. Johnson J, Clifton RG, Roberts JM, et al. Pregnancy outcomes with weight gain above or below the 2009 Institute of Medicine guidelines. Obstet Gynecol. 2013;121:969–75.
10. Vesco KK, Sharma AJ, Dietz PM, et al. Newborn size among obese women with weight gain outside the 2009 Institute of Medicine recommendation. Obstet Gynecol. 2011;117:812–8.
11. Siega-Riz AM, Viswanathan M, Moos MK, et al. A systematic review of outcomes of maternal weight gain according to the Institute of Medicine recommendations: birthweight, fetal growth and postpartum weight retention. Am J Obstet Gynecol. 2009;201:339.e1–14.
12. Goldstein RF, Abell SK, Ranasinha S, et al. Association of gestational weight gain with maternal and infant outcomes: a systematic review and meta-anlaysis. JAMA. 2017;317:2207–25.
13. Sagedal LR, Overby NC, Bere E, et al. Lifestyle intervention to limit gestational weight gain: the Norwegian fit for delivery randomised controlled trial. Br J Ob Gyn. 2017;124:97–109.
14. Skouteris H, McPhie S, Hill B, et al. Health coaching to prevent excessive gestational weight gain: a randomized-controlled trial. Br J Health Psychcol. 2016;21:31–51.
15. Poston L, Bell R, Croker H, et al. Effect of a behavioural intervention in obese pregnant women (the UPEAT study): a multicentre. randomised controlled trial Lancet Diabetes Endocrinol. 2015;3:76–7.
16. Dodd JM, Turnbull D, McPhee AJ, et al. Randomised trial group. Antenatal lifestyle advice for women who are overweight or obese: LIMIT randomised trial. BMJ. 2014;348g:1285.
17. Walsh JM, McGowan CA, Mahoney R, Foley ME, McAuliffe FM. Low glycaemic index diet in pregnancy to prevent macrosomia (ROLO study): randomised control trial. BMJ. 2012;345:35605–13.
18. Farah N, Murphy M, Ramphul M, O'Connor N, Kennelly MM, Turner MJ. Comparison in maternal body composition between Caucasian Irish and Indian women. J Obstet Gynaecol. 2011;31:483–5.
19. Fattah C, Farah N, Barry S, O'Connor N, Stuart B, Turner MJ. Maternal weight and body composition in the first trimester of pregnancy. Acta Obstet Gyn Scan. 2010;89:952–5.
20. World Health Organization. Division of non-communicable diseases. Obesity: preventing and managing the global epidemic. Report of a WHO consultation on obesity. WHO technical report series 894, Geneva: World Health Organization; 2000.
21. Institute of Obstetricians and Gynaecologists, Royal College of Physicians in Ireland. Clinical Practice Guideline: The management of pre-gestational and gestational diabetes mellitus. HSE. Dublin, 2010.
22. Ali FM, Farah N, O'Dwyer V, O'Connor C, Kennelly MM, Turner MJ. The impact of new national guidelines on screening for gestational diabetes mellitus. Irish Med J. 2013;106:57–8.
23. Ohadike CO, Cheikh-Ismail L, Ohuma EO, et al. Systematic review of methodological quality of studies aimed at creating gestational weight gian charts. Adv Nutr. 2016;7:313–22.
24. Alberico S, Montico M, Barresi V, et al. The role of gestational diabetes, pre-pregnancy body mass index and gestational weight gain on the risk of newborn macrosomia: results from a prospective multicenter study. BMC Pregnancy Childbirth. 2014;14:23.
25. Ferraro ZM, Barrowman N, Prud'homme D, et al. Excessive gestational weight gain predicts large for gestational age neonates independent of maternal body mass index. J Matern Fetal Neonatal Med. 2012;25:538–42.
26. Truong YN, Yee LM, Caughey AB, Cheng YW. Weight gain in pregnancy: does the Institute of Medicine have it right? AJOG. 2015;212:362.e1–8.
27. O'Dwyer V, O'Toole F, Darcy S, Farah N, Kennelly MM, Turner MJ. Maternal obesity and gestational weight gain. J Obstet Gynaecol. 2013;33:671–4.
28. Oken E. Secular trends in birthweight. Nestle Nutr Inst Workshop Ser. 2013; 71:103–14.
29. Turner MJ, Farah N. Gestational weight gain and birthweight. Irish Med J. 2010;103:293–4.
30. Oteng-Ntim E, Varma R, Croker H, Poston L, Doyle P. Lifestyle interventions for overweight and obese pregnant women to improve pregnancy outcome: systematic review and meta-analysis. BMC Med. 2012;10:47.
31. Thangaratinam S, Rogozinska E, Jolly K, et al. Effects of interventions in pregnancy on maternal weight and obstetric outcomes: meta-analysis of randomised evidence. BMJ. 2012;344:e2088–22.
32. Kent E, O'Dwyer V, Fattah C, Farah N, O'Connor C, Turner MJ. Correlation between birthweight and maternal body composition. Obstet Gynecol. 2013;121:46–50.

11

Do elevated symptoms of depression predict adherence and outcomes in the UPBEAT randomised controlled trial of a lifestyle intervention for obese pregnant women?

Emma Molyneaux[1*], Shahina Begum[2], Annette L. Briley[2], Paul T. Seed[2], Louise M. Howard[1], Lucilla Poston[2] and on behalf of the UPBEAT consortium

Abstract

Background: Lifestyle interventions for obese pregnant women have been widely researched but little is known about predictors of low adherence or poor outcomes. This study evaluated the prospective associations between elevated symptoms of antenatal depression and gestational diabetes, adherence and gestational weight gain in a large RCT of a behavioural intervention for obese pregnant women. The effect of the intervention on symptoms of depression at follow-up was also examined.

Methods: The UPBEAT RCT randomised 1555 obese pregnant women to receive a dietary and physical activity lifestyle intervention or standard care. Symptoms of antenatal depression were assessed with the Edinburgh Postnatal Depression Scale at baseline (15^{+0}–18^{+6} weeks' gestation) and follow-up (27^{+0}–28^{+6} weeks' gestation). Gestational diabetes was assessed with an oral glucose tolerance test at 27^{+0}–28^{+6} weeks' gestation. Adherence was pre-defined as receiving at least 5 of 8 intervention sessions. Gestational weight gain was calculated as the difference between pre-pregnancy weight (estimated as measured baseline weight minus 1.25 kg) and last measured weight at 34^{+0}–36^{+0} weeks' gestation. Due to substantial missing data in certain variables, multiple imputation was used to impute missing data. Women who were no longer pregnant at 27^{+0}–28^{+6} weeks' gestation were excluded from the sample for these analyses.

Results: One thousand five-hundered twenty-six women were included in these analyses following multiple imputation; 797 (52.2%) had complete data. 13.4% had elevated symptoms of antenatal depression at baseline. There was no evidence for associations between antenatal depression status and gestational diabetes (adjusted OR 0.80, 95%CI 0.52 to 1.22, $p = 0.30$), adherence (adjusted OR 1.16, 95%CI 0.63 to 2.15, $p = 0.63$) or gestational weight gain (adjusted regression coefficient 0.52, 95%CI -0.26 to 1.29, $p = 0.19$). The intervention was not associated with change in depressive symptoms at follow-up (regression coefficient 0.003, 95%CI -0.49 to 0.49, $p = 0.99$). Similar results were obtained in complete case analyses.

(Continued on next page)

* Correspondence: emma.molyneaux@kcl.ac.uk
[1]Section of Women's Mental Health, Institute of Psychiatry, Psychology & Neuroscience at King's College London, London, England
Full list of author information is available at the end of the article

(Continued from previous page)

Conclusions: Elevated symptoms of antenatal depression did not predict gestational diabetes, adherence or gestational weight gain in this large RCT of a lifestyle intervention for obese pregnant women. The intervention also did not influence symptoms of depression at follow-up. Obese pregnant women with elevated symptoms of depression should not be excluded from lifestyle interventions.

Keywords: Obesity, Depression, Pregnancy, Lifestyle intervention, Gestational diabetes, Gestational weight gain

Background

In recent years, there has been an abundance of research examining lifestyle interventions for obese pregnant women that aim to improve diet, increase physical activity and reduce gestational weight gain. However, these interventions often have limited effectiveness, and low adherence or high drop-out rates are common [1, 2]. There has been little research into predictors of adherence or outcomes in these interventions for pregnant women, but studies of weight management interventions for non-pregnant adults have found that elevated symptoms of depression can be associated with higher attrition and lower adherence [3]. Depression is common during pregnancy and systematic review evidence has demonstrated that obese pregnant women are more likely to experience depression than normal weight women [4]. In addition, antenatal depression has been associated with excessive gestational weight gain in some, although not all, observational studies [5–7]. It is important to identify whether depression is a risk factor for poorer outcomes in lifestyle interventions for obese women during pregnancy.

Amongst the few previous studies examining these associations in pregnancy, one found no evidence that symptoms of depression predicted adherence to the intervention or gestational weight gain in a randomised controlled trial (RCT) of a diet and exercise intervention among 205 obese pregnant women [8]. However, this study was underpowered to examine clinical outcomes of interest such as gestational diabetes, and requires replication. It is also necessary to examine whether taking part in a lifestyle intervention influences symptoms of depression among pregnant women. The few findings on this topic to date have been inconsistent [8–10].

This study examined the prospective associations between elevated symptoms of antenatal depression and 1) gestational diabetes, 2) intervention adherence, and 3) gestational weight gain in the UPBEAT trial, a large RCT of a complex behavioural intervention for obese pregnant women. The effect of the intervention on symptoms of depression at follow-up was also examined.

Methods

The UPBEAT trial

The UPBEAT trial (UK Pregnancies Better Eating and Activity Trial) is a multicentre randomised controlled trial of a complex behavioural intervention for obese pregnant women [11]. The intervention focused on improving diet and increasing physical activity with the aim of reducing the risk of gestational diabetes among obese pregnant women, and of delivery of large for gestational age infants [11]. Women randomised to the intervention attended up to eight weekly group sessions delivered by health trainers, and received an intervention handbook, a DVD of pregnancy-specific exercise routines, a pedometer and a log book for recording weekly goals. Women in the control group received standard antenatal care according to the provision in their local area.

For the UPBEAT trial, obese pregnant women (body mass index [BMI] ≥30 kg/m^2 at their first antenatal appointment) with a singleton pregnancy were recruited between 15^{+0} and 18^{+6} weeks' gestation. Exclusion criteria for the trial were lack of informed consent, BMI < 30 kg/m^2, ≤16 years old, multiple pregnancy, currently being prescribed metformin, and pre-existing medical conditions including diabetes mellitus, hypertension requiring treatment, thyroid disease or current psychosis. In addition, women with known miscarriage, termination, fetal death in utero or preterm birth prior to the first follow-up interview (27^{+0} to 28^{+6} weeks' gestation) were excluded from the sample for these analyses.

Women were recruited from eight NHS hospital trusts in the UK between March 2009 and June 2014. Ethical approval for the study was obtained in all centres (UK integrated research application system reference: 09/H0802/5) and the trial was registered with Current Controlled Trials (ISCRTN89971375). Randomisation was performed online using the MedSciNet™ secure data management system, minimised based on age, ethnicity, BMI and centre of recruitment. Given the nature of the intervention, study staff and participants were not blinded to intervention status.

Measures

Antenatal depression

Symptoms of antenatal depression were assessed during the baseline visit (15^{+0} to 18^{+6} weeks' gestation) and the first follow-up visit (27^{+0} to 28^{+6} weeks' gestation) using the Edinburgh Postnatal Depression Scale (EPDS [12]).

A validated cut-off score of ≥13 was used to indicate elevated symptoms of antenatal depression [13]. The difference between EPDS score at baseline and follow-up was calculated to indicate change in depressive symptoms.

Gestational diabetes

All women were given an oral glucose tolerance test (75 g load) at 27^{+0} to 28^{+6} weeks' gestation and the International Association of Diabetes and Pregnancy Study Groups criteria were used to diagnose gestational diabetes (fasting venous capillary glucose ≥ 5.1 mmol/L and/or 1 h venous glucose ≥10 mmol/L and/or 2 h venous glucose ≥8.5 mmol/L) [14]. All women in the study who met the diagnostic criteria for gestational diabetes were referred for antenatal diabetic services at their local centre.

Adherence

High adherence was defined as receiving at least five out of eight intervention sessions (as recommended in the UPBEAT trial protocol [15]) in person, over the phone or via email. Previous analyses in UPBEAT found no evidence that mode of session delivery influenced the primary outcomes [11]. There was also no difference in the proportion of women attending sessions in person, compared with receiving them over the phone or via email, based on depression status ($p = 0.89$).

Gestational weight gain

Gestational weight gain (in kg) was calculated as the difference between estimated pre-pregnancy weight and last objective pregnancy weight measured between 34^{+0} to 36^{+0} weeks' gestation. As pre-specified in the protocol, estimated pre-pregnancy weight was calculated from weight measured at trial entry with 1.25 kg deducted for first trimester weight gain (1.25 kg is the midpoint of the first trimester weight gain range specified by the Institute of Medicine guidelines [16]).

Confounders

Baseline BMI (calculated from measured height and weight at 15^{+0} to 18^{+6} weeks' gestation), study centre, socio-demographic factors and parity were included as potential confounders in this study. Details of the assessment and coding of the socio-demographic variables (age, ethnicity, relationship status, highest educational level, household income, and index of multiple deprivation) are given in Table 1. All socio-demographic factors except age were self-reported during the baseline interview.

Main analyses

All analyses were conducted in Stata 14 (StataCorp, 2015, College Station, Texas). There was no missing data for the majority of baseline variables; however income and EPDS score were missing for 15.5% and 12.6% of participants respectively. There was also missing data in the outcome variables, with approximately 15% missing for GDM and over 20% missing for EPDS at follow-up and gestational weight gain (see Additional file 1). Missing data reduces statistical power in complete case analysis and can lead to bias if participants with missing data differ from those with complete data. Based on the assumption of missing at random, which was plausible in this dataset (see Additional files 1, 2 and 3), multiple imputation by chained equations was used to impute missing data [17]. All analysis variables were included in the imputation model alongside other relevant auxiliary variables to improve the prediction of missing values and increase the plausibility of missing at random [18]. The number of imputed datasets was based on the proportion of missing data as simulation studies have

Table 1 Assessment of socio-demographic confounders

Variable	Description
Age	Participants reported their age when they were approached to participate in the study in early pregnancy.
Ethnicity	Participants reported their main ethnicity (European, Indian, Pakistani, Bangladeshi, Afro Caribbean, African, Middle Eastern, Far East Asian, South East Asian or Other) which was classified as White, Black, Asian or Other.
Relationship status	Relationship status was indicated by whether or not participants were currently living with their partner. This was used instead of marital status, which provided limited information on relationship status in this sample as the majority of women reported having never been married.
Highest educational level	Highest educational level was self-reported as none, GCSE or equivalent vocational qualification, A level or equivalent, first degree or higher degree. This was coded for analyses as none/GCSE, A level/vocational or degree level. GCSEs are public exams usually taken in school at 15–16 years; A levels are public exams usually taken in school at 17–18 years, and are generally required for University entrance.
Household income	Household income (participant and partner, pre-tax per year) was recorded as <£12,688, £12,688–£17,628, £17,629–£23,452, £23,453–£32,500 or > £32,500.
Index of multiple deprivation	Index of multiple deprivation [27] is assessed at the lower layer super output area (LSOA) level. Women were given an index of multiple deprivation score based on their postcode. Based on data for all LSOAs in England and Scotland, each LSOA was defined based on its quintile group [28].
Parity	Parity was self-reported and defined as the number of previous pregnancies going beyond 20 weeks' gestation.

suggested that the number of imputed datasets should be greater than the proportion of participants with missing data [19]. Sixty imputed datasets were produced. Statistical analyses were then carried on each imputed dataset separately and combined using Rubin's rules [20]. Full details of the imputation are provided in the Additional files 1, 2 and 3.

Using the imputed data, characteristics of the study sample were summarised for socio-demographic variables, BMI, parity and centre of recruitment. Characteristics of women with EPDS scores ≥13 and EPDS scores < 13 were presented as frequencies or means (with standard deviations (SD)) and compared using univariate regression analyses. The relationship between antenatal depression at 15^{+0} to 18^{+6} weeks' gestation (independent variable) and gestational diabetes (dependent variable) was then examined using univariate logistic regression. The interaction of depression and intervention group on risk of gestational diabetes was tested and if this was found to be significant, subgroup analyses were performed to examine the intervention and control groups separately. If the interaction effect was not significant, the association between antenatal depression and gestational diabetes was examined in the sample as a whole. The relationship between EPDS score (as a continuous variable) and gestational diabetes was also examined using unadjusted logistic regression. In addition, fasting blood glucose levels (mmol/L) and gestation at the time of the oral glucose tolerance test were compared between women with and without elevated symptoms of antenatal depression (EPDS < 13 and EPDS ≥13). Multiple logistic regression was then used to examine the association between depression (EPDS≥13) and gestational diabetes adjusted for potential confounders (BMI, age, ethnicity, relationship status, educational level, household income, index of multiple deprivation, parity and study centre). The association between antenatal depression and high adherence (receiving five or more intervention sessions out of a possible total of eight) was then examined for women in the intervention group only, using logistic regression with and without adjusting for confounders (as above). The relationship between EPDS score, as a continuous variable, and adherence was also examined. Next, the association between antenatal depression and gestational weight gain was examined using linear regression, again with adjustment for confounders. Assumptions of linear regression were checked (normality of residuals, homoscedasticity and independence of predictors) and one outlier for gestational weight gain was removed prior to imputation. The relationship between EPDS score, as a continuous variable, and gestational weight gain was also examined. Finally, the effect of the intervention on the change in symptoms of depression from baseline to follow-up was examined using linear regression. The main unadjusted and adjusted analyses were then repeated using complete case analysis, for comparison with the imputed data.

Results

In total, 1555 women were recruited into the UPBEAT trial. One participant was excluded after enrolment in another trial, leaving 1554 participants. The CONSORT diagram is given in Fig. 1. The number of participants

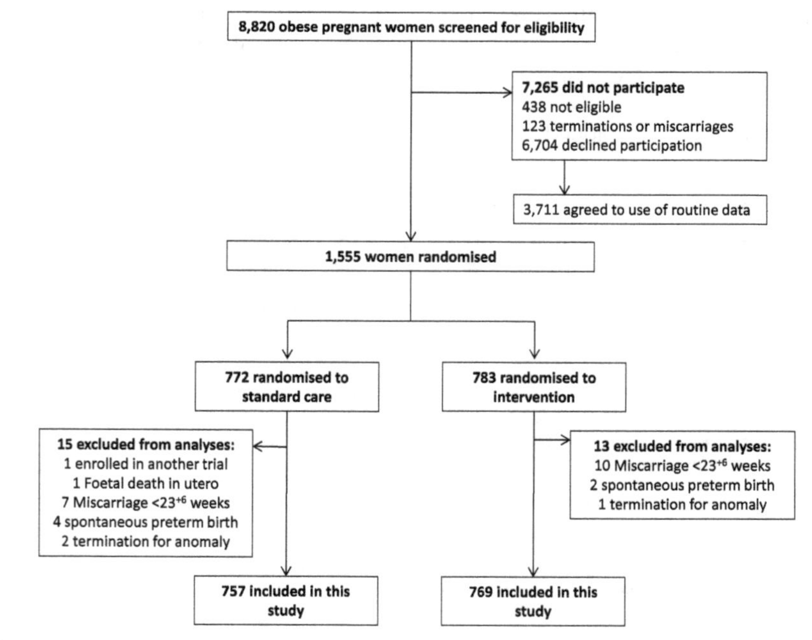

Fig. 1 Participant flow diagram

included in the trial represented 19% of the 8259 eligible women approached to participate (8820 women with BMI ≥30 kg/m^2 were approached, of whom 561 were not eligible to participate). Women with known miscarriage, termination, fetal death in utero or preterm birth prior to 27^{+0} to 28^{+6} weeks' gestation ($n = 28$) were also excluded from the sample for these analyses. One thousand five hundred twenty-six women were therefore included in this study (757 randomised to standard antenatal care and 769 randomised to the intervention).

Among the 1526 women included in this study, 797 (52.2%) had complete data for all analysis variables. In total, 47.87% ($n = 729$) of participants had missing data for at least one analysis variable but only 5.0% ($n = 76$) had missing data for more than three analysis variables. Overall, 6.2% of the total observations in the analysis variables were missing. 12.6% of women were missing EPDS score at baseline but there was complete data for most other baseline characteristics except for household income, which was missing for 15.5% of women (see Additional file 1). The pattern of missing data was examined and the assumption of missing at random was plausible (see Additional file 2). Multiple imputation by chained equations [17] was therefore performed (see Additional file 3) with 60 imputed datasets produced. Overall, characteristics of the imputed data were similar to the observed data (see Additional file 3). For example, 13.1% of women scored ≥13 on the EPDS at baseline in the observed data, and 13.4% in the imputed data. The mean length of follow-up was 10.9 weeks (SD 1.6) both for women with EPDS scores < 13 at baseline and for women with EPDS scores ≥13.

Sample characteristics

Characteristics of the sample (based on the imputed data) are given in Table 2. Approximately half of the sample was recruited from hospital trusts in London (49.3%). The mean age of the sample was 30.5 years (±5.5) and 43.3% of women were nulliparous. The majority of women (63.0%) were of white ethnicity, and 25.5% of black ethnicity. Just over three quarters of participants (77.1%) were living with a partner. One fifth (20.5%) of participants had no qualifications beyond GCSEs or equivalent. A quarter of participants (24.6%) reported a household income of £12,688 or less per year, whilst 37.8% reported a household income greater than £32,500 per year. The majority of participants (77.8%) lived in areas in the highest or second highest quintiles of deprivation.

At 15^{+0} to 18^{+6} weeks' gestation, the median EPDS score was 6 (IQR 3–10). Elevated symptoms of antenatal depression (≥13 on the EPDS) were observed in 13.4% of the sample. The proportion of women with elevated symptoms of antenatal depression did not differ between

Table 2 Characteristics of the sample and associations with antenatal depression status

		Total sample %	Antenatal depression status		
			EPDS < 13	EPDS ≥ 13	*p* value
Total; %		–	86.6	13.4	–
Centre; %	Guys' and St Thomas'[1]	24.4	84.2	15.8	0.21
	King's College Hospital[1]	17.8	84.5	15.5	
	Newcastle	15.7	89.9	10.1	
	Glasgow	17.0	89.1	10.9	
	Manchester	9.1	88.5	11.6	
	Bradford	3.3	82.4	17.7	
	Sunderland	5.4	91.6	8.4	
	St Georges'[1]	7.1	83.4	16.6	
Parity; %	0	43.3	87.0	13.0	0.17
	1	33.5	88.5	11.5	
	2	15.3	82.4	17.6	
	3+	7.9	85.1	14.9	
Age; mean (sd)		30.5 (5.5)	30.5 (5.4)	30.1 (5.7)	0.33
Main ethnicity; %	White	63.0	89.4	10.6	< 0.01
	Black	25.5	82.3	17.7	
	Asian	6.0	80.7	19.3	
	Other	5.5	81.9	18.1	
Relationship status; %	Not cohabiting	22.9	79.8	20.2	< 0.01
	Cohabiting	77.1	88.7	11.3	
Highest educational level[2]; %	None/GCSE	20.5	83.8	16.2	0.02
	A level/ Vocational	39.7	85.6	14.4	
	Degree	39.8	89.1	10.9	
Household income; %	<£12,688	24.6	78.5	21.5	< 0.01
	£12,688–17,628	13.5	83.2	16.8	
	£17,629-23,452	10.1	87.2	12.9	
	£23,453-32,500	14.1	90.4	9.7	
	>£32,500	37.8	91.7	8.3	
Index of multiple deprivation quintiles; %	1 (least)	4.1	94.0	6.0	0.03
	2	6.7	85.1	15.0	
	3	11.4	88.6	11.4	
	4	34.3	88.9	11.2	
	5 (most)	43.5	84.0	16.0	
BMI (kg/m^2); %	30–35	49.7	86.7	13.3	0.92
	35–40	32.1	86.3	13.7	
	≥40	18.2	87.1	12.9	

Sample characteristics based on imputed data. [1]London. [2]GCSEs: public exams usually taken in school at 15–16 years; A levels: public exams usually taken in school at 17–18 years the intervention groups (control group: 13.2%, intervention group 13.5%; $p = 0.90$). However, the prevalence of antenatal depression was associated with the majority of other sample characteristics (see Table 2). Elevated symptoms of depression were least common among white women (10.6%) and more common among all other ethnic groups (17.7–19.3%). The prevalence was also higher among women who were not cohabiting (20.2 vs. 11.3%). In addition, the prevalence of elevated symptoms of antenatal depression differed by all indicators of socio-economic status. For example, 21.5% for women with household income less than £12,688 scored ≥13 on the EPDS, compared with 8.3% for women with household income over £32,500. Finally, elevated symptoms of antenatal depression were reported most often in Bradford (17.7%) followed by the three London study sites (15.5–16.6%) and least often in Sunderland (8.4%) and Newcastle (10.1%).

Gestational diabetes

The overall prevalence of gestational diabetes, based on imputed data, was 28.2%. 26.3% of women with elevated symptoms of antenatal depression developed gestational diabetes compared with 28.5% of women without elevated symptoms of depression. Fasting blood glucose levels did not differ between women with and without elevated symptoms of depression (EPDS ≥13: mean 4.6 mmol/L (SD 0.6); EPDS< 13: mean 4.7 mmol/L (SD 0.6); $p = 0.25$), nor did gestational age at the time of the oral glucose tolerance test (EPDS ≥13: mean 27^{+6} weeks; EPDS < 13: mean: 28^{+0} weeks; $p = 0.26$), based on observed data.

Using unadjusted logistic regression, there was no evidence of an association between elevated symptoms of antenatal depression and gestational diabetes (OR 0.89, 95%CI 0.58–1.32, $p = 0.56$), no evidence for an interaction of depression status and intervention group on risk of gestational diabetes ($p = 0.41$), and no evidence of an association between EPDS score (as a continuous predictor) and gestational diabetes (OR 0.99, 95%CI 0.96–1.01, $p = 0.37$). Finally, there was also no evidence for an association between elevated symptoms of antenatal depression and gestational diabetes after adjusting for confounders (OR 0.80, 95%CI 0.52–1.22, $p = 0.30$).

Adherence

Among women in the intervention group, 81.1% received at least five of the eight intervention sessions (the pre-defined threshold for adherence). Examining adherence by antenatal depression status, 80.0% of women with elevated symptoms of depression were adherent compared with 81.3% of women without elevated symptoms. Elevated antenatal depression symptoms were not associated with high adherence before or after adjusting for confounders (unadjusted OR 0.92, 95%CI 0.54–1.57, $p = 0.76$; adjusted OR 1.16, 95%CI 0.63–2.15, $p = 0.63$). There was also no evidence of an association between EPDS score (as a continuous predictor) and adherence (OR 1.00, 95%CI 0.96–1.04, $p = 0.99$).

Gestational weight gain

Mean gestational weight gain was 7.41 kg. Based on antenatal depression status, mean gestational weight was 7.58 kg among women with elevated symptoms of depression, compared with 7.39 kg among women without elevated symptoms. There was no evidence for a difference in the total period of time over which gestational weight gain was assessed, based on baseline antenatal depression status (EPDS < 13: 18.1 weeks (SD 3.3); EPDS ≥13: 18.5 weeks (SD 5.9), $p = 0.23$).

There was no association between antenatal depression status and gestational weight gain in the unadjusted regression analysis (regression coefficient 0.19, 95%CI -0.59 to 0.97, $p = 0.63$), no evidence for an interaction of depression and intervention group on gestational weight gain ($p = 0.41$), and no evidence of an association between EPDS score (as a continuous predictor) and gestational weight gain (regression coefficient 0.04, 95%CI -0.02 to 0.09, $p = 0.22$). There was also no significant association between elevated symptoms of antenatal depression and higher gestational weight gain after adjusting for confounders (adjusted regression coefficient 0.52, 95%CI -0.26 to 1.29, $p = 0.19$).

Change in depressive symptoms

At follow-up, the median EPDS score was 5 (IQR 2–9). 11.1% of women in the intervention group scored ≥13 on the EPDS at follow-up compared with 11.6% in the control group. The mean reduction in EPDS score from baseline to follow-up was 0.77 points in both the intervention and control groups. There was no association between intervention group and change in EPDS symptoms (regression coefficient 0.003, 95%CI -0.49 to 0.49, $p = 0.99$).

Complete case analysis

For the complete case analyses, sample size varied based on the amount of missing data in the included variables. There was no evidence for an association between elevated symptoms of antenatal depression and gestational diabetes in the unadjusted (OR 0.72, 95%CI 0.47–1.12, $p = 0.14$; $n = 1143$) or adjusted analyses (OR 0.70, 95%CI 0.42–1.17, $p = 0.17$; $n = 972$), and no evidence for an interaction of depression status and study group on gestational diabetes ($p = 0.29$). There was also no evidence for an association between elevated antenatal depression symptoms and high adherence in the unadjusted (OR 0.84, 95%CI

0.49–1.43 $p = 0.51$; $n = 679$) or adjusted (OR 0.99, 95%CI 0.49–2.00, $p = 0.98$; $n = 567$) analyses. Elevated symptoms of antenatal depression and gestational weight gain were not associated in the unadjusted analysis (regression coefficient 0.62, 95%CI -0.26 to 1.50, $p = 0.17$; $n = 948$) but there was a significant association after adjusting for confounders (regression coefficient 1.11, 95%CI 0. Fifteen to 2.07, $p = 0.02$; $n = 805$). There was no evidence for an interaction between antenatal depression status and intervention group on total gestational weight gain ($p = 0.75$). Finally, there was no evidence for an association between intervention group and change in severity of symptoms of depression at follow-up (regression coefficient - 0.10, 95%CI -0.58 to 0.38, $p = 0.68$, $n = 1140$).

Discussion

Elevated symptoms of antenatal depression (EPDS score ≥ 13) were reported by almost one in seven (13.4%) obese pregnant women participating in the UPBEAT trial. However, elevated depressive symptoms did not predict risk of gestational diabetes, adherence or gestational weight gain. There was also no evidence that receiving the dietary and physical activity lifestyle intervention during pregnancy influenced symptoms of depression at follow-up.

Our findings are in keeping with a previous RCT of a lifestyle intervention for obese pregnant women which found no association between symptoms of antenatal depression and intervention adherence or gestational weight gain (Bogaerts et al. [8]). In this study, we extended previous research by examining gestational diabetes, which many previous trials have been underpowered to assess, but again found no association with antenatal depression. We also found no interactions between depression status and intervention group, meaning that the effectiveness of the intervention for the outcomes examined did not differ between women with and without antenatal depression. Future studies could examine whether antenatal depression is associated with differences in diet or physical activity in lifestyle interventions for obese pregnant women.

The intervention in the UPBEAT RCT was found to have no effect on symptoms of antenatal depression at follow-up. Previous findings on this topic are mixed. One small study from Spain, conducted by Perales et al. (2015), found that overweight and obese pregnant women randomised to an exercise programme had a lower prevalence of depression in late pregnancy than women in the control group [10]. Bogaerts et al., in contrast, found that their intervention had no effect on symptoms of antenatal depression, but symptoms of anxiety were reduced compared with controls [8]. Anxiety symptoms were not assessed in the UPBEAT study so this could not been examined here. However, in an large RCT of a lifestyle advice intervention for overweight and obese pregnant women ($n = 2212$), Dodd et al. [9] also found no effect of the intervention on symptoms of depression or anxiety at follow-up, including follow-up at 4 months postpartum. Considering our results in the context of these previous findings it appears that lifestyle interventions during pregnancy, including the extra contact received and any lifestyle change occuring as a result of these interventions, do not reduce symptoms of depression for the majority of obese women. It may be that structured exercise interventions, as used by Perales et al., have more effect on mental health than lifestyle interventions providing counselling around diet and exercise. However more high quality RCTs of structured exercise interventions for pregnant women are needed to conclude whether these are effective and feasible in routine clinical practice. It is important to ensure that mental health services are available for all women who require treatment for depression during pregnancy. No data were available on mental health interventions received by women in the UPBEAT trial, which is a limitation of these analyses.

The UPBEAT RCT included over 1500 obese pregnant women. This large sample size is a key strength of the study, and enabled clinical outcomes such as gestational diabetes to be assessed. The main findings of the UPBEAT trial (reported elsewhere [11]) showed that the intervention was not effective in preventing gestational diabetes (the primary maternal outcome), although it did improve diet quality and physical activity, reduce gestational weight gain and reduce maternal adiposity. The assessment of gestational diabetes was a particular strength of this study; the International Diabetes and Pregnancy Study Groups criteria [14] were used to diagnose gestational diabetes and all women were given a glucose tolerance test at 27^{+0} to 28^{+6} weeks' gestation rather than relying on clinical records to obtain outcome data.

A number of limitations of this study must also be taken into account. Only 19% of the 8259 eligible women approached about the UPBEAT RCT agreed to participate. This is similar to recruitment rates in other studies of lifestyle interventions for overweight or obese pregnant women [21–23] but limits the representativeness of the sample and the likely generalisability of the findings. Routine data (collected from non-participants who gave permission) showed that women who did not participate were younger, more likely to be of black ethnicity and had slightly lower BMI. Routine data from non-participants could not be collected on depression status but women with depression might be expected to be less likely to participate. The prevalence of elevated symptoms of antenatal depression observed in the

UPBEAT sample at baseline (approximately 13% of women scored ≥13 on the EPDS) is similar to other prevalence estimates during pregnancy [24]. However, the UPBEAT study included obese and largely low-income women, and both of these characteristics have been associated with increased risk of antenatal depression [25, 26], which may suggest that women with depression were underrepresented in the sample. It is also important to note that the EPDS is a screening measure which identifies women with elevated symptoms of depression rather than those meeting diagnostic criteria, meaning that conclusions cannot be drawn about women with depressive disorders from this study. However, the EPDS is widely used to assess antenatal depression in research and clinical practice and has been validated to indicate probable depression during pregnancy [13]. The main analyses were conducted using the EPDS as a dichotomous variable, but additional analyses using the EPDS as a continuous predictor gave similar findings.

Finally, missing data is a common problem in longitudinal studies including the UPBEAT RCT, leading to loss of statistical power and potential bias. This study included 1526 women, of whom only 52% ($n = 797$) had complete data for all analysis variables. However, the amount of missing data for each participant was generally low, with 95% of participants missing three or fewer variables. The main analyses for this paper were conducted using multiple imputation to impute missing data, which gives unbiased estimates based on the assumption that data are missing at random (i.e. that missing values can be predicted as a function of the observed data). It is not possible to conclusively test whether data are missing at random, but this was highly plausible in this sample. There were rich baseline data available on sample characteristics, the majority of which had no missing data, and these characteristics predicted missing data in the follow-up interviews. It is often argued that data on mental health is unlikely to be missing at random as participants with poor mental health may be more likely to have missing data [18]. However, in this study the vast majority of missing baseline EPDS data occurred during a short period of the study in which this variable was not recorded, so this missing data is not related to unmeasured participant characteristics and can be characterised as missing at random.

Our conclusions are also strengthened by a complete case analysis which gave very similar findings. The only difference observed between the complete case and imputed analyses is that elevated symptoms of antenatal depression were significantly associated with increased gestational weight gain after adjustment for confounders in the complete case analysis, which was not the case in the imputed analyses. However, it is plausible that this association in the complete case analyses was the result of bias from the exclusion of participants with missing data. A previous study on this topic also found no association between symptoms of antenatal depression and gestational weight gain [8], in keeping with the results of the imputed analyses.

Conclusions

Elevated symptoms of depression are common among obese pregnant women. In the UPBEAT RCT there was no association between elevated symptoms of antenatal depression at baseline and adherence to the intervention, risk of gestational diabetes, or gestational weight gain among obese pregnant women. There was also no evidence that the effectiveness of the intervention differed based on antenatal depression status, or that the intervention influenced symptoms of depression at follow-up. We conclude that obese pregnant women with elevated symptoms of depression should not be excluded from lifestyle interventions due to concerns about intervention adherence and effectiveness, or concerns about impact on depressive symptomatology. Awareness of depression among health professionals providing care for obese pregnant women nonetheless remains crucial for detection and treatment of this disorder.

Additional files

Additional file 1: Missing data for participants included in these analyses ($n = 1526$). The data in this section describe the proportion of missing data for each analysis variable.

Additional file 2: Mechanisms of missing data. The data in this section describe the patterns of missing data and examine the association of participant characteristics with missing data.

Additional file 3: Multiple imputation by chained equations. This section provides detailed information on the methods of the multiple imputation, and presents data comparing the characteristics of observed and imputed data.

Abbreviations

95% CI: 95% confidence interval; BMI: Body mass index; EPDS: Edinburgh Postnatal Depression Scale; OR: Odds ratios; RCT: Randomised controlled trial; SD: Standard deviation; UPBEAT: UK Pregnancies Better Eating and Activity Trial

Acknowledgements

We thank all staff in the UPBEAT consortium and the participants in the trial.

Funding

The UPBEAT study was funded by the UK's National Institute for Health Research (NIHR) under its grants for applied research programme (RP-PG-0407-10452), which supported the design of the study, collection, analysis and interpretation of data, and the writing of the manuscript. Contributions to funding, which supported the design of the study, collection and analysis of data, were also provided by the Chief Scientist Office Scottish Government Health Directorates (Edinburgh) (CZB/A/680), Guys and St Thomas' Charity, Tommy's Charity, and the NIHR Biomedical Research Centre at Guy's and St Thomas' NHS Foundation Trust and King's College London. EM was supported by a PhD studentship funded by the Medical Research Council and Tommy's Charity. This funding supported the analysis and interpretation of data and the writing of the manuscript. The work was supported through salary support to

LM Howard by the National Institute for Health Research NIHR Research Professorship (NIHR-RP-R3–12-011) and the NIHR Mental Health Biomedical Research Centre at South London and Maudsley NHS Foundation Trust and King's College London. This funding supported the interpretation of data and writing of the manuscript. The views expressed in this publication are those of the authors and not necessarily those of the NHS, the National Institute for Health Research or the Department of Health.

Authors' contributions

LP, AB and PTS contributed substantially to the original conception and design of the UPBEAT RCT. EM, LMH and LP conceived and designed the analyses reported here. EM and SB conducted the statistical analyses. EM, SB, AB, PTS, LMH and LP contributed to interpretation of data and the drafting of the manuscript. All authors read and approved the final manuscript.

Competing interests

The authors declare that they have no competing interests. The funders were not involved in the interpretation of results, decision to publish or preparation of the manuscript.

Author details

[1]Section of Women's Mental Health, Institute of Psychiatry, Psychology & Neuroscience at King's College London, London, England. [2]Department of Women and Children's Health, King's College, London, England.

References

1. Oteng-Ntim E, Varma R, Croker H, Poston L, Doyle P. Lifestyle interventions for overweight and obese pregnant wogxmen to improve pregnancy outcome: systematic review and meta-analysis. BMC Med. 2012;10:47.
2. Nascimento S, Surita F, Parpinelli M, Siani S, e Silva JP. The effect of an antenatal physical exercise programme on maternal/perinatal outcomes and quality of life in overweight and obese pregnant women: a randomised clinical trial. BJOG Int J Obstet Gynaecol 2011, 118(12): 1455–1463.
3. Moroshko I, Brennan L, O'Brien P. Predictors of dropout in weight loss interventions: a systematic review of the literature. Obes Rev. 2011;12(11): 912–34.
4. Molyneaux E, Poston L, Ashurst-Williams S, Howard LM. Obesity and mental disorders during pregnancy and postpartum: a systematic review and meta-analysis. Obstet Gynecol. 2014;123(4):857–67.
5. Hill B, Skouteris H, Fuller-Tyszkiewicz M, Kothe EJ, McPhie S. A path model of psychosocial and health behaviour change predictors of excessive gestational weight gain. J Reprod Infant Psychol. 2016;34(2):139–61.
6. Webb JB, Siega-Riz AM, Dole N. Psychosocial determinants of adequacy of gestational weight gain. Obesity. 2009;17(2):300–9.
7. Molyneaux E, Poston L, Khondoker M, Howard LM. Obesity, antenatal depression, diet and gestational weight gain in a population cohort study. Arch Womens Ment Health. 2016;19(5):899–907.
8. Bogaerts A, Devlieger R, Nuyts E, Witters I, Gyselaers W, Van den Bergh B. Effects of lifestyle intervention in obese pregnant women on gestational weight gain and mental health: a randomized controlled trial. Int J Obes. 2013;37(6):814–21.
9. Dodd JM, Newman A, Moran LJ, Deussen AR, Grivell RM, Yelland LN, et al. The effect of antenatal dietary and lifestyle advice for women who are overweight or obese on emotional well-being: the LIMIT randomized trial. Acta Obstet Gynecol Scand. 2016;95(3):309–18.
10. Perales M, Cordero Y, Vargas M, Lucia A, Barakat R. Exercise and depression in overweight and obese pregnant women: a randomised controlled trial. Archivos de medicina del deporte: revista de la Federación Española de Medicina del Deporte y de la Confederación Iberoamericana de Medicina del Deporte. 2015;167:156–63.
11. Poston L, Bell R, Croker H, Flynn AC, Godfrey KM, Goff L, et al. Effect of a behavioural intervention in obese pregnant women (the UPBEAT study): a multicentre, randomised controlled trial. Lancet Diabetes Endocrinol. 2015; 3(10):767–77.
12. Cox JL, Holden JM, Sagovsky R. Detection of postnatal depression. Development of the 10-item Edinburgh postnatal depression scale. Br J Psychiatry. 1987;150(6):782–6.
13. Murray D, Cox JL. Screening for depression during pregnancy with the Edinburgh depression scale (EDDS). J Reprod Infant Psychol. 1990;8(2):99–107.
14. Metzger B, Gabbe S, Persson B. International association of diabetes and pregnancy study groups consensus panel. International Association of Diabetes and Pregnancy Study Groups recommendations on the diagnosis and classification of hyperglycemia in pregnancy. Diabetes Care. 2010;33(3): 676–82.
15. Briley AL, Barr S, Badger S, Bell R, Croker H, Godfrey KM, et al. A complex intervention to improve pregnancy outcome in obese women; the UPBEAT randomised controlled trial. BMC Pregnancy Childbirth. 2014;14:74.
16. Rasmussen KM, Yaktine AL. Weight gain during pregnancy: reexamining the guidelines. Washington (DC): National Academies Press; 2009.
17. Van Buuren S, Oudshoorn K. Flexible multivariate imputation by MICE. Leiden: TNO Prevention and Health (TNO Publication No. PG/VGZ/99.054); 1999.
18. Sterne JA, White IR, Carlin JB, Spratt M, Royston P, Kenward MG, et al. Multiple imputation for missing data in epidemiological and clinical research: potential and pitfalls. BMJ Br Med J. 2009;338:b2393.
19. Bodner TE. What improves with increased missing data imputations? Struct Equ Model Multidiscip J. 2008;15(4):651–75.
20. Rubin DB. Multiple imputation for non-response in surveys. New York: John Wiley & Sons; 1987.
21. Vinter CA, Jensen DM, Ovesen P, Beck-Nielsen H, Jørgensen JS. The LiP (lifestyle in pregnancy) study: a randomized controlled trial of lifestyle intervention in 360 obese pregnant women. Diabetes Care. 2011;34(12): 2502–7.
22. Renault KM, Nørgaard K, Nilas L, Carlsen EM, Cortes D, Pryds O, et al. The Treatment of Obese Pregnant Women (TOP) study: a randomized controlled trial of the effect of physical activity intervention assessed by pedometer with or without dietary intervention in obese pregnant women. Am J Obstet Gynecol. 2014;210(2):134. e131–134. e139
23. Dodd JM, Turnbull D, McPhee AJ, Deussen AR, Grivell RM, Yelland LN, et al. Antenatal lifestyle advice for women who are overweight or obese: LIMIT randomised trial. BMJ. 2014;348:g1285.
24. Howard LM, Molyneaux E, Dennis C-L, Rochat T, Stein A, Milgrom J. Non-psychotic mental disorders in the perinatal period. Lancet. 2014;384(9956): 1775–88.
25. Lancaster CA, Gold KJ, Flynn HA, Yoo H, Marcus SM, Davis MM. Risk factors for depressive symptoms during pregnancy: a systematic review. Am J Obstet Gynecol. 2010;202(1):5–14.
26. Molyneaux E, Pasupathy D, Kenny L, McCowan L, North R, Dekker G, et al. Socio-economic status influences the relationship between obesity and antenatal depression: data from a prospective cohort study. J Affect Disord. 2016;202:124–7.
27. Department for Communities and Local Government. The English Indices of Deprivation 2010. London: Department for Communities and Local Government; 2011.
28. Payne RA, Abel GA. UK indices of multiple deprivation - a way to make comparisons across constituent countries easier. Health Stat Q. 2012;53:22–37.

12

Effects of maternal obesity on the success of assisted vaginal delivery in Chinese women

Hongying Wu and Jiayi Yue*

Abstract

Background: We examined the influence of pre-pregnancy body weight on the rates of attempted and successfully assisted-vaginal delivery.

Methods: We used 2008–2016 inpatient records including 3408 women who had singleton gestations and needed operative delivery assistance to conduct a retrospective cohort study. Patients were categorized based on pre-pregnancy BMI (normal weight = 18.5 to less than 25 or obese = 30 or greater). We used logistic regression to estimate odds ratios and 95% confidence intervals of attempted and successful forceps or vacuum-assisted vaginal delivery by body weight adjusted for marital status, age, gestational age, induction of labor, episiotomy, diabetes, and birth weight.

Results: The proportion of women with attempted either vacuum or forceps was lower among women who were obese pre-pregnancy compared to women who were normal weight. Women with excessive gestational weight gain, large for gestational age neonates, and diabetes were less likely to have a vacuum-assisted or forceps-assisted vaginal delivery attempted. Conversely, women who received labor augmentation or induction, used epidural anesthesia, gained inadequate weight, and delivered a small for gestational age infant were more likely to have a vacuum-assisted or forceps-assisted vaginal delivery attempted. Compared to normal weight women, obese women who received forceps-assisted vaginal delivery were more likely to have a successful vaginal delivery.

Conclusion: Women who had normal weight had higher likelihood to attempt assisted vaginal delivery compared to women who had pre-pregnancy obesity. However, when assisted vaginal delivery was attempted, success rates were higher when forceps-assisted delivery was used compared to vacuum-assisted delivery.

Keywords: Maternal obesity, Vacuum, Forceps, Assisted-vaginal delivery

Background

Delivery methods generally include vaginal delivery and cesarean section [1–3]. As an alternative delivery method, cesarean section rate usually ranges between 10 to 15%. However, in China it is as high as 50%, which is one of the highest rates in the world. Intrinsic risk is associated with cesarean sections, which not only increase the costs of postpartum care, but also cause psychological distress [4–6], and a likely lifetime risk to women in subsequent pregnancies. Hence, the Chinese National Health and Family Planning Commission has formulated a series of policies to reduce excessive cesarean section and promote vaginal delivery [7, 8].

* Correspondence: yuejiayiwww@126.com
Department of Gynaecology and Obstetrics, Liaocheng People's Hospital, Liaocheng 252000, Shandong Province, People's Republic of China

Assisted vaginal delivery is an important measure to promote vaginal delivery of infants by using tools including forceps and vacuum extractor during the second stage of labor [9, 10]. Assisted vaginal delivery (AVD) is often considered when immediate or potential fetal compromise is expected, when there is a need to shorten the second stage of labor for maternal benefit, or when there is an inadequate progress during second stage of labor [11, 12]. It has been shown that assisted vaginal delivery can significantly lower the rate of cesarean delivery and increase both pediatric and maternal benefits, such as reducing postpartum hemorrhage, postpartum sepsis and fetal birth asphyxia [5, 10, 12, 13]. Therefore, studies on how to implement assisted vaginal delivery methods will be critical to achieve the goal of reducing excessive cesarean section and promoting vaginal delivery.

In developing Asian countries, women generally have a lower body mass index (BMI) and a smaller gestational weight gain (GWG) than those reported in developed countries in Europe and North America [14]. However, the increases in the prevalence of obesity in pregnant women has been reported in recent years in developing countries. In addition, little information has been obtained to interpret the influence of maternal pre-pregnancy GWG and/or BMI in developing Asian countries, such as China. According to the gestational weight gain recommendations issued by Institute of Medicine (IOM) in 2009, over 50% percent of childbearing-aged women who live in northern China had excessive GWG [15, 16], which is a great public health concern in China. Until now, while there are a few studies examining the influence of maternal obesity on the outcomes of delivery in Chinese women [15–18], there are no studies on the effects of maternal obesity on vaginal delivery, even though it has been shown that maternal obesity is associated with an increased rate of cesarean delivery. Further, while studies have shown that the vacuum extractor is the preferred method because it is considered as safe for the fetus and has less likelihood to cause maternal morbidity [10, 19, 20], forceps-assisted vaginal delivery is still routinely used in many areas of China, including our hospital. However, there is lack of studies on how maternal obesity affects the rates of attempted and successful vacuum extraction and/or forceps assisted vaginal delivery. Hence, our study was designed to investigate the effects of obesity status of the childbearing-aged women on attempted and successful rates of assisted vaginal delivery in China.

Methods

Study design

This was a retrospective study. We used data from the medical records of women who delivered from January 2008 to December 2016 in Liaocheng People's Hospital, Liaocheng, Shandong Province in China. Data was also validated with manual chart for delivery mode, cervical dilation, and fetal station. The institutional review board approved this study.

Exclusion criteria

- Planned cesarean deliveries for malpresentation
- Spontaneous vaginal delivery
- Prior history of uterine surgery
- Prior cesarean delivery
- Pregnancy terminations
- Intrauterine fetal demises
- Penatal- and postnatal-diagnosed congenital anomalies
- Maternal human immunodeficiency virus.
- No documented pre-pregnancy weight, height, delivery mode, dilation, station, or potential confounders of interest including maternal age, marital status, current smoking status, race–ethnicity, primary language, parity, episiotomy, diabetes status, hypertension, receipt of prenatal care, oxytocin induction or augmentation, delivery gestational age, and neonatal birth weight (small for gestational age, appropriate for gestational age, or LGA).
- More than one pregnancy during the study period.

Inclusion criteria

- Singleton gestations
- 34 weeks of gestation or greater
- Eligible for a vacuum or forceps delivery
- Require operative assistance

Abstraction of medical records

Body mass index was calculated from pre-pregnancy weight and height obtained from the medical record. Pre-pregnancy BMI was categorized as normal weight (18.5 to less than 25) or obese (30 or greater) [21]. Gestational weight gain was calculated by subtracting pre-pregnancy weight from admission weight at delivery admission or last documented prenatal visit weight. Gestational weight gain was categorized as inadequate, appropriate, or excessive considering gestational age at delivery and using the 2009 Institute of Medicine's guidelines (Pre-pregnancy BMI-specific recommended trajectories of ranges of gain achieved by the 40th week of gestation): 25–35 pounds for women of normal weight, and 11–20 pounds for obese women [21].

We also collected Apgar score less than 7 at 1 and 5 min, and neonatal intensive care unit admission outcomes. The distribution of potential confounders by pre-pregnancy obesity status was analyzed using Chi-squared test for categorical variables and analysis of variance for continuous variables. Logistic regression models were used to estimate odds ratios (ORs) and 95% confidence intervals (CIs) for attempted and successful vacuum or forceps assisted vaginal delivery. Variables associated with delivery mode at $p < 0.10$ were included in adjusted regression models. The rates of adverse maternal and neonatal outcomes by delivery type were also compared using crude logistic regression models. All analyses were conducted using SAS 9.1.3.

Results

During 2008 and 2016, there were a total of 21,759 deliveries in our hospital. We excluded 18,451 based on our exclusion and inclusion criteria. As a result, we analyzed a total of 3408 women who were normal weight, over weighted or obese pre-pregnancy and required operative delivery assistance (Fig. 1). The characteristics of the analyzed cohort are shown in Table 1. Women were

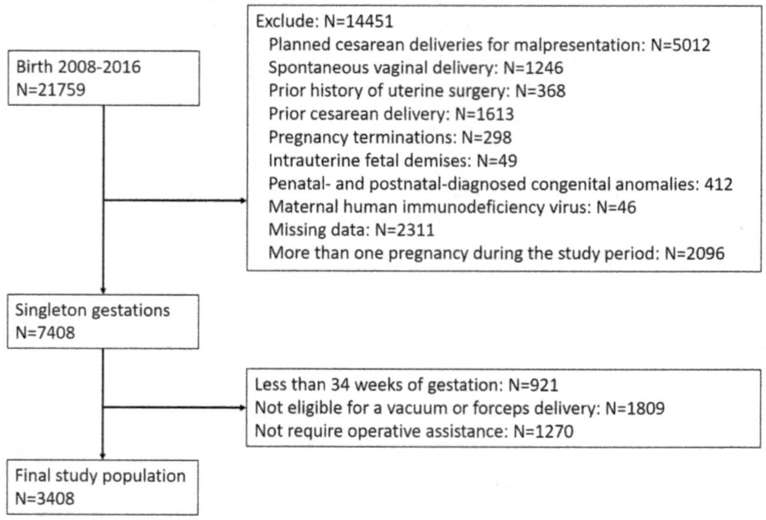

Fig. 1 Patient Enrollment Criteria

Table 1 Characteristics of laboring women who require operative delivery assistance, N (%) ($N = 3408$)

	Normal weight ($N = 2059$) Average BMI = 20.5	Over weight ($N = 360$) Average BMI = 26.3	Obese ($N = 629$) Average BMI = 31.2	*P*-value
Age (years)				
< 20	166 (8.1)	22 (6.1)	34 (5.5)	0.282
20–24	327 (15.9)	61 (16.9)	109 (17.3)	
25–29	580 (28.2)	109 (30.3)	187 (29.8)	
30–35	634 (30.8)	102 (28.5)	177 (28.1)	
> 35	348 (16.9)	66 (18.2)	121 (19.3)	
Smoking	187 (9.1)	12 (12.0)	72 (11.5)	0.018
Diabetes (Type I, II or GDM)	92 (4.6)	22 (6.1)	80 (12.8)	< 0.001
Hypertension: PIH, Chronic & Preeclampsia	148 (7.3)	29 (8.1)	125 (19.9)	< 0.001
Received prenatal care	2028 (98.5)	356 (99.1)	624 (99.2)	0.578
Induction	1466 (71.2)	249 (69.2)	513 (81.5)	< 0.001
Epidural Anesthesia	1812 (88.0)	308 (85.7)	560 (89.1)	0.719
Adherence to 2009 IOM guideline				
Inadequate	331 (16.1)	55 (15.2)	127 (20.2)	< 0.001
Appropriate	679 (33.0)	106 (29.5)	94 (14.9)	
Excessive	1052 (51.1)	176 (48.9)	412 (65.5)	
Gestational age				
EGA ≥34 –< 37 weeks	88 (4.3)	19 (5.2)	27 (4.3)	0.747
EGA 37+ weeks	1966 (95.5)	334 (92.9)	602 (95.7)	
Neonate weight				
LGA	222 (10.8)	39 (11.0)	41 (6.5)	0.001
AGA	1700 (82.6)	303 (84.2)	517 (82.3)	
SGA	132 (6.4)	33 (9.1)	71 (11.2)	

GDM (Gestational Diabetes Mellitus), EGA (Estimation of Gestational Age), IOM (Institute of Medicine), SGA (Small for Gestational Age), AGA (Appropriate of Gestational Age), LGA (Large for Gestational Age)

predominantly married (82%) and non-smokers (89%) and nulliparous (89%). The majority of women received prenatal care (99%). Nearly half (56%) of women were normal pre-pregnancy weight, and 21% were obese. We also found that the most common comorbid conditions were hypertensive disease of pregnancy (12%) and combined pre-gestational and gestation DM (8%), with higher occurrence among obese women.

Among the women who required operative delivery assistance, 36% ($n = 1226$) had an attempted vacuum assisted vaginal delivery, 31% ($n = 1056$) had an attempted forcep-assisted vaginal delivery, and 33% ($n = 1126$) had a cesarean delivery without a trial of either assisted delivery, among which, 621 of women attempted vacuum assisted vaginal delivery and 505 of women attempted forceps assisted vaginal delivery. The proportion of women with attempted either vacuum or forceps was lower among women who were obese pre-pregnancy compared to women who were normal weight (Table 2). Women with excessive gestational weight gain, large for gestational age neonates, and diabetes were less likely to have a vacuum-assisted or forceps-assisted vaginal delivery attempted. Conversely, women who received labor augmentation or induction, used epidural anesthesia, gained inadequate weight gain, and delivered a small for gestational age infant were more likely to have a vacuum-assisted or forceps-assisted vaginal delivery attempted (Table 2).

Among the women who had either a vacuum-assisted or forceps-assisted vaginal delivery attempt, the majority had successful assisted vaginal delivery, regardless of methods (Table 3). Compared to normal weight women, obese women who received forceps-assisted vaginal delivery were more likely to have a successful vaginal delivery. Among women who required operative assistance, there were no differences in infant 1-min and 5-min Apgar score < 7 or Neonatal Intensive Care Unit (NICU) admissions between vacuum assisted vaginal delivery, forceps assisted vaginal delivery, cesarean delivery without vacuum or forceps attempt, or failed vacuum or forceps delivery leading to cesarean (Table 4).

Discussion

We found that pre-pregnancy obesity reduced the likelihood in Chinese women to attempt vacuum or forceps-assisted vaginal delivery. Further, we observed higher success rates only when forceps-assisted delivery was attempted. In addition, we found that among women requiring operative delivery assistance, Apgar scores or NICU admissions were not affected by vacuum or forceps-assisted vaginal delivery, relative to cesarean delivery without assisted-vaginal delivery attempt or cesarean delivery after failed assisted vaginal delivery. These results suggested that attempting vacuum or forceps assisted vaginal delivery might not be a risky factor in certain delivery outcomes. However, it has been shown that obese women have increased risks of large for gestational age neonates and associated shoulder dystocia [18]. Also, perineal lacerations and shoulder dystocia are known risks of vacuum-assisted vaginal delivery [16, 17]. Studies have shown that women who underwent a vacuum assisted vaginal delivery had the risk rates of 3rd or 4th degree laceration (12.3%) and shoulder dystocia (2.5%) and risk rates increased relative to those who had cesarean delivery without attempted vaginally delivery [22]. Hence, clinician may always need to consider these complications deterring vacuum-or forceps assisted vaginal delivery attempts. However, this concern would need to be balanced against the significant morbidity accompanying cesarean delivery in women with obesity.

Our finding of lower odds of attempted assisted vaginal delivery in obese women is consistent with a recent study but is contradicted with previous studies [23, 24]. One of the possible reasons is the different rates of cesarean delivery. A recent prospective cohort study of Norwegian women found 50% higher rates of vacuum-assisted vaginal delivery among women with class III obesity compared to normal weight women [25]. However, a recent study in US showed lower odds of attempted assisted vaginal delivery in obese women, similar to our findings [26]. It should be noted that rates of cesarean delivery in Norway were much lower than those in the US and China during the study period [27]. Therefore, it is possible that physicians may prefer to use assisted vaginal deliveries in women with obesity, when the rate of cesarean deliveries is low. Also, obesity is associated with several health conditions, including hypertensive disease of pregnancy, chronic hypertensive disease, and gestational diabetes, which are known risk factors that are associated with higher cesarean rates. In our study, 21% of women were obese, which is similar to that in US study (18%), but much higher than that in Norway study (8%).

Another interesting finding of our study is that obese women have higher chances of success with forceps compared to normal weight women. Previous study showed that the use of forceps was associated with a higher success rate than the vacuum, for both occiput anterior and posterior positions [28]. It has previously been found that obese and short women are at greater risk of having more difficult labors [29, 30] and of occiput posterior delivery [31–33]. Hence, it is likely that forceps assisted vaginal delivery is particularly effective for obese women with occiput posterior position.

Our study has several limitations. We did not collect adequate information from medical comorbidities. Particularly, some comorbidities are associated with recommendations to shorten second stage labor, such as

Table 2 Attempted assisted vaginal delivery in relation to pre-pregnancy body weight and participant characteristics among laboring women in need of operative delivery assistance ($N = 2282$). Percentage represents the total number for each category in the final study group

Characteristics	Attempted vacuum			Attempted Forceps		
	N (%)	Crude OR [95% CI]	Adjusted OR [95% CI]	N (%)	Crude OR [95% CI]	Adjusted OR [95% CI]
Pre-pregnancy BMI (kg/m^2)						
Normal Weight (18.5 to < 23.0)	777 (37.7)	Reference	Reference	623 (30.2)	Reference	Reference
Overweight (23.0–27.5)	145 (40.2)	0.87 [0.72–0.99]	0.88 [0.69–0.98]	131 (36.3)	0.79 [0.69–0.99]	0.76 [0.68–0.98]
Obese (≥27.5)	304 (48.3)	0.43 [0.36–0.67]*	0.42 [0.32–0.72]*	302 (48.1)	0.38 [0.31–0.59]*	0.34 [0.29–0.52]*
Age (years)						
< 20 years	88 (39.6)	1.08 [1.02–1.14]	1.15 [1.08–1.44]	78 (35.1)	0.99 [0.87–1.13]	1.08 [0.98–1.13]
20–24 years	202 (40.6)	Reference	Reference	174 (35.8)	Reference	Reference
25–29 years	354 (40.4)	0.99 [0.84–1.20]	0.97 [0.79–1.31]	305 (34.8)	0.92 [0.76–1.10]	0.93 [0.85–1.03]
30–35 years	368 (40.3)	0.88 [0.69–1.14]	0.89 [0.74–1.12]	315 (34.5)	0.89 [0.79–1.09]	0.88 [0.77–1.12]
> 35 years	214 (39.8)	0.98 [0.77–1.31]	0.98 [0.79–1.18]	184 (34.4)	0.99 [0.84–1.03]	0.98 [0.85–1.09]
Smoking Cigarettes						
No smoking	1135 (40.7)	0.98 [0.66–1.24]		969 (34.9)	0.89 [0.67–1.16]	
Smoking	91 (34.8)	Reference		87 (32.5)	Reference	
Diabetes (Type 1, 2, GDM)						
Not Diabetes	1128 (39.7)	Reference	Reference	981 (34..6)	Reference	Reference
Diabetes	98 (50.5)	0.51 [0.33–0.75]*	0.55 [0.35–0.88]*	75 (38.6)	0.68 [0.56–0.78]*	0.64 [0.54–0.76]*
Hypertension (chronic, pregnancy-induced, preeclampsia)						
Not hypertension	1150 (37.7)	Reference		987 (40.6)	Reference	
Hypertension	79 (38.3)	0.88 [0.62–1.15]		74 (37.2)	0.83 [0.61–1.16]	
Received Prenatal care						
No	17 (45.0)	1.48 [0.44–4.09]		19 (39.0)	1.48 [0.49–5.01]	
Yes	1212 (40.2)	Reference		1042 (38.2)	Reference	
Induction						
No	401 (44.7)	Reference	Reference	304 (34.2)	Reference	Reference
Yes	828 (54.9)	1.61 [1.08–2.81]*	1.77 [1.00–2.87]*	757 (45.5)	1.63 [1.08–2.83]*	1.71 [1.00–2.87]*
Epidural Anesthesia						
No	205 (15.5)	Reference	Reference	135 (10.7)	Reference	Reference
Yes	1024 (30.9)	1.26 [0.86–1.68]*	1.62 [1.12–2.39]*	926 (28.6)	1.31 [0.96–1.78]*	1.78 [1.02–2.44]*
Adherence to 2009 IOM guideline						
Inadequate	108 (88.3)	1.65 [1.10–2.41]*	1.81 [1.15–2.83]*	87 (88.1)	1.69 [1.10–2.53]*	1.88 [1.11–2.92]*
Appropriate	746 (82.1)	Reference	Reference	716 (83.1)	Reference	Reference
Excessive	345 (25.1)	0.62 [0.41–0.79]*	0.72 [0.59–1.05]*	268 (20.3)	0.61 [0.51–0.87]*	0.69 [0.59–1.01]*
Estimated Gestational age (weeks)						
EGA ≥34 – < 37	61 (51.2)	Reference		58 (47.1)	Reference	
EGA 37+	1168 (50.1)	0.89 [0.50–1.31]		1003 (48.9)	0.91 [0.60–1.51]	
Neonate weight						
LGA	182 (50.7)	3.11 [1.81–5.25]*	3.24 [1.93–6.33]*	156 (48.1)	3.28 [1.80–5.49]*	3.55 [1.91–6.03]*
AGA	982 (38.8)	Reference	Reference	859 (39.6)	Reference	Reference
SGA	65 (23.1)	0.22 [0.18–0.41]*	0.25 [0.18–0.40]*	46 (19.3)	0.29 [0.20–0.40]*	0.28 [0.18–0.45]*

Adjusted for: age category, smoking, hypertension, prenatal care, epidural, adherence to GWG, race, marital status, parity, diabetes, induction, augmentation, and estimated gestational age

*Significant Odds Ratios at the $p < 0.05$ level

GDM (Gestational Diabetes Mellitus), GWG (Gestational Weight Gain), IOM (Institute of Medicine), SGA (Small for Gestational Age), AGA (Appropriate of Gestational Age), LGA (Large for Gestational Age)

Table 3 Successful assisted vaginal delivery in relation to participant characteristics among women ($N = 1987$)

Characteristics	Successful Vacuum			Successful Forceps		
	N (%)	Crude OR [95% CI]	Adjusted OR* [95% CI]	N (%)	Crude OR [95% CI]	Adjusted OR* [95% CI]
Pre-pregnancy BMI (kg/m^2)						
Normal Weight (18.5 to < 25.0)	791 (85.6)	Reference	Reference	703 (85.6)	Reference	Reference
Obese (≥30.0)	262 (86.3)	1.19 [0.59–2.28]	1.09 [0.58–2.34]	231 (96.3)	1.69 [1.07–3.18]*	1.79 [1.11–3.53]*
Age (years)						
< 20	17 (89.4)	1.11 [1.02–1.23]		11 (84.6)	0.97 [0.01–1.11]	
20–24	98 (94.2)	Reference		88 (88.8)	Reference	
25–29	312 (88.9)	0.97 [0.74–1.22]		271 (87.5)	0.85 [0.76–1.12]	
30–35	512 (84.9)	0.91 [0.69–1.21]		441 (88.6)	0.87 [0.74–1.18]	
> 35	114 (75.1)	0.99 [0.77–1.31]		123 (87.2)	0.95 [0.71–1.23]	
Smoking Cigarettes						
No Smoking	974 (85.7)	0.88 [0.68–1.06]		874 (87.9)	0.92 [0.72–1.09]	
Smoking	79 (84.0)	Reference		60 (89.5)	Reference	
Diabetes (Type 1, 2, GDM)						
Not Diabetes	994 (87.8)	Reference	Reference	889 (90.1)	Reference	Reference
Diabetes	59 (60.8)	0.49 [0.31–0.74]*	0.45 [0.27–0.68]*	45 (60.1)	0.40 [0.26–0.71]*	0.44 [0.24–0.66]*
Hypertension (chronic, pregnancy-induced, preeclampsia)						
Not hypertension	985 (85.7)	Reference		867 (87.8)	Reference	
Hypertension	68 (86.1)	0.92 [0.72–1.12]		67 (90.1)	0.85 [0.91–1.18]	
Received Prenatal Care						
No	15 (88.2)	1.08 [0.74–1.49]		17 (89.4)	1.05 [0.79–1.31]	
Yes	1038 (85.6)	Reference		917 (88.2)	Reference	
Induction						
No	345 (86.1)	Reference	Reference	265 (87.1)	Reference	Reference
Yes	708 (85.5)	1.01 [0.78–1.61]	1.07 [0.80–1.67]	668 (88.2)	1.03 [0.78–1.63]	1.01 [0.80–1.57]
Epidural						
No	185 (90.2)	Reference	Reference	115 (85.2)	Reference	Reference
Yes	868 (84.8)	1.06 [0.85–1.58]	1.07 [0.82–1.39]	819 (88.6)	1.01 [0.76–1.68]	1.08 [0.82–1.44]
Adherence To 2009 IOM Guideline						
Inadequate	94 (87.3)	1.05 [0.80–1.41]		78 (89.6)	1.09 [0.78–1.53]	
Appropriate	659 (84.9)	Reference		619 (87.7)	Reference	
Excessive	300 (86.9)	0.92 [0.71–1.12]		237 (88.4)	0.95 [0.71–1.47]	
Estimated Gestational Age						
EGA < 37	52 (85.2)	Reference		50 (86.2)	Reference	
EGA 37+	1001 (85.7)	0.99 [0.70–1.31]		884 (88.1)	0.95 [0.69–1.44]	
Neonate weight						
SGA	75 (91.7)	3.21 [1.84–5.55]*	3.14 [1.96–6.03]*	137 (87.7)	3.08 [1.89–5.79]*	3.05 [1.99–5.53]*
AGA	918 (93.0)	Reference	Reference	758 (88.2)	Reference	Reference
LGA	65 (92.3)	0.26 [0.15–0.45]*	0.24 [0.16–0.44]*	39 (84.8)	0.28 [0.17–0.44]*	0.29 [0.16–0.47]*

Adjusted for: age category, smoking, hypertension, prenatal care, epidural, adherence to GWG, race, marital status, parity, diabetes, induction, augmentation, and estimated gestational age

*Significant Odds Ratios at the $p < 0.05$ level

GDM (Gestational Diabetes Mellitus), GWG (Gestational Weight Gain), IOM (Institute of Medicine), SGA (Small for Gestational Age), AGA (Average for Gestational Age), LGA (Large for Gestational Age)

Table 4 Neonatal complications of interest by mode of delivery

	NICU Admission		Apgar Score at 1 min < 7		Apgar Score at 5 min < 7	
	N (%)	OR (95% CI)	N (%)	OR (95% CI)	N (%)	OR (95% CI)
VAVD	40 (2.7)	0.98 (0.68–1.78)	217 (20.1)	1.05 (0.75–1.38)	41 (2.9)	1.10 (0.56–2.85)
FAVD	34 (3.2)	1.03 (0.71–1.86)	221 (21.3)	1.01 (0.68–1.15)	39 (2.4)	1.15 (0.66–2.95)
CD	11 (2.9)	Ref.	88 (19.7)	Ref.	11 (2.6)	Ref.
CD after failed VAVD	3 (3.8)	1.42 (0.39–5.15)	21 (28.8)	1.33 (0.74–2.93)	4 (5.2)	1.43 (0.65–6.87)
CD after failed FAVD	2 (3.1)	1.32 (0.39–5.15)	24 (29.6)	1.43 (0.84–2.83)	5 (5.8)	1.40 (0.61–6.79)

CD (Cesarean Delivery), VAVD (vacuum-assisted vaginal delivery), FVAD (forceps-assisted vaginal delivery), NICU (Neonatal Intensive Care Unit)

valvular disease and chronic obstructive pulmonary disease [16]. We might misclassify the pre-pregnancy weight status, because it was either self-reported or was measured during early prenatal care. However, it should be noted that studies shave reported that self-reported pre-pregnancy weight is highly correlated with clinically measured pre-pregnancy weight ($r = 0.99$) [34, 35], indicating that the rate of misclassification of the pre-pregnancy weight status would be low, if there is any in our study, and unlikely to alter our findings. Further our studies did not classify obesity status. A larger sample of obese women in our follow-up study will evaluate the relationship of classes of obesity and rates to attempt and of successful assisted-vaginal delivery. Finally, both vacuum and forceps extractors are safe instruments and have been used routinely for assisted-vaginal delivery. In clinical practice, while women were selected on an individualized basis and decision was made based on individual physician, the skills of operators would certainly also have an influence on the decision of women to attempt an assisted-vaginal delivery and the choice of vacuum or forceps instrument. The forceps-assisted vaginal delivery has been adopted in our hospital for a much longer time than vacuum-assisted vaginal delivery. Hence, it should be noted that the experience and skills of operators may also help increase the success rate of forceps-assisted vaginal delivery.

Conclusion

In conclusion, our study reported that among Chinese women in need of operative delivery assistance, pre-pregnancy obesity may reduce the likelihood of an attempt to have assisted vaginal delivery. However, if assisted vaginal delivery was attempted, forceps-assisted vaginal delivery was associated with higher rate of success. This is consistent with previous reports that forceps are more likely to be used in primigravidas and less likely to fail [13, 28]. However, the risks accompanying forceps and even vacuum extraction should also be considered. Particularly, forceps-assisted vaginal delivery is reported to be associated with increased maternal morbidity and enhanced risks for facial nerve palsies and minor facial abrasions [13]. When in the clinical practice, the application of vacuum or forceps-assisted vaginal delivery in obese population should also be balanced with the higher surgical risk and morbidity of cesarean delivery [18, 24]. Hence, a more comprehensive guideline will be critical for clinicians to choose operative assistance for clinically appropriate laboring women with obesity. Future perspective studies will be necessary to examine the effects of such guidelines on the safety and efficacy in promoting vaginal delivery in a larger population.

Abbreviations

cis: Confidence intervals; ors: Odds ratios

Acknowledgements

Not applicable.

Funding

Not applicable.

Authors' contributions

HW, JY performed the experiments, analyzed and interpreted the data, wrote the manuscript. All authors read and approved the final manuscript.

Competing interests

The authors declare that they have no competing interests.

References

1. Neu J, Rushing J. Cesarean versus vaginal delivery: long-term infant outcomes and the hygiene hypothesis. Clin Perinatol. 2011;38:321–31.
2. Zhang J, Liu Y, Meikle S, Zheng J, Sun W, Li Z. Cesarean delivery on maternal request in Southeast China. Obstet Gynecol. 2008;111:1077–82.
3. Klemetti R, Che X, Gao Y, Raven J, Wu Z, Tang S, Hemminki E. Cesarean section delivery among primiparous women in rural China: an emerging epidemic. American Journal of Obstetrics & Gynecology. 2010;202(65):e61–65. e66.
4. Weiss JL, Malone FD, Emig D, Ball RH, Nyberg DA, Comstock CH, Saade G, Eddleman K, Carter SM, Craigo SD. Obesity, obstetric complications and cesarean delivery rate–a population-based screening study. American Journal of Obstetrics & Gynecology. 2004;190:1091–7.
5. Souza JP, Gülmezoglu A, Lumbiganon P, Laopaiboon M, Carroli G, Fawole B, Ruyan P. Caesarean section without medical indications is associated with an increased risk of adverse short-term maternal outcomes: the 2004-2008 WHO global survey on maternal and perinatal health. BMC Med. 2010;8:71.
6. Gibbons L, Belizán JM, Lauer JA, Betrán AP, Merialdi M, Althabe F. The global numbers and costs of additionally needed and unnecessary caesarean sections performed per year: overuse as a barrier to universal coverage. World health report. 2010;30:1–31.
7. Feng XL, Wang Y, An L, Ronsmans C. Cesarean section in the People's republic of China: current perspectives. Int J Women's Health. 2014;6:59.

8. Attane I. China's family planning policy: an overview of its past and future. Stud Fam Plan. 2002;33:103–13.
9. Hannah ME, Hannah WJ, Hewson SA, Hodnett ED, Saigal S, Willan AR, Collaborative TBT. Planned caesarean section versus planned vaginal birth for breech presentation at term: a randomised multicentre trial. Lancet. 2000;356:1375–83.
10. O'Mahony F, Hofmeyr GJ, Menon V. Choice of instruments for assisted vaginal delivery. Cochrane Libr. 2010;10(11):CD005455.
11. Bailey P, Roosmalen J, Mola G, Evans C, Bernis L, Dao B. Assisted vaginal delivery in low and middle income countries: an overview. BJOG Int J Obstet Gynaecol. 2017;124:1335–44.
12. Gei AF. Prevention of the first cesarean delivery: the role of operative vaginal delivery. In: Seminars in perinatology: Elsevier; 2012. p. 365–73.
13. Goetzinger KR, Macones GA. Operative vaginal delivery: current trends in obstetrics. Women's Health. 2008;4:281–90.
14. Yazdani S, Yosofniyapasha Y, Nasab BH, Mojaveri MH, Bouzari Z. Effect of maternal body mass index on pregnancy outcome and newborn weight. BMC research notes. 2012;5:34.
15. Li N, Liu E, Guo J, Pan L, Li B, Wang P, Liu J, Wang Y, Liu G, Baccarelli AA, et al. Maternal prepregnancy body mass index and gestational weight gain on pregnancy outcomes. PLoS One. 2013;8:e82310.
16. Liu L, Hong Z, Zhang L. Associations of prepregnancy body mass index and gestational weight gain with pregnancy outcomes in nulliparous women delivering single live babies. Sci Rep. 2015;5:12863.
17. Liu Y, Dai W, Dai X, Li Z. Prepregnancy body mass index and gestational weight gain with the outcome of pregnancy: a 13-year study of 292,568 cases in China. Arch Gynecol Obstet. 2012;286:905–11.
18. Yang S, Zhou A, Xiong C, Yang R, Bassig BA, Hu R, Zhang Y, Yao C, Zhang Y, Qiu L. Parental body mass index, gestational weight gain, and risk of macrosomia: a population-based case–control study in China. Paediatr Perinat Epidemiol. 2015;29:462–71.
19. Hehir MP, Reidy FR, Wilkinson MN, Mahony R. Increasing rates of operative vaginal delivery across two decades: accompanying outcomes and instrument preferences. European Journal of Obstetrics and Gynecology and Reproductive Biology. 2013;171:40–3.
20. Ali UA, Norwitz ER. Vacuum-assisted vaginal delivery. Rev Obstet Gynecol. 2009;2:5.
21. Doherty DA, Magann E, Francis J, Morrison J, Newnham J. Pre-pregnancy body mass index and pregnancy outcomes. Int J Gynecol Obstet. 2006;95: 242–7.
22. Ding G, Tian Y, Zhang Y, Pang Y, Zhang JS, Zhang J. Application of a global reference for fetal-weight and birthweight percentiles in predicting infant mortality. BJOG. 2013;120:1613–21.
23. Olson C, Strawderman M, Hinton P, Pearson T. Gestational weight gain and postpartum behaviors associated with weight change from early pregnancy to 1 y postpartum. Int J Obes. 2003;27:117.
24. Zhou B-F. Predictive values of body mass index and waist circumference for risk factors of certain related diseases in Chinese adults--study on optimal cut-off points of body mass index and waist circumference in Chinese adults. Biomedical and environmental sciences: BES. 2002;15:83–96.
25. Wang Y, Mi J, Shan X, Wang QJ, Ge K. Is China facing an obesity epidemic and the consequences? The trends in obesity and chronic disease in China. Int J Obes. 2007;31:177.
26. Ramos SZ, Waring ME, Leung K, Amir NS, Bannon AL, Moore Simas TA. Attempted and successful vacuum-assisted vaginal delivery by prepregnancy body mass index. Obstet Gynecol. 2017;129:311–20.
27. Council NR. Weight gain during pregnancy: reexamining the guidelines: National Academies Press; 2010.
28. Damron DP, Capeless EL. Operative vaginal delivery: a comparison of forceps and vacuum for success rate and risk of rectal sphincter injury. Am J Obstet Gynecol. 2004;191:907–10.
29. Cedergren MI. Maternal morbid obesity and the risk of adverse pregnancy outcome. Obstet Gynecol. 2004;103:219–24.
30. Ovesen P, Rasmussen S, Kesmodel U. Effect of prepregnancy maternal overweight and obesity on pregnancy outcome. Obstet Gynecol. 2011;118: 305–12.
31. Cheng YW, Shaffer BL, Caughey AB. Associated factors and outcomes of persistent occiput posterior position: a retrospective cohort study from 1976 to 2001. J Matern Fetal Neonatal Med. 2006;19:563–8.
32. Ponkey SE, Cohen AP, Heffner LJ, Lieberman E. Persistent fetal occiput posterior position: obstetric outcomes. Obstet Gynecol. 2003;101:915–20.
33. Lieberman E, Davidson K, Lee-Parritz A, Shearer E. Changes in fetal position during labor and their association with epidural analgesia. Obstet Gynecol. 2005;105:974–82.
34. Choo V. WHO reassesses appropriate body-mass index for Asian populations. Elsevier. 2002.
35. Deierlein AL, Siega-Riz AM, Adair LS, Herring AH. Effects of pre-pregnancy body mass index and gestational weight gain on infant anthropometric outcomes. J Pediatr. 2011;158:221–6.

13

A qualitative study of gestational weight gain goal setting

Shaniece Criss[1], Emily Oken[2], Lauren Guthrie[2] and Marie-France Hivert[2*]

Abstract

Background: Gestational weight gain (GWG) is an important predictor of short and long-term pregnancy outcomes for both mother and child, and women who set a GWG goal are more likely to gain within recommended ranges. Little information is available regarding potentially modifiable factors that underlie a woman's GWG goals. Our aims were to explore women's perceptions regarding factors that affect GWG, their understanding of appropriate GWG, their goal-setting experiences including patient-health care provider (HCP) conversations, and supportive interventions they would most like to help them achieve the recommended GWG.

Methods: We conducted nine in-depth interviews and seven focus groups with a total of 33 Boston, Massachusetts (MA) area women who were pregnant and had delivered within the prior 6 months. We recorded and transcribed all interviews. Two investigators independently coded resulting transcripts. We managed data using MAXQDA2 and conducted a content analysis.

Results: Perceived factors that contributed to GWG goal-setting included the mother's weight control behaviors concerning exercise and diet—including a "new way of eating for two" and "semblance of control", experiences during prior pregnancies, conversations with HCPs, and influence from various information sources. Women focused on behaviors with consistent messaging across multiple sources of information, but mainly trusted their HCP, valued one-to-one conversations with them about GWG, preferred that the HCP initiate the conversation about GWG goals, and would be open to have the conversation started based on visual aid based on their own GWG progression.

Conclusions: Pregnant women highly value discussions with their HCP to set GWG goals. Pregnant women view their clinicians as the most reliable source of information and believe that clinicians should open weight-related discussions throughout pregnancy.

Keywords: Gestational weight gain, Goal-setting, Pregnancy, Body mass index

Background

Excessive gestational weight gain (GWG) is associated with adverse health outcomes in both mothers and children. In mothers, excessive GWG increases the risk of post-partum weight retention and thus accumulation of additional excess weight later in life [1–3]. Overweight women are at greater risk of excessive GWG, setting them doubly at risk of type 2 diabetes and other cardiovascular risk factors [4, 5]. Children born to mothers who experienced excessive GWG are more likely to have greater adiposity and adverse cardiometabolic profiles in childhood and later in life [6–12].

In 2009, the Institute of Medicine (IOM) published revised recommendations about the amount of GWG a woman should achieve according to her pre-pregnancy body mass index (BMI). GWG is an on-going challenging issue with 40 to 78 % of pregnant women gaining above the recommended range in various populations of pregnant women in the United States [13–15]. Determinants of GWG are multiple; one major factor is whether a woman has set a GWG goal for herself and whether that goal is within the recommended range [16]. Goal-setting is a key concept in behavioral approaches

* Correspondence: mhivert@partners.org
[2]Obesity Prevention Program, Department of Population Medicine, Harvard Medical School and Harvard Pilgrim Health Care Institute, 401 Park Drive Suite 401E, Boston, MA, USA02215
Full list of author information is available at the end of the article

necessary in weight management. In a previous survey, we showed that only about 40 % of pregnant women had a goal consistent with IOM recommendations, another 20 % had discordant goals, and 40 % did not have a goal [17]. Those with no goal were more likely to gain outside the recommended amount of weight, either inadequate or excessive weight gain.

In this study, we focused on factors that contribute to GWG goal-setting of pregnant women. Our study is based on the Ecological Model for Health Promotion [18], which builds upon the social ecological model, to examine various levels of influence of GWG goal-setting: individual (e.g., personal attitudes), interpersonal (e.g., clinician interaction; family conversations), organizational (e.g., a GWG chart; availability of specialized health professionals for interventions), and community (e.g., media). The aims of this qualitative study using detailed interviews and focus groups in pregnant women receiving care at Atrius Harvard Vanguard Medical Associates, a large multi-center clinical practice in the greater Boston Area, USA were to:

1) Explore women's perceptions of factors that affect GWG, including diet, exercise, and information sources and content;
2) Explore pregnant women's understanding of appropriate GWG, GWG goal-setting, and weight control behavior;
3) Describe women's experiences with health care providers (HCP) and advice they have received regarding GWG; and
4) Generate feedback about the development of tools or supportive interventions they would most like to help them achieve recommended GWG.

Methods

Recruitment

We recruited participants for this study from the greater Boston area in spring 2011 (Round 1) and fall 2014 (Round 2) for focus groups and interviews. We targeted women who were at least 16 weeks pregnant or who had delivered <6 months prior so that they recently had an opportunity to interact with their HCP around GWG goals and tracking.

In Round 1, we recruited participants by means of newspaper advertisement and posted flyers in obstetric waiting rooms. Interested women contacted the study research assistant by telephone or email. The research assistant confirmed eligibility, and scheduled the focus group or interview session. In Round 2, we included only pregnant women with pre-pregnancy BMI ≥ 25 kg/m^2 to enrich our population with women with excess weight. Clinic staff informed study staff when an eligible woman had her appointment, and then recruitment would occur on-site in the obstetric waiting room after the appointment.

Study design and sample

We conducted seven focus groups and nine individual interviews for a total of 33 participants. We conducted separate focus groups with participants who had normal pre-pregnancy BMI (two groups) and those who were overweight or obese (BMI ≥ 25 kg/m^2,five groups). One study staff member conducted all of the individual interviews (Round 1, $n = 9$ participants) with eligible participants unable to attend a focus group, another conducted four focus groups (Round 1, $n = 14$ participants), and a third conducted three focus groups (Round 2, $n = 10$ participants). All interviewers were trained and experienced in qualitative interview techniques. The Harvard Pilgrim Health Care Human Studies Committee approved the study and all participants provided written informed consent.

Interview guide

We developed the interview guide based on a review of the literature, Ecological Model for Health Promotion [18], and previous experience with this population. Table 1 shows the topic domains. We structured open-ended questions to determine: 1) insights about attitudes and behaviors about factors that affect GWG, 2) GWG goal-setting, 3) HCP interaction and advice about GWG, and 4) tools and resources for GWG management.

Data collection and analysis

All interviews and focus groups were conducted at a central Boston clinic location, and lasted 60 to 90 min. We conducted focus groups in the evening to maximize participation, and provided dinner. Participants received a $25 gift card and transportation reimbursement.

To protect the privacy of participants, we made every effort to capture audio recordings with no identifying information. All audio recordings were digitally recorded, transferred to a secure computer, transcribed, and de-identified. Members of the research team immersed themselves in the data, coded, identified themes, reviewed the results, and continued discussion until a consensus was met [19]. Specifically, a study team member read the transcripts to get an overall impression of potential themes, and developed the codebook based on the interview guide and the major themes identified in each of the transcripts. Three reviewers evaluated the codebook to ensure accuracy and clarity of code definitions. Round 1 transcripts were then independently coded by two reviewers using MAXQDA2, a qualitative software management program. In addition, a third reviewer coded and completed a content analysis on Round 1 and Round 2 transcripts.

Table 1 Gestational weight gain goal setting interview guide domains and question examples

Domain	Question Examples
Diet related to pregnancy	How have you changed your diet since you found out that you are pregnant? Why have you made these changes?
	What makes it hard for you to eat the way you would like to be eating?
Physical activity related to pregnancy	What impact does your exercise have on your baby?
	What concerns do you have about risks related to exercising during pregnancy?
Gestational weight gain (GWG)	How important do you think the amount of weight you gain during pregnancy is for the health of your pregnancy?
	How much do you worry about your pregnancy weight gain?
Weight gain goal	What is your weight gain goal?
	How did you decide on this goal? Is this something you decided upon on your own or in consultation with your OB or someone else?
Patient-Clinician Conversations	Has your OB discussed weight gain during pregnancy with you? How and when did s/he raise the topic?
	During the course of this pregnancy, have any of your OB providers told you whether you are gaining about the right amount, too much, or too little?
Information sources	Where have you heard information about weight gain during pregnancy? How much do you trust this source?
Weight control behavior	How much control do you feel that have over how much weight you gain during pregnancy? What factors make you feel that you are not in control?
	Are you actively trying to influence the amount of weight you gain during your pregnancy? What are you doing to influence your weight gain?
Tools and resources for GWG management	Imagine that you were gaining too much weight during your pregnancy. What do you think would be most helpful for you to help you get back on track?
	How would you feel about seeing a graph of your weight gain during pregnancy? Who would you like to get this graph from, your doctor, nurse, midwife, or someone else?
	Have you used pregnancy-related applications on your smart phone? Which ones? What do you like about them? What do you use the apps for?

Results

The participants ($n = 33$) were on average 34 years old and at a mean of 23 weeks of gestation. Two-thirds of participants were of European descent, 15 % were African-American, and the remainder from other ethnic backgrounds. More than 80 % (27 out of 33) had completed a college degree or higher level of education. About half of the participants (17 out of 33) reported having pre-pregnancy BMI ≥ 25 kg/m^2. The following themes were consistent among all groups, unless otherwise indicated.

Perceived factors that affect GWG

Diet

A new way of eating for two Many women shared stories of friends and family urging them to "eat for two," yet they did not feel that they needed to overindulge in eating. Here is how one participant revised the concept:

> "Because now I'm not only eating for myself, I'm eating for two, only not quantity-wise. Every time I say that I always think of people saying, 'Oh, you're eating for two. You can indulge.' And I say, 'Yes, technically I am.' But it doesn't mean that I'm going to go overboard. Or go and buy snacks that I wish I could have, but I know I can't."

Several women indicated that they felt that what they ate affected the baby: "I mean, you have to feed yourself and remember that also goes to the baby. If you're eating crap now, you're giving that crap to the baby." Some women with previous pregnancies indicated that their child likes to eat what they ate in pregnancy. In contrast, some women did not think their current eating would cause any issues for the baby, and nutrition was important once s/he is born. Participants indicated barriers that prevented them from having a nutritious diet, including cost of healthy food, lack of time for food preparation (e.g., taking care of another child), not feeling like cooking, and the continuous availability of unhealthy food.

Physical activity

Several women reported that physical activity was important, but it was more challenging during pregnancy. One participant said, "The second I got pregnant, my first trimester, I went to the gym, and my inner body alarm clock was just screaming at me- don't do it." Most women reported that they were not currently exercising during pregnancy, although those who were participated in a variety of activities ranging from walking to belly dancing.

Exercise for mom, not baby Many women did not see a clear link between physical activity and the health of the baby, but many reported that exercise could ease labor and enhance their own mental/emotional health.

One participant said, "I pay more importance to diet, and I think exercise is just more important for myself, like for my feeling good and like, but I don't think it affects baby much." A few women said that modeling exercise to their born child would be more important.

The women listed numerous barriers to physical activity in pregnancy, including: reduced energy levels/being tired, trouble breathing, pain, lack of time due to professional and/or personal life (e.g., other children), inclement weather being a safety concern (e.g., falling on ice), and the expense of exercise classes.

Understanding appropriate GWG, GWG goal-setting, and weight control behavior

Appropriate GWG

Many women shared the belief that excessive GWG can increase risks of gestational diabetes and preeclampsia, and that women need to closely monitor their weight if they have gestational diabetes. A few participants indicated that if the mother gained too much weight, then the child could be overweight or obese. Several participants were unable to identify specific health-related issues for the baby resulting from excessive GWG. In contrast, many participants reported that gaining too little weight is an issue because underweight babies can have health problems.

Weight gain goals

Several participants set GWG goals and reported ranges between 15 to 49 lb. Several women, including participants with BMI ≥25 kg/m^2, stated that they did not have a GWG goal and they assumed that their HCP would discuss GWG with them if it was an issue: "I don't have a goal. I just, I've gained already 35 lb, and I still have 2 more months left." Many participants reported that they felt "conscious" of their weight. One woman said, "oh my gosh- my body's changing so much. So for me, it's already a little bit weird to be gaining weight like this. I'm always thinking, OK, you don't wanna be gaining too much." Other participants were not as concerned about weight gain because they felt that they would be able to "shed the pounds" post-partum based on losing weight with previous pregnancies or motivation to be active for their child.

Weight control behavior

Semblance of control Most women reported that they felt as though they had "some" control over their weight gain, but the control varied based on needing more calories for pregnancy, mother and baby's cravings, stress, trimester, and the way the body processes the nutrients. One participant said:

> "I feel like I have some semblance of control...I feel like I could be more controlling of how much weight I was gaining if I weren't pregnant. So I could be like, 'Well, you know, I feel like I gorged the last two days so I'll kind of chill out and just eat fruits and salads for the next couple of days.' But I feel like I'd be cheating my baby if I did that right now."

Concerning cravings, a participant said, "I have some control, but not much. Because sometimes I feel hungry and I've wanted some specific food that it's hard to resist...you should eat it, because it means you lack something in the food." Similarly, a woman stated, "If I feel the urge to eat... I kind of feel like that's the baby that wants more. And I feel like I don't want to deprive the baby of eating more." One participant indicated that she had control and said, "I know ultimately it's my fault. I cannot blame anyone else for my weight gain." In contrast, another participant expressed she lacked control because heartburn and indigestion limited her options.

Patient-HCP conversations and advice regarding GWG

Provider conversations

Most participants reported that they highly ranked their HCP's advice concerning GWG. Specifically, the participants stated that they "trusted" their clinician. One participant said, "I trust my doctor more because she works with patients every day." Another participant said, "If my doctor said, 'This is what you have to do,' then I would do it." Participants reported receiving information about GWG in different ways, which is highlighted in the next sections.

Patient-initiated Many participants reported that they specifically had to ask their HCP about appropriate weight gain based on curiosity or a prior health issue (e.g., diabetes), but that their HCP did not often offer this information spontaneously. Women also reported that they assumed that "no news was good news" if the doctor or midwife did not discuss weight. One participant reported, "So I sort of think, in general, unless you have a specific question, it doesn't tend to come up in conversation." Some participants did not ask their clinicians about weight gain because they thought their obstetrician or midwife would discuss weight gain with them if it was an issue. Several participants reported that discussing weight gain guidelines in the beginning of the first trimester would have been helpful.

HCP-initiated Participants reported that HCP-initiated conversations typically stemmed from the patient being overweight or having health issues. One woman said, "Yeah, it [goal weight] came up pretty immediately. Because I was overweight when I got pregnant...other than that, it hasn't been a drastic weight gain, so no one's been talking about it." Some participants shared that their HCP gave the weight recommendation during an early appointment. Throughout their appointments, several participants would say that the HCP would say that they're "on track." Several participants commented that if they heard their HCP advise them about their weight gain, then it would be an "impetus for actually changing something."

HCP advice Several women expressed that their provider has given recommendations about nutrition, physical activity, and/or weight gain, but the HCP did not explain why it was an issue or how to make the change. One participant stated, "[the doctor] never told me what I should be eating– just to make sure that I was eating enough. But I don't know what 'enough' is." Another woman stated, "too much weight gain doesn't mean anything to me. If there were vital signs...that were showing that my body was having a hard time [then my provider should explain]."

Participants gave examples of HCP advice they liked: "We want to see the baby grow, we don't want to see you grow" and "feed yourself–think about it as if the baby's sitting in front of you...it's sort of stuck in my head (laughs). So now when I eat a 4th Girl Scout cookie, I think, would I really shove that in a kid's face? Probably not." Some women reported that they did not like the way the provider gave weight-related advice: "the WIC lady that I see has said I'm like above the norm...who says that to a woman? It's not helpful, especially because I'm pregnant."

Referral to nutritionists Most women reported that they would be open to meet with a nutritionist, especially if excessive GWG was an issue. Some participants stated that would prefer a nutritionist to talk about diet because they "studied" this area. Some women who had visited a nutritionist said that the information, ideas, and recipes were helpful. A few participants did not think the nutritionist's visit was helpful because the person just handed out pamphlets or had an unpleasant demeanor. One person mentioned that her WIC nutritionist was "just not therapeutic...she just says her opinion and then moves on [and] doesn't really have a discussion or anything."

Tools and resources for GWG management

Information sources

The main information sources for participants about GWG were HCP, family, friends, pregnancy websites, books, and magazines. Most participants reported that the HCP's recommendations were the most trusted source. Participants reported that family would either say to "eat what they want" or "not to gain too much weight." For instance, one woman stated, "my mom also told me [when I first got pregnant], 'don't get fat. There's no need to get fat'" and another participant shared that her mother had said, "So-and-so gained hardly any weight. She's really skinny. And all her kids are fine. I'm like, 'Mom. Not helpful'." Participants reported that their friends would typically be encouraging about their appearance and would give them helpful advice about their pregnancy, like "try to lose a little weight before pregnancy" or "I had gestational diabetes, so be careful." Several participants reported reading pregnancy websites, apps, and weekly emails. Women trusted pregnancy-related websites from national medical organizations, but most did not trust comment sections on such websites or Facebook.

Potential interventions

Most participants said that they would be willing to attend information sessions to learn more about GWG if accessible and available at different times of the day. Some participants reported preferring group nutrition/cooking and exercise classes (e.g., walking in the park; yoga). Other participants indicated they would prefer more personalized attention. Several participants reported that they would be amendable to a health coach emailing and texting them, but felt that women with high-risk pregnancies would be better candidates for real-time conversations. Most participants reported receiving packets and would prefer to have a discussion with their HCP about the information because "I don't think handing people packets [handouts] is educating them at all," and reported that discussing weight gain guidelines in the beginning of the first trimester would be helpful, including that pregnant women only need an additional 300 calories a day. Some participants with BMI >25 kg/m^2 stated that a handout with specific daily meal plans for pregnant women for breakfast, lunch, and dinner "would be perfect."

GWG Chart

During the interviews and focus groups, we shared with the participants a chart that gives a visual display of GWG progression aligned with the IOM recommendation. Nearly all participants said that it was "useful" and "helpful." Some people said the graph would be a good discussion starter and motivate them to modify their food intake and exercise; whereas, a few people said that they would not "pay too much attention to it," they would not "want to know the number," and they would "not want another piece of paper." A few women requested that the GWG chart be available on the patient online system.

Discussion

Using the McLeroy et al.'s ecological model [18], we elucidated the nuances associated with GWG and goal-setting for weight gain. Our qualitative analyses of semi-structured interviews and focus groups in pregnant women showed that factors that might influence GWG include mother's beliefs concerning diet and exercise and experience during prior pregnancies (individual), conversations with HCPs (interpersonal), interest in clinics utilizing GWG charts (organizational), and influence of information sources (community). Women focused on behaviors that messages were consistent across multiple sources of information, but mainly trusted their HCP. Women highly valued one-to-one conversations with their HCP about GWG, especially if they have weight issues prior or during pregnancy.

Implications for Practice and/or Policy

Indeed, one of the major points that we highlighted in our observations is that pregnant women rank highly clinician advice concerning GWG. Many points throughout the interviews and focus groups supported this conclusion. First, women considered clinicians the most reliable source of information and verified with their provider information found from other sources. This is in line with qualitative studies where women also reported that clinicians were the most credible source of information [20, 21], and a quantitative study that found that discordant clinician advice was directly associated with excessive GWG [22]. In addition, clinician input seems to also be an important adjunct to the use of educational tools about GWG. Women in our study reported having received many handouts, but felt that was not sufficient per se and that their providers need to discuss the content with them if the specific matter is an important health issue for the pregnancy. Similarly, pregnant women from a large academic medical center in Wisconsin also reported receiving handouts for nutritional education during pregnancy but underlined the fact that the material was rarely reviewed during the medical encounter [23]. In our study, when we presented a graphic tool to chart GWG during pregnancy, women stated that the tool would be useful if accompanied by a discussion with their provider, highlighting once again the importance of clinician's input about GWG in women's opinion.

We and others have shown that women whose provider recommended weight gains consistent with IOM recommendations were more likely to have a concordant GWG goal compared to women whose providers recommended gains inconsistent with recommendations or no clear GWG recommendations [17, 24]. Previous interviews found that most clinicians reported discussing appropriate GWG with their patients at the beginning of pregnancy [25]. Many women reported receiving a GWG goal, but this was not consistent across all participants; unfortunately, many overweight women reported not receiving a specific GWG goal. Similarly, Stengel et al. reported that nine out the 24 overweight/obese women they interviewed were not given a goal, and many were given vague goals or goals outside the IOM recommendations [21].

In the current analysis, women stated that they would like their providers to open the conversation and give them a goal for GWG early in pregnancy. In our previous qualitative study among obstetric providers, clinicians reported that they felt that weight is a sensitive issue for women and often wait for women to ask questions – or only bring up weight gain as a topic if GWG reaches out of the expected range [25]. This HCP behavior seems to be fairly common in obstetric providers since the theme also emerged from a systematic review in the UK [26] and in other US practitioners' qualitative studies on GWG [27, 28]. Women in our study and in other reports [23, 29] felt that GWG should be addressed up front by their provider if this is important and not wait for women to bring up the topic of weight gain to the providers, an approach sometimes called 'reactive' counseling [23, 28]. It is striking that both parties feel like the other one should open the conversation: clinicians believe that weight is sensitive and usually wait until women raised the issue or when GWG was concerning, and women felt as though their provider should and would raise that discussion if that is something that is important for their health.

Providers' confidence level in their own counseling skills is associated with higher adherence to guidelines for prenatal clinical care of obese pregnant women [30]. Consequently, the clinicians' difficulty in opening the discussion might also derive from the fact that providers do not feel adequately prepared and feel uncertain about the impact of their counseling effort, as we and others reported based on interviews with obstetric providers [25, 27, 28, 31]. This situation is not unique to clinicians in obstetric care, since a few studies have reported that physicians often feel ill-prepared and lack confidence to provide adequate lifestyle counseling, particularly in the fields of physical activity, nutrition, and weight management [32, 33]. Multidisciplinary approaches and referral to appropriate health professionals are likely part of adequate weight management in obese women during pregnancy, but providers need to have confidence in their knowledge and skills about lifestyle counseling to open the discussions.

Strengths and limitations

Strengths of our study include the use of standardized moderator guides, recording of the group discussions and interviews, and analyzing the transcripts using established qualitative methods. Our study also has limitations. We interviewed women of diverse race/ethnicity in the greater Boston, MA area, and most had college or graduate degrees, so results may not be generalizable to pregnant women living elsewhere or with lower education. In order to build upon this study, future studies will include a quantitative survey on a larger population. GWG goals are based on self-report and may have been over or underreported. Women who participated in the study are likely interested in weight related issues and so our results might overestimate the frequency of GWG goal-setting.

Conclusion

Pregnant women highly value advice and the information about GWG provided by their HCP. Women hope to receive goals for appropriate GWG early in pregnancy from their primary HCP. To achieve the set GWG goals, women focused on behaviors that were consistently promoted from different sources of information, but mainly if the information was provided or confirmed by their HCP. Women believed that HCPs should proactively address GWG and related behaviors along the course of pregnancy – not just in a 'reactive' fashion. Based on our study and other studies [20–22, 29], it seems important to find ways to facilitate early conversations about GWG between pregnant women and HCP in clinical settings.

Abbreviations

BMI: Body mass index; GWG: Gestational weight gain; HCP: Health care provider; IOM: Institute of Medicine.

Acknowledgments

Thank you to the study team and study participants.

Funding

This project was supported by the Centers for Disease Control and Prevention (200-2010-M-33818), the National Institutes of Health (, K24 HD069408, P30 DK092924), and by a Faculty Grant (Department of Population Medicine) from the Harvard Pilgrim Health Care Institute. Funding support for S. Criss was also provided by training grants from the Harvard T.H. Chan School of Public Health and the Dana-Farber Cancer Institute NIH Award # 3R25CA057711, the Initiative to Maximize Student Diversity Award # GM055353-13, and Maternal and Child Health Bureau Award #T03MC07648. Its contents are solely the responsibility of the authors and do not necessarily represent the official views of the listed funding sources. The funding bodies did not participate in the design of the study; collection, analysis, and interpretation of data; or in writing the manuscript.

Authors' contributions

EO and MH designed of the study; all authors participated in collection, analysis, and interpretation of data; and SC, LG, and MH participated in writing the manuscript. All authors read and approved the final manuscript.

Competing interests

The authors declare that they have no competing interest.

Consent for publication

Not applicable.

Author details

[1]Department of Health Sciences, Furman University, 3300 Poinsett Hwy, Greenville, SC 29613, USA. [2]Obesity Prevention Program, Department of Population Medicine, Harvard Medical School and Harvard Pilgrim Health Care Institute, 401 Park Drive Suite 401E, Boston, MA, USA02215.

References

1. Nehring I, Schmoll S, Beyerlein A, Hauner H, Von Kries R. Gestational weight gain and long-term postpartum weight retention: a meta-analysis. Am J Clin Nutr. 2011;94:1225–31.
2. Oken E, Kleinman KP, Belfort MB, Hammitt JK, Gillman MW. Associations of gestational weight gain with short-and longer-term maternal and child health outcomes. Am J Epidemiol. 2009;170:173–80.
3. Walter JR, Perng W, Kleinman KP, Rifas-Shiman SL, Rich-Edwards JW, Oken E. Associations of trimester-specific gestational weight gain with maternal adiposity and systolic blood pressure at 3 and 7 years postpartum. Am J Obstet Gynecol. 2015;212:499. e1–499. e12.
4. Al Mamun A, Mannan M, O'callaghan MJ, Williams GM, Najman JM, Callaway LK. Association between gestational weight gain and postpartum diabetes: evidence from a community based large cohort study. PLoS ONE. 2013;8:e75679. doi:10.1371/journal.pone.0075679.
5. Fraser A, Tilling K, Macdonald-Wallis C, Hughes R, Sattar N, Nelson SM, Lawlor DA. Associations of gestational weight gain with maternal body mass index, waist circumference, and blood pressure measured 16 y after pregnancy: the Avon Longitudinal Study of Parents and Children (ALSPAC). Am J Clin Nutr. 2011;93:1285–92.
6. Fraser A, Tilling K, Macdonald-Wallis C, Sattar N, Brion M-J, Benfield L, Ness A, Deanfield J, Hingorani A, Nelson SM. Association of maternal weight gain in pregnancy with offspring obesity and metabolic and vascular traits in childhood. Circulation. 2010;121:2557–64.
7. Hivert MF, Rifas-Shiman SL, Gillman MW, Oken E. Greater early and mid-pregnancy gestational weight gains are associated with excess adiposity in mid-childhood. Obesity. 2016;24(7):1546–53.
8. Hochner H, Friedlander Y, Calderon-Margalit R, Meiner V, Sagy Y, Avgil-Tsadok M, Burger A, Savitsky B, Siscovick DS, Manor O. Associations of maternal prepregnancy body mass index and gestational weight gain with adult offspring cardiometabolic risk factors the Jerusalem Perinatal Family Follow-up Study. Circulation. 2012;125:1381–9.
9. Karachaliou M, Georgiou V, Roumeliotaki T, Chalkiadaki G, Daraki V, Koinaki S, Dermitzaki E, Sarri K, Vassilaki M, Kogevinas M. Association of trimester-specific gestational weight gain with fetal growth, offspring obesity, and cardiometabolic traits in early childhood. Am J Obstet Gynecol. 2015;212:502. e1–502. e14.
10. Oken E, Rifas-Shiman SL, Field AE, Frazier AL, Gillman MW. Maternal gestational weight gain and offspring weight in adolescence. Obstet Gynecol. 2008;112:999.
11. Oken E, Taveras EM, Kleinman KP, Rich-Edwards JW, Gillman MW. Gestational weight gain and child adiposity at age 3 years. Am J Obstet Gynecol. 2007;196:322. e1–8.
12. Parker M, Rifas-Shiman SL, Oken E, Belfort MB, Jaddoe VW, Gillman MW. Second trimester estimated fetal weight and fetal weight gain predict childhood obesity. J Pediatr. 2012;161:864–870. e1.
13. Durie DE, Thornburg LL, Glantz JC. Effect of second-trimester and third-trimester rate of gestational weight gain on maternal and neonatal outcomes. Obstet Gynecol. 2011;118:569–75.
14. Ferrari RM, Siega-Riz AM. Provider advice about pregnancy weight gain and adequacy of weight gain. Matern Child Health J. 2013;17:256–64.
15. Park S, Sappenfield WM, Bish C, Salihu H, Goodman D, Bensyl DM. Assessment of the Institute of Medicine recommendations for weight gain during pregnancy: Florida, 2004–2007. Matern Child Health J. 2011;15:289–301.
16. Cogswell ME, Scanlon KS, Fein SB, Schieve LA. Medically advised, mother's personal target, and actual weight gain during pregnancy. Obstet Gynecol. 1999;94:616–22.
17. Tovar A, Guthrie LB, Platek D, Stuebe A, Herring SJ, Oken E. Modifiable predictors associated with having a gestational weight gain goal. Matern Child Health J. 2011;15:1119–26.

18. Mcleroy KR, Bibeau D, Steckler A, Glanz K. An ecological perspective on health promotion programs. Health Educ Behav. 1988;15:351–77.
19. Green J, Willis K, Hughes E, Small R, Welch N, Gibbs L, Daly J. Generating best evidence from qualitative research: the role of data analysis. Aust N Z J Public Health. 2007;31:545–50.
20. Criss S, Woo Baidal JA, Goldman RE, Perkins M, Cunningham C, Taveras EM. The Role of Health Information Sources in Decision-Making Among Hispanic Mothers During Their Children's First 1000 Days of Life. Matern Child Health J. 2015;19:2536–43.
21. Stengel MR, Kraschnewski JL, Hwang SW, Kjerulff KH, Chuang CH. "What my doctor didn't tell me": examining health care provider advice to overweight and obese pregnant women on gestational weight gain and physical activity. Women's Health Issues. 2012;22:e535–40.
22. Herring SJ, Nelson DB, Davey A, Klotz AA, Oken E, Foster GD. Determinants of excessive gestational weight gain in urban, low-income women. Women's Health Issues. 2012;22:e439–46.
23. Duthie EA, Drew EM, Flynn KE. Patient-provider communication about gestational weight gain among nulliparous women: a qualitative study of the views of obstetricians and first-time pregnant women. BMC Pregnancy Childbirth. 2013;13:231.
24. Stotland NE, Haas JS, Brawarsky P, Jackson RA, Fuentes-Afflick E, Escobar GJ. Body mass index, provider advice, and target gestational weight gain. Obstet Gynecol. 2005;105:633–8.
25. Oken E, Switkowski K, Price S, Guthrie L, Taveras EM, Gillman M, Friedes J, Callaghan W, Dietz P. A qualitative study of gestational weight gain counseling and tracking. Matern Child Health J. 2013;17:1508–17.
26. Campbell F, Johnson M, Messina J, Guillaume L, Goyder E. Behavioural interventions for weight management in pregnancy: a systematic review of quantitative and qualitative data. BMC Public Health. 2011;11:491.
27. Chang T, Llanes M, Gold KJ, Fetters MD. Perspectives about and approaches to weight gain in pregnancy: a qualitative study of physicians and nurse midwives. BMC Pregnancy Childbirth. 2013;13:47.
28. Stotland NE, Gilbert P, Bogetz A, Harper CC, Abrams B, Gerbert B. Preventing excessive weight gain in pregnancy: how do prenatal care providers approach counseling? J Women's Health. 2010;19:807–14.
29. Mills A, Schmied VA, Dahlen HG. 'Get alongside us', women's experiences of being overweight and pregnant in Sydney, Australia. Matern Child Nutr. 2013;9:309–21.
30. Herring SJ, Platek DN, Elliott P, Riley LE, Stuebe AM, Oken E. Addressing obesity in pregnancy: what do obstetric providers recommend? J Women's Health. 2010;19:65–70.
31. Stewart ZA, Wallace E, Allan C. Weight gain in pregnancy: a survey of current practices in a teaching hospital. Aust N Z J Obstet Gynaecol. 2012;52:208–10.
32. O'loughlin J, Makni H, Tremblay M, Lacroix C, Gervais A, Déry V, Meshefedjian G, Paradis G. Smoking cessation counseling practices of general practitioners in Montreal. Prev Med. 2001;33:627–38.
33. Rogers LQ, Gutin B, Humphries MC, Lemmon CR, Waller JL, Baranowski T, Saunders R. Evaluation of internal medicine residents as exercise role models and associations with self-reported counseling behavior, confidence, and perceived success. Teach Learn Med. 2006;18:215–21.

14

Maternal nutrition, inadequate gestational weight gain and birth weight: results from a prospective birth cohort

Anke Diemert[1*], Susanne Lezius[2], Mirja Pagenkemper[1], Gudula Hansen[1], Alina Drozdowska[1], Kurt Hecher[1], Petra Arck[1†] and Birgit C. Zyriax[3†]

Abstract

Background: The aim of our study was to examine maternal weight gain as well as nutrient intake in pregnancy throughout each trimester compared to current recommendations in a low-risk population and its correlation to birth weight. Additionally, we have investigated the association of maternal nutrition with gestational weight gain and birth weight in an economically unrestricted population.

Methods: Our analysis was carried out in a population-based prospective birth cohort in Hamburg, Germany. 200 pregnant women and 197 infants born at term were included in the analysis. Maternal body weight, weight gain throughout gestation, and birth weight, macro- and micronutrients were assessed based on a 24 h dietary recall in each trimester. Our main outcome measures were weight gain, birth weight, and self-reported dietary intake in each trimester in comparison to current recommendations.

Results: One third of the women were characterized by an elevated pre-pregnancy BMI, 60 % did not comply with current weight gain recommendations. Particularly overweight and obese women gained more weight than recommended. In a multivariate analysis birth weight correlated significantly with maternal BMI ($p = 0.020$), total weight gain ($p = 0.020$) and gestational week ($p < 0.001$). Compared to guidelines mean percentage of energy derived from fat ($p = 0.002$) and protein ($p < 0.001$) was significantly higher, whereas carbohydrate ($p = 0.033$) intake was lower. Mean fiber intake was significantly lower ($p < 0.001$). Saturated fat and sugar contributed largely to energy consumption. Gestational weight gain correlated significantly with energy ($p = 0.027$), carbohydrates ($p = 0.008$), monosaccharides and saccharose ($p = 0.006$) intake. 98 % of the pregnant women were below the iodine recommendation, while none of the women reached the required folate, vitamin D, and iron intake.

Conclusions: During gestation appropriate individual advice as to nutrient intake and weight gain seems to be of high priority. Pregnancy should be used as a 'window of opportunity' for behavioral changes.

Keywords: Pregnancy, Gestational weight gain, Birth cohort, Diet, Nutrient intake, Overweight, Obesity

Background

An increased body-mass-index (BMI) at the beginning of pregnancy and inadequate gestational weight gain (GWG) represent a substantial health burden for mother and child. Normal weight for women at childbearing age should be strived for. However, the global obesity epidemic has resulted in an increasing number of overweight and obese women entering pregnancy. Data from cross-sectional studies indicate that at present about 20 % of the German women aged 20–39 are overweight, another 9–14 % are obese and up to 18 % are affected by central obesity [1, 2]. In addition a substantial proportion of pregnant women seems to be characterized by an inadequate GWG according to the recommendations of the US Institute of Medicine (IOM) [3, 4]. Both extremes, excessive or inadequate GWG can lead to adverse pregnancy outcomes. Maternal complications

* Correspondence: a.diemert@uke.de
†Equal contributors
[1]Department of Obstetrics and Fetal Medicine, University Medical Center Hamburg-Eppendorf, Martinistrasse 52, Hamburg 20246, Germany
Full list of author information is available at the end of the article

arising from excessive GWG include an increased rate of caesarean section, hypertensive disorders, diabetes, weight retention and abdominal adiposity. The latter conditions determine a women's lifetime risk for cardiovascular disease [5–11]. Fetal risks includes stillbirth, miscarriage, malformation, macrosomia, as well as an increased risk of premature death and transgenerational obesity [12–17].

Adherence to a balanced diet throughout pregnancy, influences maternal body weight as well as short- and long-term health of mother and child [18–20]. Data of the 'German National Nutrition Survey II' indicate, that average nutrient intake in women of childbearing age is at least in parts inadequate [21]. During gestation the need for certain micronutrients increases more than energy requirement [22]. Thus, deficiencies in micronutrients may occur frequently, leading to adverse outcomes for mother and child. However, information as to dietary intake throughout gestation is limited [23, 24]. Most birth cohorts did not evaluate maternal dietary habits. Nutritional data for pregnant women derive mainly from cross-sectional studies where pregnant women represent a minority. Furthermore, in previous studies nutrient intake was measured only once during pregnancy. Considering the fact that pregnancy constitutes a unique opportunity to change dietary behavior in order to preserve maternal and fetal health more research on this topic is warranted.

The aim of this paper was therefore to evaluate maternal weight gain and nutrient intake throughout pregnancy in an economically unrestricted prospective birth cohort comprising mostly normal pregnancies and to compare the nutrient intake to current guidelines and birth weight. Additionally, we have investigated the association of maternal nutrition with gestational weight gain and birth weight.

Methods

Design and Recruitment

From 2011–2013 200 healthy low risk women aged 18 years and older with singleton spontaneously conceived pregnancies presented at the University medical Centre Hamburg-Eppendorf to participate in this study between gestational age 12 + 0 to 14 + 6 weeks. Exclusion criteria were risk factors according to menstrual- (such as unknown last menstrual period), obstetrical- (such as history of IUGR or preeclampsia) and medical history (other diseases), drug usage (such as alcohol or tobacco) or chronic medication.

At 3 time points (once per trimester (gestational week 12 + 0 to 14 + 6, 22 + 0 to 24 + 6 and 34 + 0 to 36 + 6) participants presented for a detailed fetal ultrasound examination, psychometric and lifestyle questionnaires (24 hours-recall) and maternal blood draw. Additionally a morphology scan was performed at gestational week 20–24 and birth weight and pregnancy outcome was collected. Sociodemographic data such as familial status and education were also reported to ensure no constraints regarding dietary options.

Data collection

Assessment of anthropometric data

The maternal height and weight - light clothing, but no shoes allowed - were measured to the nearest 0.5 cm or 0.1 kg respectively, and taken with the same instruments (scale and yardstick) that were calibrated in regular intervals for the whole population at each visit. The body mass index (BMI) was calculated as BMI = weight (kg)/height $(m)^2$.

Pregnancy weight gain was compared with current S3 guideline on gestational diabetes derivated from the recommendation of the US Institute of Medicine (IOM), depending on BMI classes: 12.5–18 kg for underweight women, 11.5–16 kg for normal weight women, 7–11.5 kg for overweight women and 5–9 kg for obese women [25, 26].

Nutritional counseling and assessment of nutrition

Pregnant women included in our study were counseled on guideline recommended nutrition during pregnancy by physicians certified for nutritional medicine. Information about nutrition was obtained by using a 24 h dietary recall in each trimester based on the nutritional software EBISpro System based on the national food composition table (BLS 3.01). Recommendations for dietary intake of energy, macro- and micronutrients during pregnancy were based on the D-A-CH reference value of the German, Swiss and Austrian society for nutrition [22].

Data analysis/Statistical methods

Continuous variables are presented as means (± standard deviations). Categorical variables are presented as absolute numbers and rates. Mean nutrition values are derived by patient-individual averaging.

Comparisons to guidelines or recommendations are performed using the one-sample *t*-test.

Time trends were determined with random effects models allowing for autoregression with a random intercept for the individual patients and adjusted for education level und maternal age. Associations with maternal weight gain and birth weight were analyzed using ANOVA models adjusted for maternal age, maternal BMI at the beginning of pregnancy, education level and in case of birth weight additionally for gestational week. Further adjustments are stated separately.

Not normally distributed parameters were log transformed where necessary. All analyses were two-sided with α = 0.05. No alpha adjustment for multiple testing was applied.

All calculations are performed using SPSS Version 21 (SPSS Inc., Cary, NC, USA).

Results

Baseline characteristics

Baseline characteristics of the study population are listed in Table 1. All women were married or living in a stable relationship. The study population consisted of 191 Caucasian, seven Asian, one African and one Latin American women. 78 % of the participants had a high educational level and two-thirds a normal weight at the beginning of pregnancy. One third were overweight (defined as BMI > =25 but lower than 30) or obese (defined as BMI > =30). 57 % of study subjects were primipara.

Table 1 Baseline characteristics of the PRINCE birth cohort. Depicted is either the mean value or the percentage value. Values are given as mean ± 1 standard deviation (SD) or as absolute and relative frequencies ([a]n = 197, [b]n = 196)

Characteristics	Total n = 200
Clinical characteristics	
Maternal age (years)	31.0 (±3.5)
Height (cm)	168 (±6)[a]
Weight	
Weight at the beginning of pregnancy (kg)	69.9 (±13.9)[a]
BMI (kg/m^2)	24.7 (4.6)[a]
BMI <18,5 (kg/m^2)	4 % (n = 8)
BMI 18,5 - <25 (kg/m^2)	63 % (n = 124)
BMI 25 - <30 (kg/m^2)	21 % (n = 41)
BMI ≥30 (kg/m^2)	12 % (n = 24)
Parity	
First pregnancy	57 % (n = 114)
Former pregnancy	43 % (n = 86)
1 living child	49 % (n = 41)
≥2 living children	13 % (n = 11)
Delivery	
Gestational age at delivery (weeks)	40.0 (±1.5)[a]
Fetal weight at delivery (g)	3457 (±497)[b]
<3rd percentile	2 % (n = 3)
>97th percentile	2 % (n = 4)
Life birth	197 (98 %)
Pregnancy discontinued (termination, miscarriage)	3 (2 %)
Lifestyle characteristics	
Education level [b]	
No high school diploma	22 % (n = 44)
High school or vocational diploma	34 % (n = 66)
College or higher education	44 % (n = 86)
Smoking habits	
Current non-smokers	100 %
Alcohol use	
Alcohol abstinence	100 %

Energy and macronutrient intake

During gestation the average daily energy intake in our study population increased from 1987 kcal (±505) in the first trimester to 2068 kcal (±463) in the second and 2151 kcal (±472) in the last trimester ($p = 0.001$ for increase between first and 3rd trimester). Protein intake increased significantly from 76 g (±24) in the first trimester to 80 g (±21) in the second ($p = 0.037$) and 82 g (±23) in the third trimester ($p = 0.003$ for increase between first and 3rd trimester). Major sources for protein were animal products (data not shown). With regard to the fat consumption daily intake increased significantly from 77 g (±29) to 82 g (±27) and 86 g (±28) over the trimesters ($p = 0.003$ for increase between first and 3rd trimester). Saturated fatty acids (SAFA) contributed mainly to mean total fat consumption (SAFA = 36 g ±10 of total fat 81 g ± 19), whereas the intake of monounsaturated fatty acids (26 g ± 7) and polyunsaturated fatty acids (13 g ±4) was much lower. Mean intake of docosahexaenoic acid (DHA), derivated from marine sources was 221 mg (±243). Throughout gestation carbohydrate intake raised from 239 g (±65) in the first trimester to 245 g (±66) in the 2nd trimester to 254 g (±66) in the last trimester non-significantly ($p = 0.152$). Monosaccharide and saccharose contributed largely to the carbohydrate consumption (43 %), while mean fiber intake was low (24 g ±6). When additionally adjusted for total energy no significant changes in macronutrient intake throughout pregnancy were observed.

If macronutrient intake was calculated in percentage of energy intake this was 16 % from protein, 36 % from fat, and 49 % from carbohydrates. In comparison to current recommendations the overall mean protein and fat intake of the participants was significantly higher than recommended (protein 16 vs. 15 %, $p < 0.001$ and fat 36 vs. 35 %, $p = 0.002$). In addition, the percentage of saturated fat intake with regard to total fat consumption was much higher than recommended (45 % vs. 10 %, $p < 0.001$), whereas mean carbohydrate intake was significantly lower than recommended (49 vs. 50 %, $p = 0.033$) (DACH Referenzwerte, 2015).

When categories instead of mean values were taken into account 38 % of the pregnant women reported a protein intake below the recommended 15 % of energy intake. Within the study population 58 % of the pregnant women reported a fat intake above the upper threshold of 35 % of energy predominately characterized by a high consumption of saturated fat, while 62 % of the women did not fulfill the criteria of a sufficient intake of docosahexaenoic acid. As to carbohydrate intake 56 % of the women were below the recommendation of 50 % of energy. The percentage of women consuming less than 30 g fiber per day was 84 %. In each trimester mean dietary intake of protein, fat, carbohydrates and fiber differed significantly from the recommendation with the exception of fat and carbohydrate intake during the first trimenon.

Micronutrient intake

Mean intake of vitamins and minerals from food increased slightly between the first and the last trimester (Table 2). However, most changes were not significant, particularly when additionally adjusted for energy intake (data not shown). In each trimester mean dietary intake of certain micronutrients differ significantly from the recommendation (Table 2).

Vitamins

Compared to current recommendations mean dietary intake of vitamin A, E, B_1, B_2, and B_{12} seems to be adequate (Table 2) [22]. However, on the average a considerable amount of the women did not reach the recommendation on vitamin A (37 %), vitamin E (55 %), vitamin B_1 (48 %), vitamin B_2 (28 %) and vitamin B_{12} (73 %) intake (Fig. 1). In addition 23 % of the pregnant women did not reach the recommended intake of vitamin C, while 67 % reported an insufficient intake of vitamin B_6 (Fig. 1). With regard to folate and vitamin D mean daily intake from food was much lower than recommended (folate 288 μg (±126) vs 550 μg, $p < 0.001$; vitamin D 2.6 μg (±3.6) vs 20 μg, $p < 0.001$) (Table 2). (DACH Referenzwerte, 2015). None of the pregnant women fulfilled on average the recommendation as to folate or vitamin D intake (Fig. 1).

Minerals

An iron requirement of 30 mg throughout pregnancy is recommended, whereas mean daily iron intake in the study population was only 12 mg (±2 $p < 0.001$) (Table 2) (DACH Referenzwerte, 2015). Thus, in 100 % of the pregnant women iron supply in each trimester was inadequate (Fig. 1). For iodine the mean daily intake was 123 μg (±48) which is significantly less than the recommendation of 230 μg ($p < 0.001$) (Table 2) (DACH Referenzwerte, 2015). On the average 98 % of the women were below the recommended threshold (Fig. 1).

Mean daily intake of calcium, magnesium and zinc seems to be adequate in comparison to the recommendation (calcium 1179 mg (±324) vs 1000 mg; magnesium 378 mg (±76) vs 310 mg, zinc 11 mg (±2) vs 10 mg). However, as to calcium, 32 % of the pregnant women ingested less than recommended, while 18 % of the women were below the recommendation of magnesium and 26 % below the recommended zinc intake (Fig. 1).

Besides the intake of micronutrients from food, 96 % ($n = 192$) of the women reported to use supplements. However, evaluation of the obtained data is difficult as various products were reported and most supplements were not used continuously (data not published).

Table 2 Intake of micronutrients during pregnancy compared with current recommendations (DACH Referenzwerte, 2015) [22]. Values are given as mean ± 1 standard deviation (SD)

Critical-micronutrients	1. trimenon	2. trimenon	3. trimenon	mean intake	recommendation	*p*-value
Iron (mg)	12 ± 4	13 ± 3	12 ± 3	12 ± 2	30	<0.001
Iodine (μg)	115 ± 62	130 ± 86	123 ± 67	123 ± 48	230	<0.001
Vit D (μg)	2.5 ± 3.7	2.4 ± 2.3	2.8 ± 4.4	2.6 ± 2.1	20	<0.001
Folat (μg)	273 ± 124	291 ± 119	296 ± 133	287 ± 81	550	<0.001
-Other-micronutrients						
Vit A (mg)	1.4 ± 1.7	1.7 ± 1.5	1.5 ± 1.4	1.5 ± 0.9	1.1	<0.001
Vit E (mg)	13 ± 7	14 ± 7	14 ± 8	13.5 ± 5.0	13	n.s.
Vit B1 (mg)	1.3 ± 0.5	1.4 ± 0.6	1.4 ± 0.6	1.3 ± 0.4	1.3	n.s.
Vit B2 (mg)	1.5 ± 0.7	1.7 ± 0.6	1.8 ± 0.7	1.7 ± 0.4	1.4	<0.001
Vit B6 (mg)	1.7 ± 0.7	1.8 ± 0.7	1.9 ± 0.8	1.8 ± 0.5	1.9	0.002
Vit B12 (μg)	4.7 ± 4.7	4.6 ± 2.3	4.9 ± 2.7	4.7 ± 2.2	3.5	<0.001
Vit C (mg)	146 ± 90	158 ± 94	166 ± 105	158 ± 67	105	<0.001
Calcium (mg)	1133 ± 487	1193 ± 457	1227 ± 502	1179 ± 324	1000	<0.001
Magnesium (mg)	359 ± 103	388 ± 99	386 ± 106	378 ± 76	310	<0.001
Zinc (mg)	11 ± 4	12 ± 3	11 ± 3	11 ± 2	10	<0.001

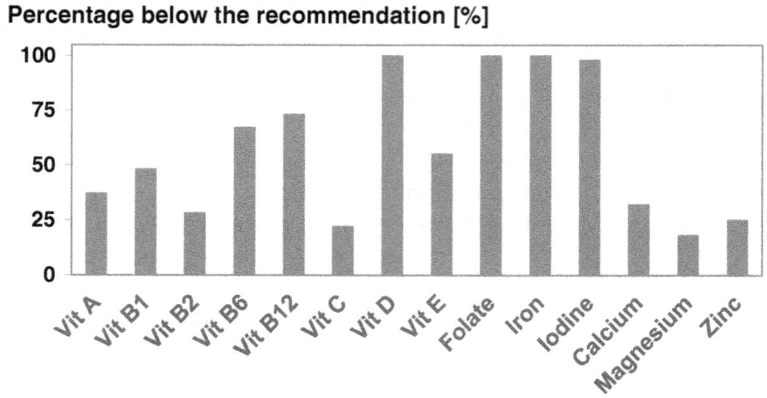

Fig. 1 Percentage of women below the recommended dietary intake of vitamins and minerals (DACH Referenzwerte, 2015) [22]

Maternal BMI and gestational weight gain

Mean maternal BMI at the beginning of pregnancy was 24.7 (±4.6), with 63 % of the women being normal weight, 4 % being underweight, 21 % overweight and 12 % obese at this time. In the second trimester maternal weight reached a BMI of 26.7 (±4.6), while in the third trimester mean BMI was 28.5 (±4.5).

Mean maternal weight gain in our study cohort was 11.2 kg (±3.9). Compared to current guidelines only 40 % of our pregnant women gained weight during gestation appropriately, 22 % more than recommended and 38 % less than recommended. Particularly underweight and overweight women did not follow gestational weight gain recommendations. In a multivariate model no association could be determined between GWG and maternal age, education, parity or fetal sex, whereas pre-pregnancy BMI ($p = 0.003$) was a significant predictor for the amount of weight gained during pregnancy

Within each BMI categories significant deviations from the recommendation were observed. According to maternal BMI at the beginning of pregnancy 86 % of the underweight women gained less weight than suggested, whereas only 14 % gained within the recommended range (Fig. 2). Of the normal weight participants every second woman (52 %) gained less than recommended, 38 % appropriate and only a small minority (10 %) above the recommendation. The opposite distribution was noted in the overweight population: every second woman (50 %) gained weight above the recommendation, 47 % according to the recommendation, whereas in 3 % gestational weight gain was insufficient. In obese women 50 % gained above and 50 % according to the recommendation.

In separate analyses total gestational weight gain correlated significantly with energy intake ($p = 0.036$). Per each 100 cal increment maternal weight increased by 195 g (95 % CI 13–378). A positive association was also found, when carbohydrate intake or consumption of monosaccharide and saccharose was taken into account. An increase of 1 g carbohydrate was related to an increment of 17 g in weight during pregnancy (95 % CI 5–29;

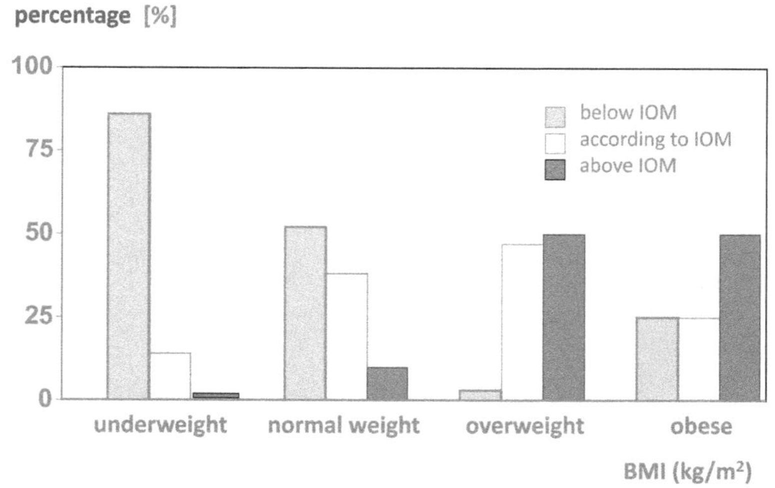

Fig. 2 Gestational weight gain according to the recommendation of the Institute of Medicine (IOM) (Institute of Medicine, 2009) [4]

$p = 0.008$), while 1 g sugar was associated with an increase of 26 g weight (95 % CI 8–44; $p = 0.005$). After further adjustment for energy intake, the correlation between sugar consumption and gestational weight gain remained significant ($p = 0.049$) whereas the association between carbohydrates and weight gain lost significance ($p = 0.097$). After adjustment for energy intake other macronutrients or fiber intake were not associated with gestational weight gain.

Birth weight

Two women terminated the pregnancy due to fetal malformations and one aborted spontaneously. Of the 197 births (birth weight was available in $n = 196$ cases), mean birth weight was 3457 g (±497), 24 (12 %) of the children were characterized by a birth weight > 4000 g. Newborn's weight was lower in normal weight mothers compared to overweight, obese and underweight mothers. In a multivariate analysis birth weight correlated significantly with maternal BMI at the beginning of pregnancy ($p = 0.020$), total weight gain ($p = 0.020$) and gestational week ($p < 0.001$) For each unit increment in pre-pregnancy BMI birth weight increased by 17 g (95 % CI 3–32), whereas each kilogram weight gained during pregnancy leads to an increase in birth weight by 20 g (95 % CI 3–36). An increase in birth weight by 138 g was observed per gestational week (95 % CI 89–187). All the other nutrients tested in this analysis were not associated significantly with birth weight.

Discussion

Main Findings

The aim of this analysis was to evaluate maternal weight gain as well as nutrient intake throughout each trimester of pregnancy compared to international recommendations and birth weight in a low risk population. Currently information as to weight development and dietary habits in pregnant women is limited.

A principal finding of our prospective birth cohort is that approximately two third of pregnant women did not comply regarding to gestational weight gain to current guidelines [4]. This has been previously described for other countries [26]. Every second woman with overweight or obesity and more than one third of the normal weight women gained more weight than recommended, whereas the majority of underweight women failed to gain sufficient weight. After adjustment for education, maternal age, baseline BMI and duration of the pregnancy a significant correlation between total weight gain and birth weight persisted

In addition a substantial proportion of women were characterized by poor dietary habits throughout the whole pregnancy although our population represents a rather educated (78 % higher education) and socioeconomically unrestricted population, which are factors associated with a better diet. As to macronutrients, more than every second women reported a fat consumption above the recommendation, characterized by a high intake of saturated fat, while the intake of polyunsaturated fatty acids, namely docosahexaenoic acid was insufficient. Compared to current guidelines the consumption of carbohydrates and fiber was mostly too low, and nearly half of the carbohydrates were obtained from sugar. Energy, as well as carbohydrate and sugar intake correlated significantly with total gestational weight gain even after adjustment for education and maternal age. The observed association between weight gain and monosaccharides and saccharose consumption remained significant even after further adjustment for energy intake.

With regard to micronutrient requirement a sustainable number of pregnant women fail to comply with the recommended daily intake. On the average none of the women reached the recommendation as to iron, folate and vitamin D and almost all participants reported an iodine intake below the guideline were independent from education levels or BMI categories.

Strengths and Limitations

To our knowledge our study is one of the first population–based ones evaluating not only gestational weight gain but also detailed dietary habits in a sample of German pregnant women. Data was collected prospectively, whereas most existing birth cohorts have recruited women in the course of pregnancy. Mean maternal age and rates of overweight and obesity are representative of the German population. Weight and nutrient intake was assessed in each trimester and compared to current recommendations.

However there are limitations that need to be addressed. First, our findings are confined to those women who voluntarily chose to take part in this study. Second, the sample is rather small and consisted of married women with a higher educational level. Third, we recorded maternal weight at the beginning of pregnancy in the first trimester. This did not differ significantly to recorded pre-pregnancy weight gain in our cohort (data not shown) and is widely used for these analysis as a true pre-pregnancy weight can only be obtained by patient recall. However we could draw the conclusion that in fact pregnancy weight gain could be even higher. Finally, nutrient assessment was obtained from only three 24 h recalls per women, one in each trimester. Further research is needed to confirm our results. In spite of these limitations, our data provides information as to weight gain and nutrient intake throughout pregnancy, findings that will have important implications for clinical practice.

Interpretation

Mean maternal age in the PRINCE cohort is representative of the German population (mean maternal age at delivery of the first child is 30.2 years in Germany [27]. One third of the women were characterized by overweight or obesity, which is in line with findings from the German National Nutrition Survey II and the German DEGS-Study in women of childbearing age [1, 2]. Some studies reported, that maternal weight at the beginning of pregnancy seems to have a greater impact on health of mother and child than weight gained throughout pregnancy [19, 28]. However, inadequate gestational weight gain, particularly excessive weight gain is known to be associated with unfavorable pregnancy outcomes [7–9, 11]. In line with most previous research birth weight correlated significantly with maternal BMI at the beginning of pregnancy as well as with weight gain and gestational week even after further adjustment for education and age in a multivariate model. However most of the existing studies did not take into account gestational week. Excessive weight gain can be used as a potential predictor for offspring's overweight and obesity, particularly in normal weight women [3].

In addition, potential priming effects of high maternal weight gain on offsprings's overweight cannot be excluded [29]. Mean total gestational weight gain in our study was slightly below data reported from two other population-based birth cohorts [3]. Consistent with other studies two thirds of our cohort did not follow recommendations as to weight gain [3]. Weight development throughout pregnancy should also be discussed in the light of maternal post-partum weight retention, further pregnancies and lifelong cardiovascular risk for the mother. Women whose doctors recommended weight gains consistent with IOM guidelines were more likely to follow the recommendation [30]. Results from intervention studies indicate that nutrition and lifestyle counseling usually combined with supplementary weight monitoring in pregnant women reduced the rate of pregnancies with excessive gestational and weight retention at six months postpartum weight gain without increasing insufficient weight gain and seems to be safe [31–33].

Dietary habits before and throughout pregnancy influence short- and long-term health of mother and child over and beyond a potential influence on gestational weight gain. Particularly a low intake in critical micronutrients such as folate, iodine or iron leads to fetal complications. Maternal dietay habits may even play a role in terms of in utero programming of offspring appetite [34] and food preference of the offspring [35]. Up to now detailed information as to energy intake, macronutrients and micronutrient content of the diet at different stages of gestation are limited [36]. In our study population the mean energy intake increases significantly by 8 % during the course of pregnancy, which is in line with the recommended 10 % [22]. However, the individual energy need may vary substantially depending mainly on the level of physical activity. Experience has shown, that most women decrease their physical activity throughout gestation, leading to the current recommendation that additional calories in overweight and obese women should be avoided [22].

More than one out of ten women did not reach the recommended protein intake in our study, while every second women was above the recommended fat intake throughout pregnancy. Data from animal studies indicate that high fat maternal diets during pregnancy seems to have adverse effects in offspring with regard to exercise performance, hepatic lipid accumulation, insulin resistance, and development of atherosclerosis [37–39]. As to carbohydrate and fiber intake the majority of women were obviously below the recommendation.

Present findings reflect in most parts mean dietary intake of macronutrients and fiber in the women of childbearing age in the German population, leading to the assumption, that without targeted intervention "healthy" pregnant women will not change the quality of their diet [1]. Initiatives to promote a healthy lifestyle during pregnancy like the German 'Healthy Start – Young Family Network' are helpful to increase awareness, however, more individual advice is highly recommended [19]. A mismatch between dietary practice and macronutrient recommendation in pregnant women is supported by a systematic review and meta-analysis including data of developed countries [23]. The quality of fat and carbohydrate intake is also of increasing interest. In our study saturated fat contributed largely to the fat consumption, while the intake of polyunsaturated fatty acids, namely docosahexaenic acid was too low. These findings are in line with findings from other European countries [23]. Carbohydrate intake, particularly sugar seems to be an important determinate of gestational weight gain in our cohort, which is supported by data from a Danish birth cohort, analyzing the impact of added sugar on excessive weight development during pregnancy [40].

To supply adequate amounts of vitamins, minerals and other micronutrients a nutrient-dense diet is desirable, particularly in the light of an increase in the requirement of certain micronutrients. Consistent with a meta-analysis in developed countries, our findings indicate that pregnant women are at risk of suboptimal micronutrient intake [24]. On the average none of the women met the recommendation as to folate, iron, and vitamin D throughout pregnancy and almost all were below the recommendation as to iodine intake. These findings reflect in most parts mean dietary intake of vitamins and minerals in women of childbearing age in the German population. The reference values for folate, iron, iodine and vitamin D can hardly be reached through diet alone [1, 22]. Supplying micronutrients to protect deficiencies can be useful to reduce adverse outcomes, but should not replace a healthy well-balanced diet. In addition, further studies to evaluate the effect of various combination and doses of micronutrients are warranted [41].

Conclusions

In summary, our analysis contributes to the limited literature on nutrient intake and weight gain throughout pregnancy. The data clearly indicate that the majority of women do not follow current recommendations as to dietary habits and gestational weight gain. Increasing rates of obese women of childbearing age will strengthen the problem. In the light of the present study a lifestyle counseling delivered to all pregnant women is highly justified, as intervention during pregnancy are characterized by a unique treatment adherence and can prevent short-term and long-term health risk of mother and child. Dietary advice is part of the prenatal care in Germany. However, this is mostly done by gynecologists and not by nutritional experts. Often this information is given as a leaflet to the patients. This highlights the need of high quality nutritional brochures but also individual advice affect the metabolic and weight trajectory both for women and their offspring.

Abbreviations

BMI, body-mass-index; D-A-CH, Germany-Austria-Switzerland; DHA, docosahexaenoic acid; GWG, gestational weight gain; IOM, US Institute of Medicine; IUGR, intra-uterine growth restriction; SAFA, Saturated fatty acids; SPSS, Statistical Package for the Social Sciences

Acknowledgement

We are indebted to all participants of the PRINCE study for their collaboration.

Funding

Financial support of the PRINCE study was primarily given by LEXI (Landes-Exzellenz-Initiative), State of Hamburg and the DFG (german research association, KFO 296, Grant-Number: DI 2103/2-1 AOBJ: 619132).

Authors' contributions

A.D. conceived, designed and performed the experiments, analyzed the data and wrote the paper. S.L. contributed analyzing tools, analyzed the data and wrote the paper. M.P. and G.H. performed the experiments. A.Dr. analyzed the data. K.H. contributed materials and tools and designed the study. P.A. and B.Z. conceived and designed the experiment, analyzed the data and wrote the paper and contributed equally. All authors read and approved the final manuscript.

Competing interests

BZ reports fees from Bayer for lectures and a review article.

Author details

[1]Department of Obstetrics and Fetal Medicine, University Medical Center Hamburg-Eppendorf, Martinistrasse 52, Hamburg 20246, Germany. [2]Institute for Medical Biometry and Epidemiology, University Medical Center Hamburg-Eppendorf, Hamburg 20246, Germany. [3]Preventive Medicine, University Heart Center, University Medical Center Hamburg-Eppendorf, Hamburg, Hamburg.

References

1. Max Rubner Institut. Nationale Verzehrstudie II, Ergebnisbericht, Teil 1. Karlsruhe: Bundesforschungsinstitut für Ernährung und Lebensmittel; 2008.
2. Mensink GBM, Schinekiewitz M, Haftenberger M, Lampert T, Ziese T, Scheidt-Nave C. Übergewicht und Adipositas in Deutschland. Ergebnisse der Studie zur Gesundheit Erwachsener in Deutschland (DEGS1). Bundesgesundheitsblatt. 2013 Nov 24;56:786–94
3. Beyerlein A, Nehring I, Rzehak P, Heinrich J, Müller MJ, Plachta-Danielzik S, et al. Gestational weight gain and body mass index in children: results from three german cohort studies. PLoS ONE. 2012;7(3):e33205.
4. Institute of Medicine (US), National Research Council (US) Committee to Reexamine IOM Pregnancy Weight Guidelines, Rasmussen KM, Yaktine AL. Weight Gain During Pregnancy: Reexamining the Guidelines. Washington (DC): National Academies Press (US); 2009.
5. Gaillard R. Maternal obesity during pregnancy and cardiovascular development and disease in the offspring. Eur J Epidemiol. 2015 Sep 16
6. Leddy MA, Power ML, Schulkin J. The impact of maternal obesity on maternal and fetal health. Rev Obstet Gynecol. 2008;1(4):170–8.
7. Heslehurst N, Simpson H, Ells LJ, Rankin J, Wilkinson J, Lang R, et al. The impact of maternal BMI status on pregnancy outcomes with immediate short-term obstetric resource implications: a meta-analysis. Obes Rev. 2008; 9(6):635–83.
8. Guelinckx I, Devlieger R, Bogaerts A, Pauwels S, Vansant G. The effect of pre-pregnancy BMI on intention, initiation and duration of breast-feeding. Public Health Nutr. 2012;15(5):840–8.
9. Sarwer DB, Allison KC, Gibbons LM, Markowitz JT, Nelson DB. Pregnancy and obesity: a review and agenda for future research. J Womens Health (Larchmt). 2006;15(6):720–33.
10. Mosca L, Benjamin EJ, Berra K, Bezanson JL, Dolor RJ, Lloyd-Jones DM, et al. Effectiveness-based guidelines for the prevention of cardiovascular disease in women–2011 update: a guideline from the american heart association. Circulation. 2011;123:1243–62.
11. McClure CK, Catov JM, Ness R, Bodnar LM. Associations between gestational weight gain and BMI, abdominal adiposity, and traditional measures of cardiometabolic risk in mothers 8 y postpartum. Am J Clin Nutr. 2013;98(5): 1218–25.
12. Flenady V, Koopmans L, Middleton P, Frøen JF, Smith GC, Gibbons K, et al. Major risk factors for stillbirth in high-income countries: a systematic review and meta-analysis. Lancet. 2011;377(9774):1331–40.
13. Barker DJP. Mothers, babies and disease in later life. 2nd edition. Churchill Livingstone: 1998. ISBN-10: 0443061653
14. Catalano PM, McIntyre HD, Cruickshank JK, McCance DR, Dyer AR, Metzger BE, et al. The hyperglycemia and adverse pregnancy outcome study: associations of GDM and obesity with pregnancy outcomes. Diabetes Care. 2012;35(4):780–6.
15. Schellong K, Schulz S, Harder T, Plagemann A. Birth weight and long-term overweight risk: systematic review and a meta-analysis including 643,902 persons from 66 studies and 26 countries globally. PLoS ONE. 2012;7(10): e47776.
16. Reynolds RM, Allan KM, Raja EA, Bhattacharya S, McNeill G, Hannaford PC, et al. Maternal obesity during pregnancy and premature mortality from cardiovascular event in adult offspring: follow-up of 1 323 275 person years. BMJ. 2012;347:f4539–9.
17. Slyvka Y, Zhang Y, Nowak FV. Epigenetic effects of paternal diet on offspring: emphasis on obesity. Endocrine. 2015;48(1):36–46.
18. Symonds ME, Mendez MA, Meltzer HM, Koletzko B, Godfrey K, Forsyth S, et al. Early life nutritional programming of obesity: mother-child cohort studies. Ann Nutr Metab. 2012;62(2):137–45.

19. Koletzko B, Bauer CP, Bung P, Cremer M, Flothkötter M, Hellmers C, et al. German national consensus recommendations on nutrition and lifestyle in pregnancy by the 'Healthy Start - Young Family Network'. Ann Nutr Metab. 2012;63(4):311–22.
20. Smith CJ, Ryckman KK. Epigenetic and developmental influences on the risk of obesity, diabetes, and metabolic syndrome. Diabetes Metab Syndr Obes. 2014;8:295–302.
21. Max Rubner Institu. Nationale Verzehrstudie II, Ergebnisbericht, Teil 2. Karlsruhe: Bundesforschungsinstitut für Ernährung und Lebensmitte; 2008.
22. D-A-CH Referenzwerte für die Nährstoffzufuhr. Deutsche Gesellschaft für Ernährung (DGE), Österreichische Gesellschaft für Ernährung (ÖGE), Schweizerische Vereinigung für Ernährung (SGE). Umschau/Braus, Frankfurt/Main 2015, ISBN-10: 3829571143
23. Blumfield ML, Hure AJ, Macdonald-Wicks L, Smith R, Collins CE. Systematic review and meta-analysis of energy and macronutrient intakes during pregnancy in developed countries. Nutr Rev. 2012;70(6):322–36.
24. Blumfield ML, Hure AJ, Macdonald-Wicks L, Smith R, Collins CE. A systematic review and meta-analysis of micronutrient intakes during pregnancy in developed countries. Nutr Rev. 2013;71(2):118–32.
25. Kleinwechter H, Schaefer-Graf U. Gestationsdiabetes–praktische Aspekte nach der neuen S3-Leitlinie. Diabetologie und Stoffwechsel. Diabetologie und Stoffwechsel. 2011;24(3):27–40.
26. Rasmussen KM, Catalano PM, Yaktine AL. New guidelines for weight gain during pregnancy: what obstetrician/gynecologists should know. Curr Opin Obstet Gynecol. 2009;21(6):521–6.
27. Statistisches Bundesamt (2012), Fachserie 1, Reihe 1.1 – 2010, www.destatis.de
28. National Institute for Health and Clinical Excellence. Dietary Interventions and Physical Activity Interventions for Weight Management before, during and after Pregnancy. London: National Institute for Health and Clinical Excellence; 2010.
29. Fraser A, Tilling K, Macdonald-Wallis C, Sattar N, Brion M-J, Benfield L, et al. Association of maternal weight gain in pregnancy with offspring obesity and metabolic and vascular traits in childhood. Circulation. 2010;121(23):2557–64.
30. Tovar A, Guthrie LB, Platek D, Stuebe A, Herring SJ, Oken E. Modifiable predictors associated with having a gestational weight gain goal. Matern Child Health J. 2011;15(7):1119–26.
31. Tanentsapf I, Heitmann BL, Adegboye ARA. Systematic review of clinical trials on dietary interventions to prevent excessive weight gain during pregnancy among normal weight, overweight and obese women. BMC Pregnancy Childbirth. 2011;11:81.
32. Streuling I, Beyerlein A, von Kries R. Can gestational weight gain be modified by increasing physical activity and diet counseling? A meta-analysis of interventional trials. Am J Clin Nutr. 2010;92(4):678–87.
33. Rauh K, Gabriel E, Kerschbaum E, Schuster T, Kries Von R, Amann-Gassner U, et al. Safety and efficacy of a lifestyle intervention for pregnant women to prevent excessive maternal weight gain: a cluster-randomized controlled trial. BMC Pregnancy Childbirth. 2013;13:151.
34. Brion M-JA, Ness AR, Rogers I, Emmett P, Cribb V, Davey-Smith G, et al. Maternal macronutrient and energy intakes in pregnancy and offspring intake at 10 y: exploring parental comparisons and prenatal effects. Am J Clin Nutr. 2010;91(3):748–56.
35. Gugusheff JR, Ong ZY, Muhlhausler BS. The early origins of food preferences: targeting the critical windows of development. FASEB J. 2015;29(2):365–73.
36. Talai Rad N, Ritterath C, Siegmund T, Wascher C, Siebert G, Henrich W, et al. Longitudinal analysis of changes in energy intake and macronutrient composition during pregnancy and 6 weeks post-partum. Arch Gynecol Obstet. 2011;283(2):185–90.
37. Wakana N, Irie D, Kikai M, Terada K, Yamamoto K, Kawahito H, et al. Maternal high-fat diet exaggerates atherosclerosis in adult offspring by augmenting periaortic adipose tissue-specific proinflammatory response. Arterioscler Thromb Vasc Biol. 2015;35(3):558–69.
38. Benatti RO, Melo AM, Borges FO, Ignacio-Souza LM, Simino LAP, Milanski M, et al. Maternal high-fat diet consumption modulates hepatic lipid metabolism and microRNA-122 (miR-122) and microRNA-370 (miR-370) expression. Br J Nutr. 2014;111(12):2112–22.
39. Walter I, Klaus S. Maternal high-fat diet consumption impairs exercise performance in offspring. J Nutr Sci. 2014;3:e61.
40. Maslova E, Halldorsson TI, Astrup A, Olsen SF. Dietary protein-to-carbohydrate ratio and added sugar as determinants of excessive gestational weight gain: a prospective cohort study. BMJ Open. 2015;5(2):e005839.
41. Zerfu TA, Ayele HT. Micronutrients and pregnancy; effect of supplementation on pregnancy and pregnancy outcomes: a systematic review. Nutr J. 2013;12:20.

15

High risk for obstructive sleep apnea and other sleep disorders among overweight and obese pregnant women

Jayne R. Rice[1], Gloria T. Larrabure-Torrealva[2,3], Miguel Angel Luque Fernandez[1], Mirtha Grande[5], Vicky Motta[2], Yasmin V. Barrios[1], Sixto Sanchez[4,5], Bizu Gelaye[1*] and Michelle A. Williams[1]

Abstract

Background: Obstructive sleep apnea (OSA), a common and serious disorder in which breathing repeatedly stops during sleep, is associated with excess weight and obesity. Little is known about the co-occurrence of OSA among pregnant women from low and middle-income countries.

Methods: We examined the extent to which maternal pre-pregnancy overweight or obesity status are associated with high risk for OSA, poor sleep quality, and excessive daytime sleepiness in 1032 pregnant women in Lima, Peru. The Berlin questionnaire was used to identify women at high risk for OSA. The Pittsburgh Sleep Quality Index (PSQI) and Epworth Sleepiness Scale (ESS) were used to examine sleep quality and excessive daytime sleepiness, respectively. Multinomial logistic regression procedures were employed to estimate odds ratios (aOR) and 95 % confidence intervals (CI) adjusted for putative confounding factors.

Results: Compared with lean women (<25 kg/m^2), overweight women (25–29.9 kg/m^2) had 3.69-fold higher odds of high risk for OSA (95 % CI 1.82–7.50). The corresponding aOR for obese women (≥30 kg/m^2) was 13.23 (95 % CI: 6.25–28.01). Obese women, as compared with their lean counterparts had a 1.61-fold higher odds of poor sleep quality (95 % CI: 1.00–2.63).

Conclusion: Overweight or obese pregnant women have increased odds of sleep disorders, particularly OSA. OSA screening and risk management may be indicated among pregnant women in low and middle income countries, particularly those undergoing rapid epidemiologic transitions characterized by increased prevalence of excessive adult weight gain.

Background

Obesity continues to be one of the fastest growing metabolic conditions worldwide. According to the World Health Organization (WHO) the prevalence of obesity is estimated to be approximately 12 % making it one of the 21st century epidemic disease [1]. The prevalence of obesity in Andean Latin American countries has almost doubled from 9 % in 1980 to 17 % in 2008 [2]. Recent studies conducted in Peru found that more than 40 % of the adult population in the metropolitan Lima is overweight or obese [3]. Excess consumption of energy dense foods and lack of physical activity have been implicated as reasons for the rise in obesity prevalence in Peru and elsewhere. Major obesity-related chronic disorders include: cardiovascular diseases, diabetes, hypertension, and breathing difficulties [1]. During pregnancy, maternal overweight or obese status are associated with adverse perinatal and neonatal outcomes such as gestational diabetes [4], pregnancy induced hypertension, preeclampsia [5], cesarean delivery [6], miscarriage [7], large for gestational age [4], macrosomia [8], and stillbirth [9].

There is a growing body of evidence that documents the impact of obesity on sleep disorders, more specifically obstructive sleep apnea (OSA) [2, 10, 11]. OSA is a condition characterized as repeated episodes of complete or total blockage of the upper airway during sleep [12, 13]. Snoring, persistent daytime sleepiness, and

* Correspondence: bgelaye@hsph.harvard.edu
[1]Department of Epidemiology, Harvard T.H. Chan School of Public Health, 677 Huntington Ave, K501, Boston, MA, 02115 USA
Full list of author information is available at the end of the article

periods of awakening out of breath during the night are hallmark symptoms of OSA [13]. Epidemiologic studies have shown that OSA and poor sleep quality are independently associated with weight gain, cardiometabolic disorders, cognitive impairments, hypertension, psychiatric disorders and headaches [2, 14]. Accumulating evidence also documents a strong, positive and bi-directional association of obesity with high risk for OSA and other sleep disorders [2, 15]. Investigators have argued that increased fat deposits around the upper airways of overweight and obese individuals can produce obstruction of breathing, reducing the flow of oxygen leading to sleep apnea [16]. Conversely, OSA can contribute to obesity because fragmented and non-restorative sleep related to sleep apnea has been associated with increased caloric intake [15]. Sleep patterns are known to change throughout pregnancy in part due to physiological and hormonal changes [17]. Studies have reported increased snoring and narrower upper airways during the third trimester of pregnancy compared to postpartum [18].

Despite the high prevalence of sleep disorders among pregnant women [19] and despite a well-established body of evidence showing elevated BMI as a significant predictor of sleep disorders [20], few studies have investigated the risk of sleep disorders among overweight and obese pregnant women. To fill this void in the literature, we sought to assess the extent to which pre-gestational overweight and obesity status are associated with increased odds of high risk of OSA and other sleep disorders among pregnant women in Peru.

Methods

Participants, sample size and study setting

This study was conducted among pregnant women attending prenatal care clinics at the Instituto Nacional Materno Perinatal (INMP) in the city of Lima, Peru between February 2013 and March 2014. The INMP, overseen by the Peruvian Ministry of Health, is the primary referral hospital for maternal and perinatal care. Eligible women were 18 years of age or older, could speak and read Spanish, and with a gestational age between 24 to 28 weeks. Enrolled participants were invited to participate in an interview where trained research personnel used a structured questionnaire to elicit information regarding maternal socio-demographic, lifestyle characteristics, medical and reproductive histories, and sleep characteristics. Anthropometric measures and vital signs were measured by experienced midwives. Women were weighed in light clothing using the WHO standard guidelines. All participants provided written informed consent and study procedures were approved by institutional review boards of the INMP, Lima, Peru and the Harvard T.H. Chan School of Public Health Office of Human Research Administration, Boston, MA, USA.

Instruments and variable specification

The Berlin Questionnaire originated from Berlin, Germany is a widely used and validated screening instrument for assessing high risk for obstructive sleep apnea (OSA). The questionnaire consists of 11 questions separated into three sections [21, 22]. Section 1 asked participants whether they snore. Those who responded affirmatively were asked how loud their snoring was, how often it occurred, and whether their snoring bothered other people. In the present study, participants were also asked whether anyone has ever noticed cessation of their breathing during sleep. Section 2 asked participants how often they felt tired or fatigued right after sleep, how often they felt tired, fatigued, or not up to par during wake time, and whether they ever fall asleep driving a car. In section 3, participants were asked about a history of hypertension, as well as their height, weight, and age. A section was considered positive if there were two affirmative answers in either section 1 or 2, or one affirmative response in section 3. In section 3, high risk for OSA was defined when there was a history of hypertension or obesity.

The Berlin questionnaire is widely used in pregnancy [23–26]. For the purposes of this study when 2 or more sections were classified as positive, the participant was deemed to be at high risk for OSA [21, 22]. In addition, given the lack of consensus concerning the utility of this diagnostic criteria in pregnancy [23–25], we evaluated the extent to which snoring (i.e., those positive for section 1) is associated with maternal obesity status.

Sleep quality was evaluated using the Pittsburgh Sleep Quality Index (PSQI), a 19-item self-reported questionnaire that assesses sleep quality over the past month [27]. The PSQI has seven sleep components: sleep duration, disturbance, latency, habitual sleep efficiency, use of sleep medicine, daytime dysfunction due to sleepiness and overall quality of sleep. Each component produced a score ranging from 0 to 3, where a score of 3 indicates the highest level of dysfunction. A global sleep quality score is obtained by summing the individual component scores (range 0 to 21) with higher scores indicative of poorer sleep quality during the previous month. Participants with global scores that exceed 5 are classified as poor sleepers [27]. Those with a score of 5 or less were classified as good sleepers. This classification system is consistent with prior studies of pregnancy including those conducted in Peru [28–30].

Daytime sleepiness was measured using the Epworth Sleep Scale (ESS) [31]. The instrument has been widely validated globally including in Peru [32]. The ESS is an 8-item questionnaire capturing an individual's propensity to fall asleep during commonly encountered situations on a scale from 0 to 3. Overall scores range between 0 and 24. ESS scores of 10 or higher are indicative of excessive daytime sleepiness [31].

Other covariates

Maternal age at the time of interview was categorized as follows: 18–20, 20–29, 30–34, and ≥35 years. Other sociodemographic variables were categorized as follows: maternal and paternal educational attainment (≤6, 7–12, and >12 completed years of schooling); marital status (married and living with partner vs. others); access to basic foods (very hard/hard, somewhat hard, not very hard); food insecurity (yes vs. no); access to medical care (very hard/hard, somewhat hard, not very hard); and parity (nulliparous vs. multiparous). Pre-pregnancy body mass index was calculated as weight (in kilograms) divided by the square of height (in meters and used to identify lean (BMI < 25 kg/m^2), overweight (BMI: 25–29.9 kg/m^2), and obese (BMI ≥ 30 kg/m^2) women according to the World Health Organization (WHO) criteria.

Statistical analysis

We examined the distributions of maternal sociodemographic, reproductive, and medical characteristics according to pre-pregnancy BMI categories. Multivariate multinomial logistic regression models were fitted to estimate adjusted odds ratios [33] and 95 % confidence intervals (95 % CI) of sleep disorders in relation to maternal overweight and obesity status after adjusting for potential confounders. Separate models were fitted for each sleep complaint. In multivariable models we adjusted for maternal age, educational attainment, marital status, and parity. Additional adjustment for the other covariates listed in Table 1 did not substantially change odds ratios. We explored the possibility of a nonlinear relation between BMI and odds of high risk for OSA, using generalized additive logistic regression modeling procedures (GAM). Finally, on the basis of study findings reporting limited clinical utility of the total score of the Berlin questionnaire in pregnancy [25], we conducted *post-hoc* analyses to examine the extent to which maternal overweight and obesity status are associated with increased odds of snoring (as assessed using information from section 1 of the Berlin questionnaire). All analyses were performed using Stata 12.0 statistical software (Stata, College Station, TX). The GAM analyses were performed using "R" software version 3.1.2. All reported p-values are two-tailed and deemed statistically significant at $\alpha = 0.05$.

Results

The socio-demographic characteristics of the participants are presented in Table 1. A total of 1032 pregnant women between the ages of 18 and 45 years (mean age = 28.6 years, standard deviation = 6.2 years) participated in the study. The majority of participants were married or living with their partner (87.6 %) while more than half (55.5 %) reported an education attainment of 7 or more years.

Table 1 Maternal socio-demographics characteristics

Characteristic	Total sample (*N* = 1,032) n (%)
Maternal Age (years)	
<19	42 (4.1)
20–29	551 (53.4)
30–34	237 (23.0)
≥35	202 (19.5)
Maternal Age (years) Mean (SD) [Min, Max]	28.6 (6.2) [18, 45]
Marital Status	
Married or living with partner	903 (87.6)
Single or living alone/divorced	128 (12.4)
Maternal Education (years)	
>12	32 (3.10)
7–12	541 (52.4)
≤6	459 (44.5)
Paternal Education (years)	
>12	23 (2.2)
7–12	566 (55.4)
≤6	433 (42.4)
Pre-pregnancy BMI (kg/m^2)	
<25 (Normal weight)	573 (55.5)
25–29.9 (Overweight)	350 (33.9)
≥30 (Obese)	109 (10.6)
Difficulties to Pay for Basics	
Very hard/hard	153 (14.9)
Somewhat hard	351 (34.1)
Not very hard	526 (51.1)
Food Insecurity	
No	369 (35.8)
Yes	663 (64.2)
Difficulties to Access Medical Care	
Very hard/hard	199 (19.3)
Somewhat hard	714 (69.3)
Not very hard	118 (11.4)

Approximately 50 % of participants reported having difficulty paying for basics (48.9 %), while 64.2 % reported food insecurities and more than three fourth (88.6 %) reported difficulties to accessing medical care.

Table 2 shows the relationship between pre-pregnancy BMI and sleep disorders. The prevalence of high risk for OSA was 2.1 %, 8.0 % and 25.7 % for lean, overweight and obese study participants, respectively. The corresponding prevalence for poor sleep quality were 19.0 %, 21.4 %, and 28.4 %. Generally similar prevalence of excessive daytime sleepiness was noted among lean (12.7 %), overweight (13.1 %) and obese (12.9 %) study

Table 2 Odds of obstructive sleep apnea, poor sleep quality, and excessive daytime sleepiness in relation to pre-pregnancy body mass index (BMI)

	Pre-pregnancy BMI in kg/m^2			Unadjusted OR (95 % CI)		*Adjusted OR (95 % CI)	
	BMI <25 (*N* = 573)	BMI 25–29.9 (*N* = 350)	BMI ≥ 30 (*N* = 109)	BMI 25–29.9	BMI ≥30	BMI 25–25.9	BMI ≥30
Berlin Questionnaire	n (%)	n (%)	n (%)				
Low risk OSA	561 (97.9)	322 (92.0)	81 (74.3)	Reference	Reference	Reference	Reference
High risk OSA	12 (2.1)	28 (8.0)	28 (25.7)	4.06 (2.04–8.10)	16.2 (7.90–33.04)	3.69 (1.82–7.50)	13.23 (6.25–28.01)
Poor Sleep Quality							
No (PSQI ≤5)	464 (81.0)	275 (78.6)	78 (71.6)	Reference	Reference	Reference	Reference
Yes (PSQI >5)	109 (19.0)	75 (21.4)	31 (28.4)	1.20 (0.83–1.61)	1.70 (1.06–2.70)	1.16 (0.82–1.63)	1.61 (1.00–2.63)
Excessive Daytime Sleepiness							
No (ESS <10)	500 (87.3)	304 (86.9)	95 (87.1)	Reference	Reference	Reference	Reference
Yes (ESS ≥10)	73 (12.7)	46 (13.1)	14 (12.9)	1.03 (0.70–1.54)	1.00 (0.55–1.86)	1.06 (0.70–1.60)	1.07 (0.57–2.03)

*Adjusted for maternal age, education, marital status and parity; Reference group: BMI < 25
OR Odds ratio; *CI* Confidence Interval; *OSA* obstructive sleep apnea; *PSQI* Pittsburgh sleep quality index; *ESS* Epworth sleepiness scale

participants. In general, as pre-pregnancy BMI increased, the odds of sleep disorders increased. After adjusting for confounders compared with normal weight women (<25 kg/m^2), overweight women (25–29.9 kg/m^2) had 3.69-fold higher odds of experiencing high risk for OSA (assessed using the Berlin questionnaire) (95 % CI: 1.82–7.50). Obese women (≥30 kg/m^2) had a 13.2-fold higher odds of experiencing high risk for OSA (aOR = 13.23; 95 % CI: 6.25–28.01) as compared with their lean counterparts. Additionally the odds of high risk for OSA was modeled in relation to BMI expressed as continuous variable using procedures based on a general additive model. Results from these analyses confirmed a linear relationship between increasing BMI and the odds of high risk for OSA (Fig. 1).

Compared with lean women, overweight women were associated with modest elevated, and statistically non-significant, odds of poor sleep quality (aOR = 1.16; 95 % CI: 0.82–1.63). However, obese women had a statistically significant 1.61-fold increased odds of poor sleep quality (95 % CI: 1.00–2.63), as compared with lean women (Table 2). We observed no clear evidence of an association of pre-pregnancy BMI and excessive daytime sleepiness. In *post-hoc* analyses restricted to the snoring components of the Berlin questionnaire (section 1), we found that compared with lean women, obese (aOR = 1.83; 95 % CI: 1.03–3.24) and overweight women (aOR = 1.20; 95 %CI: 0.78–1.83) were more likely to report snoring during pregnancy.

Discussion

Overall, we found that pregnant women who are overweight and obese have increased odds of sleep disorders. Compared with lean women (<25 kg/m^2), overweight women (25–29.9 kg/m^2) had 3.69-fold higher odds of high risk for OSA (95 % CI 1.82–7.50). The corresponding OR for obese women (≥30 kg/m^2) was 13.23 (95 % CI: 6.25–28.01). Obese women, as compared with their lean counterparts had a 1.61-fold higher odds of poor sleep quality (95 % CI: 1.00–2.63).

In the present study, the prevalence estimates of high risk for OSA were 6.5 % (assessed using Berlin questionnaire). The prevalence of high risk for OSA found in our study is lower than estimates from other studies. In their study among predominantly Hispanic pregnant women in Houston, Texas Antony et al. found a 15.5 % prevalence of high risk for OSA assessed using Berlin questionnaire [4]. The investigators further noted that obesity was associated with a 9-fold increased odds (95 % CI 4.68–17.39) of high risk for OSA compared with normal weight women in that population. In a study of 276 pregnant women in Korea, Ko et al. [20] found a high prevalence of OSA in obese women (43.6 %) compared with non-obese women (32.6 %) ($p = 0.001$). Their findings indicating increased odds of high risk for OSA among overweight and obese pregnant women are in general agreement with our study findings. Other studies conducted among men and non-pregnant women [34–36] report findings that are in agreement with those reported by our team and others [4, 20]. For example, using data from the 2007 Sleep in America Poll of the National Sleep Foundation, Kapsimalis and Kryger [37] noted that the prevalence of high risk for OSA (determined using Berlin questionnaire) was 8.5 % among women with normal BMI while the prevalence estimates were markedly higher among overweight (21 %) and obese (62 %) women. In a recently published study of college students in Chile, Wosu et al. [15] reported, that obese students were 8.26 times-as likely to experience high risk for OSA compared with normal weight students (95 % CI:4.59–14.86) after adjusting for confounders. Another finding that merits consideration is our results that showed obese pregnant

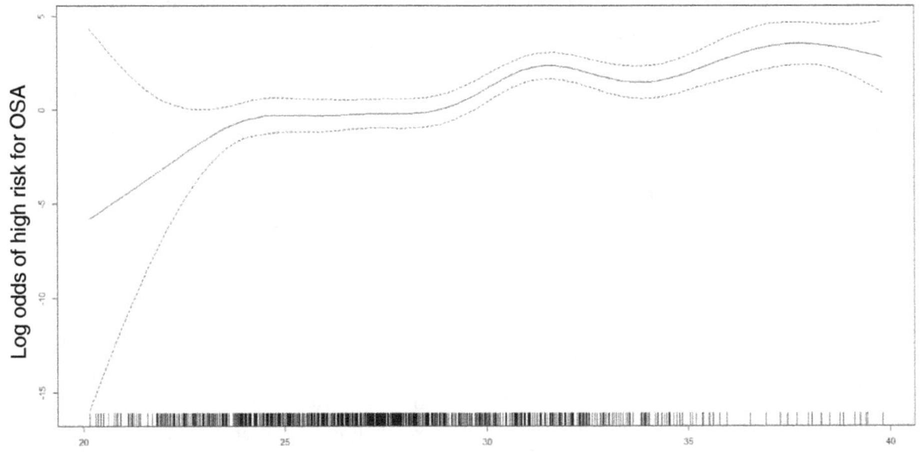

Fig. 1 Relation between log odds of high risk for obstructive sleep apnea and pre-pregnancy body mass index (solid line) with 95 % confidence interval (dotted lines)

women were 1.83-time as likely to report snoring (aOR = 1.83; 95 % CI: 1.03–3.24) during pregnancy as compared with lean women. However, this association did not reach statistical significance for overweight women (aOR = 1.20; 95 % CI: 0.78–1.83). Investigators have documented similar findings and have speculated that pregnant women are more likely to have higher BMI while carrying a lesser proportion of body fat and therefore more likely to meet the criteria of obesity used by the Berlin questionnaire [23]. Taken together, the current data indicate that the Berlin questionnaire might have limited utility in OSA screening due to the inclusion of obesity as one of the classification criteria.

In the last 50 years, the average self-reported sleep duration in the United States has decreased by 1.5 to 2 h while the prevalence estimates of obesity and diabetes have increased with Hispanics and Blacks showing marked increase [38, 39]. A large literature primarily focused on men and non-pregnant women has shown that obesity is related to sleep insufficiency and poor sleep quality [40]. For instance, Chaput et al. (2007) in Canada found that women with short sleep duration (5 to 6 h) were 1.69-times as likely (OR = 1.69; 95 % CI: 1.15–2.39) to be overweight or obese compared with normal sleepers (7 to 8 h) [41]. In Taiwan Hung et al. (2012) noted that being overweight or obese was statistically significantly associated with increased global PSQI scores ($p < 0.001$) [40]. Logue et al. (2014) in an urban family medicine center in the US reported a statistically significant association of poor sleep quality and obesity ($p = 0.005$) independent of age, gender, and ethnicity [42]. It is well established that sleep is altered during pregnancy [43]. Of note, in the second and third trimesters, pregnant women are more likely to have frequent awakenings due to fetal movements, discomfort, backaches as well as frequent urge to urinate due to an enlarged uterus [44] contributing to sleep insufficiency and fragmentation. Poor material sleep quality and other sleep disorders influence not only the mother but also their offspring to adverse cardio metabolic pathology later in life.

In the current study, we found no evidence of an association between BMI and excessive daytime sleepiness after adjustment for possible confounders. Dixon et al. (2007), in their study among 1055 Australian patients presenting for obesity surgery, also found no statistically significant association between ESS scores and BMI [45]. We do not have an explanation for these null findings although it is important to note that the ESS is a global summary score of questions on the risk of daytime sleepiness during different situations during the daytime. The ESS was originally developed to measure one construct—excessive daytime sleepiness [27, 31]. However, an emerging literature has shown that the eight items of ESS do not necessarily assess a unidimensional construct rather two or three different aspects of daytime sleepiness [46]. Hence, the summary score of the all eight items may not be the best index of excessive day time sleepiness. Future studies should look at how individual items might be influenced by obesity/overweight status.

Several plausible and compelling biological mechanisms have been proposed to explain the observed obesity/overweight-sleep disorder associations. Obesity can contribute to many physiological changes that increase the risk of OSA. For example, excessive soft tissue due to obesity, may narrow the pharyngeal airway and reduce lung volume [2]. Additionally, pregnancy induces many physiological changes. These includes enlargement of the uterus which can elevate the diaphragm and alter respiration. These alterations, for instance, may increase the tendency for collapsing the upper airway during sleep [19]. Changes in hormones also predispose pregnant women to episodes of sleep apnea. Notably, increased estrogen concentration has been linked to mucosal edema, and progesterone has been linked to increase respiratory center sensitivity to CO_2, therefore causing instability of the respiratory control mechanism [47]. Collectively, these physiological and hormonal changes may interact to increase the obesity-sleep disorders associations.

Our study has several notable strengths including a relatively large sample size, the use of cross-culturally accepted instruments to characterize sleep disorders and rigorously trained research staff administering the questionnaires. However, several important limitations must be considered when interpreting our findings. First, since this was a cross-sectional study, we cannot delineate the temporal relationship between maternal elevated BMI and sleep disorders. We also cannot determine whether sleep disturbances may be attributed to pregnancy related physiological alterations. Second, our findings are based on a population of pregnant women seeking care at a specialized maternal hospital; hence, caution is needed before generalizing the results to other populations. Third, although we used multiple validated questionnaires, these questionnaires may have contributed to some errors in the classification of participants' sleep disturbances [20]. Use of screening questionnaires for assessing sleep disorders in pregnancy is an important component of sleep health research. The success of screening however, is largely dependent on the accuracy of the questionnaires and use diagnostic procedures, used as the gold standard, to evaluate the effectiveness of screening questionnaires. The gold standard for documenting many sleep disorders including OSA is in-laboratory polysomnography (PSG) assessment. Unfortunately due to cost, complexity and participant burden, use of PSG testing is limited in large-scale epidemiologic studies. Thus use of screening questionnaires with low specificity remains the main modality for ascertaining OSA. Future studies are warranted to develop, refine and enhance the psychometric properties of screening questionnaires and improve their utility for early identification of sleep disorders in pregnancy. The fact that our findings are similar to those that used more invasive, though objective measures of sleep traits (e.g., polysomnography) [48] serve to attenuate some concerns.

Available literature suggests that maternal OSA may be associated with an increased risk of adverse perinatal outcomes [47, 49]. For instance in a meta-analysis of 9795 participants Luque-Fernandez et al. [49] found women with sleep disordered breathing had a 3-fold increased risk of gestational diabetes (OR = 3.06; 95 % CI: 1.89–4.96). Chen et al. [50] found that mothers with OSA were more likely to have low birth weight, preterm birth, and small for gestational age newborns, cesarean section, preeclampsia, gestational diabetes, and gestational hypertension as compared with unaffected mothers. Louis et al. [51] reported that OSA was associated with an increased risk of preterm delivery and maternal morbidity. Additionally, Kamysheva et al. have reported increased odds of antepartum and postpartum depression among women with symptoms of poor sleep [52].

Conclusion

In conclusion, we observed increased risks of sleep disorders amongst overweight and obese pregnant Peruvian women. These observations, when coupled with earlier report, have important clinical and public health implications because pregnant women with symptoms of OSA are at higher risk of adverse pregnancy and perinatal outcomes [47]. Collectively, our findings and those of others [14] underscore the clinical and public health implications for OSA screening and treatment among reproductive age and pregnant women in low and middle income countries, particularly those undergoing rapid epidemiologic transitions characterized by increased prevalence of excessive adult weight gain.

Competing interests

The authors declare that they have no competing interests.

Authors' contributions

MAW conceived and designed the study. JRR, MALF, BG and MAW analyzed data. JRR, BG and MAW drafted the manuscript. All authors interpreted the data, critically revised the draft for important intellectual content, and gave final approval of the manuscript to be published.

Acknowledgment

This research was supported by Roche Diagnostic Operations Inc. (project number 208617–5074547) and the National Institutes of Health (NIH), National Institute for Minority Health and Health Disparities (T37-MD000149). The funders had no role in study design; in the collection, analysis and interpretation of data; in the writing of the report; and in the decision to submit the paper for publication. The authors wish to thank the dedicated staff members of Asociacion Civil Proyectos en Salud (PROESA), Peru and Instituto Especializado Materno Perinatal, Peru for their expert technical assistance with this research.

Author details

[1]Department of Epidemiology, Harvard T.H. Chan School of Public Health, 677 Huntington Ave, K501, Boston, MA, 02115 USA. [2]Instituto Nacional Materno Perinatal de Lima, Lima, Peru. [3]Departamentos de Medicina y Ginecología y Obstetricia Universidad Nacional Universidad Nacional Mayor de San Marcos, Lima, Peru. [4]Universidad de Ciencias Aplicadas, Lima, Peru. [5]Asociación Civil de Proyectos en Salud, AC.PROESA, Lima, Peru.

References

1. Unwin N, Whiting D, Guariguata L, Ghyoot G, and Gan D, Eds., Diabetes Atlas, International Diabetes Federation, Brussels, Belgium, 5th edition, 2011.
2. Burke CCILE. The obesity epidemic: the USA as a cautionary tale for the rest of the world. Curr Epidemiol Rep. 2014;1:82–8.
3. Ortiz DM: More than 40 percent of Peruvian adults are obese or overweight. In: National. Peru; 2013.

4. Carreno CA, Clifton RG, Hauth JC, Myatt L, Roberts JM, Spong CY, et al. Excessive early gestational weight gain and risk of gestational diabetes mellitus in nulliparous women. Obstet Gynecol. 2012;119(6):1227–33.
5. Chandrasekaran S, Levine LD, Durnwald CP, Elovitz MA, Srinivas SK. Excessive weight gain and hypertensive disorders of pregnancy in the obese patient. J Matern Fetal Neonatal Med. 2014;17:1–5.
6. Weiss JL, Malone FD, Emig D, Ball RH, Nyberg DA, Comstock CH, et al. Obesity, obstetric complications and cesarean delivery rate–a population-based screening study. Am J Obstet Gynecol. 2004;190(4):1091–7.
7. Boots C, Stephenson MD. Does obesity increase the risk of miscarriage in spontaneous conception: a systematic review. Semin Reprod Med. 2011;29(6):507–13.
8. Egan AM, Dennedy MC, Al-Ramli W, Heerey A, Avalos G, Dunne F. ATLANTIC-DIP: excessive gestational weight gain and pregnancy outcomes in women with gestational or pregestational diabetes mellitus. J Clin Endocrinol Metab. 2014;99(1):212–9.
9. Chu SY, Kim SY, Lau J, Schmid CH, Dietz PM, Callaghan WM, et al. Maternal obesity and risk of stillbirth: a metaanalysis. Am J Obstet Gynecol. 2007;197(3):223–8.
10. Kohler M. Risk factors and treatment for obstructive sleep apnea amongst obese children and adults. Curr Opin Allergy Clin Immunol. 2009;9(1):4–9.
11. Pien GW, Pack AI, Jackson N, Maislin G, Macones GA, Schwab RJ. Risk factors for sleep-disordered breathing in pregnancy. Thorax. 2014;69(4):371–7.
12. Edwards N, Middleton PG, Blyton DM, Sullivan CE. Sleep disordered breathing and pregnancy. Thorax. 2002;57(6):555–8.
13. Cutler MJ, Hamdan AL, Hamdan MH, Ramaswamy K, Smith ML. Sleep apnea: from the nose to the heart. J Am Board Fam Pract. 2002;15(2):128–41.
14. Hiestand DM, Britz P, Goldman M, Phillips B. Prevalence of symptoms and risk of sleep apnea in the US population: results from the national sleep foundation sleep in America 2005 poll. Chest. 2006;130(3):780–6.
15. Wosu AC, Velez JC, Barbosa C, Andrade A, Frye M, Chen X, et al. The relationship between high risk for obstructive sleep apnea and general and central obesity: findings from a sample of Chilean college students. ISRN Obes. 2014;2014:871681.
16. Venkata C, Venkateshiah SB. Sleep-disordered breathing during pregnancy. J Am Board Fam Med. 2009;22(2):158–68.
17. Fung AM, Wilson DL, Barnes M, Walker SP. Obstructive sleep apnea and pregnancy: the effect on perinatal outcomes. J Perinatol. 2012;32(6):399–406.
18. Izci B, Vennelle M, Liston WA, Dundas KC, Calder AA, Douglas NJ. Sleep-disordered breathing and upper airway size in pregnancy and post-partum. Eur Respir J. 2006;27(2):321–7.
19. Cai XH, Xie YP, Li XC, Qu WL, Li T, Wang HX, et al. The prevalence and associated risk factors of sleep disorder-related symptoms in pregnant women in China. Sleep Breath. 2013;17(3):951–6.
20. Ko HS, Kim MY, Kim YH, Lee J, Park YG, Moon HB, et al. Obstructive sleep apnea screening and perinatal outcomes in Korean pregnant women. Arch Gynecol Obstet. 2013;287(3):429–33.
21. Netzer NC, Stoohs RA, Netzer CM, Clark K, Strohl KP. Using the Berlin questionnaire to identify patients at risk for the sleep apnea syndrome. Ann Intern Med. 1999;131(7):485–91.
22. Meerlo P, Sgoifo A, Suchecki D. Restricted and disrupted sleep: effects on autonomic function, neuroendocrine stress systems and stress responsivity. Sleep Medicine Reviews. 2008;12(3):197–210.
23. Wilson DL, Walker SP, Fung AM, O'Donoghue F, Barnes M, Howard M. Can we predict sleep-disordered breathing in pregnancy? The clinical utility of symptoms. J Sleep Res. 2013;22(6):670–8.
24. Tantrakul V, Sirijanchune P, Panburana P, Pengjam J, Suwansathit W, Boonsarngsuk V, et al. Screening of obstructive sleep apnea during pregnancy: differences in predictive values of questionnaires across trimesters. J Clin Sleep Med. 2015;11(2):157–63.
25. Olivarez SA, Ferres M, Antony K, Mattewal A, Maheshwari B, Sangi-Haghpeykar H, et al. Obstructive sleep apnea screening in pregnancy, perinatal outcomes, and impact of maternal obesity. Am J Perinatol. 2011;28(8):651–8.
26. Mindell JA, Cook RA, Nikolovski J. Sleep patterns and sleep disturbances across pregnancy. Sleep Medicine. 2015;16(4):483–8.
27. Buysse DJ, Reynolds 3rd CF, Monk TH, Berman SR, Kupfer DJ. The Pittsburgh sleep quality index: a new instrument for psychiatric practice and research. Psychiatry Res. 1989;28(2):193–213.
28. Gelaye B, Barrios YV, Zhong QY, Rondon MB, Borba CP, Sanchez SE, et al. Association of poor subjective sleep quality with suicidal ideation among pregnant Peruvian women. Gen Hosp Psychiatry. 2015. doi:10.1016/j.genhosppsych.2015.04.014.
29. Okun ML, Hanusa BH, Hall M, Wisner KL. Sleep complaints in late pregnancy and the recurrence of postpartum depression. Behav Sleep Med. 2009;7(2):106–17.
30. Zhong QY, Gelaye B, Sanchez SE, Williams MA. Psychometric Properties of the Pittsburgh Sleep Quality Index (PSQI) in a Cohort of Peruvian Pregnant Women. J Clin Sleep Med. 2015. [Epub ahead of print].
31. Johns MW. A new method for measuring daytime sleepiness: the Epworth sleepiness scale. Sleep. 1991;14(6):540–5.
32. Rose D, Gelaye B, Sanchez S, Castaneda B, Sanchez E, Yanez ND, Williams MA. Morningness/eveningness chronotype, poor sleep quality, and daytime sleepiness in relation to common mental disorders among Peruvian college students. Psychol Health Med. 2014:1–8. In press.
33. Shimizu E, Hashimoto K, Okamura N, Koike K, Komatsu N, Kumakiri C, et al. Alterations of serum levels of brain-derived neurotrophic factor (BDNF) in depressed patients with or without antidepressants. Biol Psychiatry. 2003;54(1):70–5.
34. Palla A, Digiorgio M, Carpene N, Rossi G, D'Amico I, Santini F, et al. Sleep apnea in morbidly obese patients: prevalence and clinical predictivity. Respiration. 2009;78(2):134–40.
35. Resta O, Foschino-Barbaro MP, Legari G, Talamo S, Bonfitto P, Palumbo A, et al. Sleep-related breathing disorders, loud snoring and excessive daytime sleepiness in obese subjects. Int J Obes Relat Metab Disord. 2001;25(5):669–75.
36. Mallory Jr GB, Fiser DH, Jackson R. Sleep-associated breathing disorders in morbidly obese children and adolescents. J Pediatr. 1989;115(6):892–7.
37. Kapsimalis F, Kryger M. Sleep breathing disorders in the U.S. female population. J Womens Health. 2009;18(8):1211–9.
38. Lucassen EA, Rother KI, Cizza G. Interacting epidemics? Sleep curtailment, insulin resistance, and obesity. Ann N Y Acad Sci. 2012;1264:110–34.
39. Flegal KM, Carroll MD, Kit BK, Ogden CL. Prevalence of obesity and trends in the distribution of body mass index among US adults, 1999–2010. JAMA. 2012;307(5):491–7.
40. Hung HC, Yang YC, Ou HY, Wu JS, Lu FH, Chang CJ. The Association Between Self-Reported Sleep Quality and Overweight in A Chinese Population. Obesity. 2013;21(3):486–92.
41. Chaput JP, Despres JP, Bouchard C, Tremblay A. Short sleep duration is associated with reduced leptin levels and increased adiposity: Results from the Quebec family study. Obesity. 2007;15(1):253–61.
42. Logue EE, Scott ED, Palmieri PA, Dudley P. Sleep duration, quality, or stability and obesity in an urban family medicine center. J Clin Sleep Med. 2014;10(2):177–82.
43. Lee KA. Alterations in sleep during pregnancy and postpartum: a review of 30 years of research. Sleep Medicine Reviews. 1998;2(4):231–42.
44. Kennelly MM, Fallon A, Farah N, Stuart B, Turner MJ. Effects of body mass index on sleep patterns during pregnancy. J Obstet Gynaecol. 2011;31(2):125–7.
45. Dixon JB, Schachter LM, O'Brien PE. Sleep disturbance and obesity: changes following surgically induced weight loss. Arch Intern Med. 2001;161(1):102–6.
46. Gelaye B, Lohsoonthorn V, Lertmaharit S, Pensuksan WC, Sanchez SE, Lemma S, et al. Construct validity and factor structure of the Pittsburgh Sleep Quality Index and Epworth Sleepiness Scale in a multi-national study of African, South East Asian and South American college students. PloS One. 2014;9(12):e116383.
47. Venkata C, Venkateshiah SB. Sleep-disordered breathing during pregnancy. J Am Board Fam Med. 2009;22(2):158–68.
48. Moraes W, Poyares D, Zalcman I, de Mello MT, Bittencourt LR, Santos-Silva R, et al. Association between body mass index and sleep duration assessed by objective methods in a representative sample of the adult population. Sleep Medicine. 2013;14(4):312–8.
49. Luque-Fernandez MA, Bain PA, Gelaye B, Redline S, Williams MA. Sleep-disordered breathing and gestational diabetes mellitus: a meta-analysis of 9795 participants enrolled in epidemiological observational studies. Diabetes Care. 2013;36(10):3353–60.
50. Chen YH, Kang JH, Lin CC, Wang IT, Keller JJ, Lin HC. Obstructive sleep apnea and the risk of adverse pregnancy outcomes. Am J Obstet Gynecol. 2012;206(2):136. e131-135.

Physical activity, depressed mood and pregnancy worries in European obese pregnant women: results from the DALI study

Linda de Wit[1], Judith G. M. Jelsma[1], Mireille N. M. van Poppel[1,2*], Annick Bogaerts[3], David Simmons[4], Gernot Desoye[5], Rosa Corcoy[6,7], Alexandra Kautzky-Willer[8], Jürgen Harreiter[8], Andre van Assche[9], Roland Devlieger[9], Dirk Timmerman[9], David Hill[10], Peter Damm[11], Elisabeth R. Mathiesen[11], Ewa Wender-Ozegowska[12], Agnieszka Zawiejska[12], Pablo Rebollo[13], Annunziata Lapolla[14], Maria G. Dalfrà[14], Stefano Del Prato[15], Alessandra Bertolotto[15], Fidelma Dunne[16], Dorte M. Jensen[17], Liselotte Andersen[17] and Frank J. Snoek[18,19]

Abstract

Background: The purpose of this study was to examine the association between mental health status (i.e. depressed mood and pregnancy-related worries) and objectively measured physical activity levels in obese pregnant women from seven European countries.

Methods: Baseline data from the vitamin D and lifestyle intervention for the prevention of gestational diabetes mellitus (DALI) study were used. Time spent in moderate-to-vigorous physical activity (MVPA) and sedentary behaviour was measured with accelerometers. Depressed mood was measured with the WHO well-being index (WHO-5) and pregnancy-related worries with the Cambridge Worry Scale (CWS). In addition, socio-demographic characteristics, lifestyle factors, and perceptions and attitude regarding weight management and physical activity were measured. Linear regression analyses were performed to assess the association of mental health status with MVPA and sedentary behaviour.

Results: A total of 98 obese pregnant women from Austria, Belgium, Ireland, Italy, Poland, Spain and the Netherlands were included. Women had a mean age of 31.6 ± 5.8 years, a pre-pregnancy BMI of 34.1 ± 4.3 kg/m^2, and were on average 15.4 ± 2.8 weeks pregnant. WHO-5 scores indicative of depressed mood (<50) were reported by 27.1 % of the women and most frequently endorsed pregnancy-related worries pertained to own and the baby's health. Women with good well-being spent 85 % more time in MVPA compared to women with a depressed mood ($P = 0.03$). No differences in MVPA levels were found for women with no, some, or many pregnancy worries. Depressed mood and pregnancy-related worries were not associated with sedentary behaviour.

Conclusions: These findings suggest that in pregnant women who are obese, a depressed mood, but not pregnancy-related worries, may be associated with less physical activity. The combined risk of poor mental health and low physical activity levels makes women vulnerable for pregnancy complications. Whether a depressed mood may be a barrier for improving physical activity warrants further study.

Keywords: Exercise, Mental health, Pregnancy, Obesity

* Correspondence: mnm.vanpoppel@vumc.nl
[1]Department of Public and Occupational Health, EMGO+ Institute for Health and Care Research, VU University Medical Centre, Van der Boechorststraat 7, 1081BT Amsterdam, The Netherlands
[2]Institute for Sport Science, University of Graz, Graz, Austria
Full list of author information is available at the end of the article

Background

There is compelling evidence that physical activity during pregnancy is associated with fewer complications during pregnancy and delivery, lower chance of gestational diabetes (GDM), lower rates of hypertension [1–4], and better mental health status [5–8].

The American College of Obstetrics and Gynaecologists (ACOG) recommends pregnant women to be active in moderate intensity activities (3–5 metabolic equivalents) for at least 30 min on most, and preferably all, days of the week [9]. However, adherence to these recommendations appears to be low, with less than 50 % of all women meeting the ACOG recommendations pre-pregnancy and throughout pregnancy in the USA [4, 6, 10] and in the EU [11, 12].

With the growing number of overweight (body mass index (BMI) > 25 kg/m^2) and obese (BMI > 30 kg/m^2) women of reproductive age [13], obesity during pregnancy is becoming an increasing problem. Obesity in pregnancy increases the risk of excessive weight gain, and the risk of pregnancy-related complications, such as GDM [14]. In pregnant women who are overweight and obese, physical activity is of even greater importance, since it can help improve these pregnancy outcomes [4, 15, 16].

A better understanding of the factors related to low physical activity levels in pregnant women in general is required in order to maximize acceptability and efficacy of lifestyle interventions [17, 18]. One predictor of low physical activity levels that has been well studied outside of pregnancy is poor emotional well-being signifying depression [19–21]. People with depressive symptoms are likely to be less physically active [19]. Conversely, increasing physical activity can help to reduce depressive symptoms in previously inactive people [20]. Also in pregnancy, research suggests that low levels of physical activity are associated with poorer mental health (reviewed in [18]), but the evidence is less convincing. Studies had either a small sample size [2, 8, 22] or physical activity was measured with a (non-validated) diary or questionnaire [23]. Therefore, in this study we measured physical activity levels objectively in a larger study sample, in order to provide more accurate assessment of the relationship between physical activity and mental health.

In pregnant women who are overweight or obese, a poorer mental health status has been found compared to non-obese women [24, 25]. Feelings of humiliation and medicalization of being obese and pregnant appear to have a negative impact on women's mental health status [26]. In addition, stigma towards obese individuals may lead to a lower self-esteem and may negatively impact mental health [13, 26, 27]. Pregnancy may be experienced as a distressing period, leading to anxieties. Insecurity about the baby's health, possibility of miscarriage, and concerns about giving birth are especially reported in the first trimester [28]. Women who are depressed or anxious in pregnancy have a higher risk of adverse pregnancy or birth outcomes [29, 30].

Similar to other populations, obese pregnant women with poor mental health (i.e. depressed mood and pregnancy-related worries) might be less physically active, which may further increase their risk for adverse pregnancy outcomes [18]. Moreover, poor mental health may limit the effectiveness of physical activity interventions in obese pregnant women [31]. Therefore, the aim of this study is to examine the association between mental health status and objectively measured physical activity levels of obese pregnant women. For this purpose, we employed data from the European vitamin D and lifestyle intervention for gestational diabetes mellitus prevention (DALI) study. This allows insight into the association between mental health and physical activity in obese pregnant women throughout Europe.

Methods

Participants

For this study, baseline data from the DALI project (ISRCTN70595832) were used. Baseline data were collected between October 31, 2011 and April 30, 2013. The study design and data collection of the DALI project are described in detail elsewhere [32]. In summary, this project aims to identify the best available measures to prevent GDM in an ongoing pregnancy, and therefore a randomised controlled trial was conducted in nine European countries: the United Kingdom, Ireland, the Netherlands, Belgium, Poland, Italy, Spain, Austria, Denmark (2 study centres), with women from a diverse range of socio-economic and ethnic backgrounds. For all nine countries, the study design and procedures were approved by the Medical Ethics committee of the respective centres (Cambridge, United Kingdom: National Research Ethics Service, Norwich Research Ethics Committee; Galway, Ireland: Clinical Research Ethics Committee, Galway University Hospitals; Amsterdam, the Netherlands: Ethical Committee of the VU University Medical Center; Leuven, Belgium: Commissie Medische Ethiek van de Universitaire Ziekenhuizen KU Leuven; Poznan, Poland: Komisja Bioetyczna Przy Uniwersytecie Medycznym im. Karola Marcinkowskiego W Poznaniu; Padua, Italy: Il Comitato Etico per la Sperimentazione Clinica della Provincia di Padova; Barcelona, Spain: Comité Ético de Investigación Clínica de la Fundació de Gestió Sanitaria del Hospital de la Santa Creu i Sant Pau; Vienna, Austria: Ethik Kommission Medizinische Universität Wien;

Copenhagen and Odense, Denmark: De Videnskabsetiske Komiteer D for Region Hovedstaden). Participating hospitals and surrounding midwife, obstetrician and general practices were involved in recruitment. Women were followed for about 7 months (from 10 weeks of pregnancy until delivery). Pregnant women were included if aged 18 years and older, were less than 20 weeks pregnant, had a singleton pregnancy, and had a pre-pregnancy body mass index (BMI) ≥ 29 kg/m^2 based on self-reported weight and measured height. This BMI criterion was agreed upon following a review of local obesity prevalence to ensure all sites had the potential to recruit sufficient women. In a pilot study, the lifestyle interventions (diet and/or exercise) and measurement procedures were tested in each country. Although women who were diagnosed with GDM at baseline (using International Association of the Diabetes in Pregnancy Study Groups (IADPSG) criteria defined as fasting venous plasma glucose ≥ 5.1 mmol/l and/or 1 h glucose ≥10 mmol/l and/or 2 h glucose ≥ 8.5 mmol/l) [33] were excluded from the DALI intervention study, they were not excluded for analysis presented in this paper.

Measures

Physical activity

Physical activity was objectively measured with an Actigraph GT3X, GT1M or Actitrainer accelerometer (all three devices made by ActiGraph, Pensacola, Florida, USA). Previous validation studies found physical activity estimates from the three devices very comparable [34–36]. Although the GT3X is a tri-axial accelerometer, it was analysed from the vertical plane only to standardize activity estimates across the three accelerometers. All three accelerometers are lightweight devices with a sampling frequency of 60–80 (Hz). In this study we used a 1 min epoch. Accelerations derived from participant's movements were converted into counts per minute.

Participants were asked to wear the accelerometer from waking up until going to bed, attached to the right hip by an elastic waist belt, for at least 3 days. The Actigraph accelerometer has previously gained validity and reliability in free living conditions in adults for between 3 and 5 days [37]. The participants were asked to remove the accelerometer while swimming, showering or bathing. For non-wearing intervals, participants were instructed to write down in a diary how they spent their time.

Crude data were obtained using ActiLife 6 (ActiGraph, LLC, Pensacola, Florida, USA). Periods with no counts for at least 60 min were defined as non-wear time. Days with less than 480 min activity were labelled as invalid data and excluded for analysis [38]. Only women with data for at least three valid days were included [38]. Using the Freedson cut-off points [39], the number of minutes per day in light (100–1951 counts/min), moderate (1952–5724 counts/min) and vigorous (>5724 counts/min) activity were calculated as well as time spent sedentary (<100 counts/min). These cut-off points are widely used, also in pregnancy [7, 40]. Swimming time, recorded in the diary, was added to MVPA, based on the Ainsworth cut-off points [41], a procedure recommended by Esliger *et al.* [42]. For analysis, the time spent in moderate-to-vigorous activity (MVPA) minutes per day) and in sedentary behaviour (as proportion of total wear time) were used.

Mental health

Mental health was assessed based on questionnaire data. Questionnaires were administered in the main language of the site: English (UK and Ireland), Dutch (Netherlands and Belgium), Polish, Italian, Spanish, German (Austria) and Danish.

The WHO well-being index (WHO-5) was used to assess emotional well-being [43]. This uni-dimensional questionnaire contains five statements, describing positive moods (e.g. good spirits, relaxation). Each item was rated on a 6-point Likert scale, ranging from 0 ('at no time') to 5 ('all of the time') pertaining to the past 2 weeks. Total scores were calculated and standardized, ranging from 0 to 100. A total score of 50 or above was considered as good well-being, while a score below 50 indicated depressed mood. This is not a formal depression diagnosis but signifies likely depression [44]. Cronbach's alpha was 0.83 for all items. Validated versions of the WHO-5 were available for all the languages required in the study.

Pregnancy-related worries were measured with the Cambridge Worry Scale (CWS) [28]. The CWS has good reliability and validity in pregnant women, and overall a strong association with trait anxiety [28]. This 13-item scale assesses current concerns across four domains: social-medical, socio-economic, health and relationships. Responses were scored on a 6-point Likert-scale, ranging from 0 ('not a worry) to 5 ('major worry') for each item. Total scores (0–70) and domain scores (socio-medical 0–20, socio-economic 0–15, health 0–20 and relationships 0–10) were calculated, with higher scores indicating more worrying. There is no established clinical cut-off point. We stratified total scores into tertiles: no or few worries (score ≤ 13), some worries (score 14–25) and many worries (score ≥ 26). Cronbach's alpha was 0.86 for all items. Spearman correlation between WHO-5 and total CWS was 0.44. The CWS was only available in English and was translated into all the other languages (without back-translation).

Other variables

Socio-demographic information was collected at baseline, including age, country, ethnicity, household composition, education (highest completed level) and work status. In addition, aspects such as parity and lifestyle factors at baseline, (e.g. smoking (yes/no) and alcohol consumption (yes/no)) were assessed.

Pre-pregnancy weight in kilograms divided by height in squared meters (kg/m^2) was used to calculate Body Mass Index (BMI). Pre-pregnancy weight (kg) was based on self-report, while height was measured at baseline with a stadiometer (SECA 206). Objective height measurement was obtained with an accuracy to the nearest centimeter, and the average value of two measurements was used.

Furthermore, attitude, social support and self-efficacy outcome expectancies (based on the Health Action Process Approach (HAPA) model [45] regarding weight and physical activity management during pregnancy were measured. Women indicated the extent to which they agreed with eight items; each item on a 11-point Likert-scale, ranging from 0 ('not at all') to 10 ('very much'). One attitude item pertained to current weight and one attitude item pertained managing weight. Three items pertained to self-efficacy beliefs regarding weight and physical activity management; one item pertained to social support in physical activity and two items pertained to outcome expectancies regarding weight and physical activity management.

Statistical analysis

For all variables frequencies, means, and standard deviations were calculated. Median values were presented if a continuous variable was not normally distributed. To compare distribution of variables in the different mental health categories (good emotional well-being/depressed mood and tertiles for pregnancy worries), t-tests and one-way ANOVAs were performed for normally distributed variables, non-parametric tests for not-normally distributed variables, and chi-square tests for dichotomous variables.

To analyze the association between mental health and objective physical activity, linear regression analyses were performed for the WHO-5 well-being index (dichotomised) and the Cambridge Worry Scale (in tertiles) combined in the same model. In addition, associations with the proportion of wear time spent in sedentary behavior were assessed. To test the (possible) clustering effect within countries, multilevel analysis with a random intercept were performed. The country of recruitment and the individuals were the levels in the analyses. Because of the positively-skewed distribution of MVPA (min/day), a natural log transformation was executed for the linear regression analyses. Because of the log transformed dependent variable in the regression analyses, the exponent of the beta minus 1 represents the % of change in MVPA between mental health categories.

Interactions between mental health and age, ethnicity, prepregnancy BMI, smoking, alcohol consumption, and parity were assessed, by adding the interaction terms one by one to the regression model. However, none of the interaction terms was significant ($p < 0.05$).

Factors found to be associated with both mental health and physical activity in previous research were considered potential confounders (age, ethnicity, occupational status, household composition, prepregnancy BMI, smoking, alcohol consumption, gestational age, parity). All the variables were entered in the models one by one. Confounding was defined as a change in the regression coefficient of more than 10 % [46].

After controlling for confounding, the HAPA factors (attitude, self-efficacy, social support and outcome expectancy) were added to the models, in order to assess whether these factors confounded the association between mental health and MVPA and/or sedentary behavior. Significance level of the associations in the final model was set at *P*-value 0.05. The data were analysed using SPSS 20.0 (IBM Corporation, Armonk, NY, USA).

Results

A total of 258 women were measured at baseline and 132 of them wore an accelerometer (except in the UK and Denmark). Of those who wore accelerometers, 14 had no valid data for 3 days and 20 had software problems. These excluded women ($n = 34$) had a higher pre-pregnancy BMI (mean 40.6 kg/m^2; $P < 0.01$) and were further along in their pregnancies (16.8 weeks; $P = 0.03$).

Finally, 98 women with valid data were included in the analyses. The mean age was 31.6 ± 5.8 years and most were white/Caucasian (75.5 %) and had at least a secondary education (81.6 %) (Table 1). At baseline measurement, women were 15.4 ± 2.8 weeks pregnant. Just over a quarter (27.1 %) of the total sample ($n = 26$) had a depressed mood (WHO-5 score < 50). These women reported a significantly more positive attitude towards physical activity and scored lower on perceived social support ($P < 0.05$) (Table 1). In addition, women with a depressed mood had more pregnancy-related worries, both overall and for the specific domains ($P < 0.05$) (Table 1).

Physical activity levels are displayed in Table 2. On average, women wore the accelerometer for almost 13 h (773.8 min) per day, and were sedentary 62.3 % of that time. Fifty percent of the women spent fewer than 23 min (inter quartile range 12.3–35.7) in MVPA per day. Women with a good well-being were involved in MVPA approximately 24 min per day, while women with a depressed mood spent about 13 min per day in MVPA ($P < 0.05$). The time spent in MVPA did not differ between women with more pregnancy-related worries compared to women with less worries ($P = 0.74$).

Table 3 shows the results of the linear regression analyses for mental health in association with time spent in MVPA (minutes/day) and sedentary behaviour (proportion of total

Table 1 Baseline characteristics

Characteristic	Total sample (*n* = 98)	Depressed mood[a] (*n* = 26)	Good well-being[a] (*n* = 70)
Country (n)			
Spain	20	5	15
Austria	27	5	22
Belgium	16	7	9
Poland	10	4	6
Italy	1	0	1
Ireland	7	1	6
The Netherlands	17	5	12
Age (mean ± SD)	31.6 ± 5.8	30.6 ± 6.8	32.0 ± 5.5
Pre-pregnancy BMI (mean ± SD)	34.1 ± 4.3	35.0 ± 5.7	33.8 ± 3.7
Weeks of pregnancy (mean ± SD)	15.4 ± 2.8	15.8 ± 2.7	15.4 ± 2.9
Pregnant before (% yes)	54.2	53.8	54.4
Gestational diabetes mellitus (%)	13.5	19.2	11.4
Smoking behaviour (% yes)	10.3	19.2	7.2
Any alcohol consumption (% yes)	6.3	4.0	7.2
Ethnicity (% white/Caucasian)	75.5	61.5*	81.4*
Household composition (% living with partner)	85.3	76.0	88.2
Education (% ≥ vocational education)	81.6	84.6	80.0
Occupational status (%)			
Home duties	5.2	3.8	5.8
Unemployed/not able to work	17.5	19.2	17.4
Working (fulltime/part-time)/student	77.3	76.9	76.8
Perceptions and attitude[b] (median (IQR))			
Attitude to current weight	8.0 (6–9)	8.0 (6–10)	7.0 (6–9)
Attitude to physical activity	9.0 (7–10)	10.0 (8–10)*	8.0 (7–10)*
Self-efficacy	21.0 (17–24.)	21.0 (15–24)	21.0 (17–24)
Social support	8.0 (6–10)	7.0 (5–8)*	8.5 (6–10)*
Outcome expectancy	18.0 (15–20)	18.0 (17–20)	17.0 (14–20)
Cambridge Worry Scale (total 13 items) (median (IQR))	19.0 (11–28)	28.0 (20–40)**	15.0 (10–25)**
Cambridge Worry Scale dimensions (median (IQR))			
Social-medical	5.0 (2–10)	8.5 (4–12)*	4.0 (2–9)*
Socio-economic	4.0 (1–8)	7.5 (2–10)*	4.0 (1–6)*
Health	9.0 (5–12)	13.0 (9–15)**	7.0 (4–10)*
Relationships	0.0 (0–3)	4.0 (0–5)**	0.0 (0–1)**

* $P < 0.05$; differences between depressed mood and good well-being
** $P < 0.001$; differences between depressed mood and good well-being
[a]Data from WHO-5 were missing for 2 participants
[b]Based on the HAPA model

wear time). In the adjusted model, women with good well-being spent 70 % more minutes per day in MVPA compared women with a depressed mood ($P = 0.04$). Adding a random intercept for country did not (significantly) improve the model, and was therefore not included in the models. Adding HAPA factors (self-efficacy, attitude and social support) did not reduce the association between depressed mood and physical activity. In this model (model 2), women with good well-being spent 85 % more time in MVPA compared to women with depressed mood ($P = 0.03$) (Table 3). Pregnancy-related worries were not significantly associated with MVPA in

Table 2 Physical activity levels for total sample and stratified for the different categories of the WHO-5 well-being index and Cambridge Worry Scale

		Total	WHO-5 well-being index		Cambridge worry scale		
			Depressed mood	Good well-being	Many worries	Some worries	No or few worries
Minutes of wear time per day	mean (SD)	773.8 (91.1)	771.5 (92.6)	772.2 (91.0)	775.9 (92.7)	775.1 (93.2)	759.7 (83.7)
MVPA[a] minutes per day	median (IQR)	23.1 (12.3–35.7)	13.3* (8.6–30.0)	24.4* (13.1–38.4)	21.3 (10.8–30.3)	24.0 (12.2–40.8)	24.3 (14.1–35.1)
	Proportion of total wear time (%)	3.4 (2.8)	2.4* (2.1)	3.6* (2.8)	2.9 (1.9)	3.6 (3.1)	3.6 (3.0)
Sedentary behaviour[b] minutes per day	mean (SD)	484.2 (22.3)	506.2 (96.2)	479.0 (81.1)	477.0 (79.7)	495.3 (95.3)	485.8 (86.1)
	Proportion of total wear time (%)	62.3 (9.7)	65.1 (11.2)	61.7 (8.6)	61.5 (10.0)	63.3 (9.6)	63.4 (9.0)

*$P < 0.05$; differences between depressed mood and good well-being
[a]Moderate-to-vigorous activity (≥1952 counts per minute)
[b] < 100 counts per minute

crude or corrected models (Table 3), and neither aspects of mental health were associated with sedentary behaviour (Table 3).

Discussion

To the best of our knowledge, we are the first to have studied the associations between emotional well-being and pregnancy-related worries on the one hand, and physical activity, and sedentary behavior on the other, in obese pregnant women across different European countries. Results show that in obese pregnant women, 27 % had depressed mood and these women were significantly less involved in MVPA compared to women with a good well-being. Interestingly, pregnancy-related worries did not significantly impact MVPA levels.

The fact that we measured physical activity with an accelerometer that provides objective information about intensity and duration of different physical activity in daily life [47] is a strength of the study. Previous studies regarding the association between mental health and MVPA used physical activity questionnaires or diaries that have a low correlation with objective physical activity measurement [7, 8]. In addition, these studies were mostly performed in a normal-weighted pregnant population, while our study only included women with a higher BMI who may have worse mental health and lower MVPA levels [4, 5, 24]. Despite these methodological differences, our findings corroborate earlier observations suggesting that a depressed mood is a barrier to be active or to become more active [5, 31].

In our study we operationalized mental health along two dimensions: emotional well-being (depressed mood) and pregnancy-related worries, using validated questionnaires. In our population, 27.1 % of the women had a depressed mood, indicating likely depression, which is somewhat higher than found in Sweden by Claesson and colleagues, who reported around 18 % depression in obese women who were 15 weeks pregnant [48]. In a recent meta-analyses, the median prevalence of depressive symptoms in pregnant women who were obese was 33 %, compared to 22.6 % in normal-weight pregnant women [25]. Differences in depression prevalence may be attributed to case-mix or instruments used. For instance, in the study of Claesson *et al.* [48], fewer women smoked, more women lived together with a partner, and depressive symptoms were measured with the Edinburgh Postnatal Depression Scale [49].

The CWS, used to assess pregnancy-related worries, was found to be highly correlated with trait anxiety, and especially the cognitive element [28]. Our study shows no association with MVPA, suggesting that 'anxious thoughts' are not *per se* (linear) related to physical activity. This is in line with earlier findings [2, 8]. Anxious pregnant women may be more restless and nervous, which may lead to increased activity levels. On the other hand, women who have high concerns about the baby's health and miscarriages may limit their physical activity purposively [31]. The relationship may indeed be curvilinear. Exploring the association between (extreme high and low) anxiety and physical activity behavior in pregnancy may be a fruitful area for future research.

Correction for possible confounders in analyses with MVPA and mental health led in the first step only to correction for lifestyle factors (BMI smoking behaviour, alcohol consumption). Remarkably, no interference with socio-economic factors was found, while previous studies have identified these as important predictors of both mental health and exercise behaviour [7, 17, 50, 51]. A possible explanation for our different result may be that our sample was relatively well-educated and employed (81.6 % with at

Table 3 Linear regression analyses examining the relationship of mental health with moderate-to-vigorous activity (MVPA) (minutes/day) and sedentary behaviour (% of wear time)

Ln(MVPA)	Ratio	95 % CI	*p*-value
Crude model			
Good well-being vs depressed mood	1.72	0.99 – 2.99	0.06
Many worries (ref)	1.00		
Some worries	1.27	0.72 – 2.23	0.40
No or few worries	1.18	0.64 – 2.19	0.59
Model 1			
Good well-being vs depressed mood	**1.70**	**1.02 – 2.82**	**0.04**
Many worries (ref)	1.00		
Some worries	0.97	0.58 – 1.62	0.89
No or few worries	0.92	0.52 – 1.61	0.77
Model 2			
Good well-being vs depressed mood	**1.85**	**1.06 – 3.24**	**0.03**
Many worries (ref)	1.00		
Some worries	0.94	0.55 – 1.61	0.83
No or few worries	1.01	0.57 – 1.80	0.97
Sedentary behaviour	Difference	95 % CI	*p*-value
Crude model			
Good well-being vs depressed mood	−16.82	−60.76 – 27.13	0.45
Many worries (ref)	0		
Some worries	8.05	−35.78 – 51.89	0.72
No or few worries	−18.62	−66.52 – 29.27	0.44
Model 1			
Good well-being vs depressed mood	−18.94	−63.95 – 26.08	0.41
Many worries (ref)	0		
Some worries	4.88	−40.01 – 49.76	0.83
No or few worries	−16.17	−64.86 – 32.51	0.51
Model 2			
Good well-being vs depressed mood	−36.24	−85.07 – 12.60	0.14
Many worries (ref)	0		
Some worries	1.70	−43.34 – 46.74	0.94
No or few worries	−13.43	−62.25 – 35.39	0.59

Model 1: Corrected for BMI, smoking behaviour, and alcohol consumption
Model 2: Corrected for BMI, smoking behaviour, alcohol consumption, attitude weight, attitude physical activity, self-efficacy, social support and outcome expectancies
Bold font indicates statistically significant associations ($p < 0.05$).

least vocational education and 77.3 % had work) and were interested in participating in a lifestyle intervention study.

In a second step, all HAPA factors were added to the models. Although these factors led to some change in the effect estimate, this did not reduce the strength of the associations. The measured perceptions and attitudes, although interesting in their own right, did not explain the association between mental health and physical activity.

In our analyses we did not find a clustering effect between the European countries in the association. This may imply an Europe-wide homogeneity of the associations in obese pregnant women with different cultural background. An explanation for this finding is that included countries, albeit with different cultures, were all Western societies with highly similar attitudes towards weight and physical activity in pregnancy [13, 26]. Future studies in a more culturally heterogeneous sample may shed light on the issue of perceptions and stigmas around weight gain, physical activity and obesity in pregnancy.

Some limitations of our study should be acknowledged. We included women who consented to take part in the DALI study and are therefore likely to be motivated to change their physical activity behaviour compared to women who declined to participate. Selection bias may have led to an underestimation of the studied associations.

The use of accelerometer in (obese) pregnant women has been subject of discussion [52, 53]. Due to higher waist circumference and the abdominal shape of obese pregnant women, the accelerometer may change position and measurement may be less accurate. Nevertheless, measuring MVPA by accelerometry may be the best choice in an intervention that promotes physical activity in obese pregnant women [52]. In addition, the Freedson cut-off points were used to determine different activity levels. It is arguable if these cut-off points are adequate in our obese pregnant women, because no golden standard is available and optimal cut-off points may vary across populations [7, 52]. Another concern in our study was that there were some women ($n = 34$) with not enough valid data or software problems. Additional limitations are that no data on prepregnancy physical activity or mental health were available, no data on pregnancy-related symptoms such as nausea, and that prepregnancy BMI was based on self-reported data. Furthermore, the study had a relative small sample size, and was imbalanced, in addition, with only 26 women with depressed mood.

Of course we need to be cautious in interpreting our data, as they are cross-sectional and we cannot exclude reversed causality. Low levels of physical activity may induce or maintain depressed mood and increase pregnancy-related worries. Future studies should aim to assess the association between mental health status and MVPA longitudinally and determine the causal relationship. Because worries and emotional well-being may vary over time, and physical activity levels may decrease with progressing pregnancy, associations may also change.

Conclusion

Although women with good well-being spent significantly more minutes in MVPA than those who with a depressed mood, still in our sample only 29.6 % of the women complied with the recommendations of MVPA for least 30 min per day. There is ample room for improvement in the total population of pregnant women who are obese. This is exactly the purpose of the DALI study, where pregnant women are offered lifestyle counselling based on principles of motivational interviewing [32].

However, for pregnant women who are obese and have a depressed mood there is a stronger need for improving physical activity behaviour. The combined risk of having poor mental health, obesity and low physical activity levels makes this group extra vulnerable for pregnancy complications. The short WHO-5 might be a suitable instrument for screening in clinical practice. Whether a lifestyle intervention is similarly effective in women with good well-being and those with a depressed mood remains to be seen. Possibly, poor mental health is a barrier for improving lifestyle. Therefore, longitudinal analyses of the association of mental health and changes in physical activity after lifestyle intervention are warranted. However, based on our findings there is a need for focused efforts for the promotion of physical activity among obese pregnant women with at-risk levels of depressive mood.

Competing interest

The authors declare that they have no competing interests.

Authors' contributions

JJ contributed to the analysis of the questionnaire and writing of the manuscript and took the lead in redrafting the script following editorial review. DS contributed to the data collection in the UK. RC and JA contributed to the data collection in Spain. JH and AK contributed to the data collection in Austria. AA, RD, DT contributed to the data collection in Belgium. PD and EM contributed to the data collection in Denmark. EWO and AZ contributed to the data collection in Poland. AL, MDG, SP, AB contributed to the data collection in Italy. FD contributed to the data collection in Ireland. AB, FS and MvP contributed to the conception and design of the study and reviewed the manuscript. DS, GD, RC, AK, DH, EM, PD, PR, AL, FD, DJ and LA have made substantial revisions to the draft manuscript. All of the authors have read and approved the final manuscript.

Acknowledgments

We are deeply grateful to the participants who participated in this study.

Financial support

The research leading to these results has received funding from the European Community's 7th Framework Programme (FP7/2007-2013) under Grant Agreement no 242187 and from The Netherlands Organization for Health Research and Development (ZonMw), grant number:200310013.

Author details

[1]Department of Public and Occupational Health, EMGO+ Institute for Health and Care Research, VU University Medical Centre, Van der Boechorststraat 7, 1081BT Amsterdam, The Netherlands. [2]Institute for Sport Science, University of Graz, Graz, Austria. [3]Department of Healthcare Research, PHL University College, Limburg Catholic University College, Hasselt, Belgium. [4]Institute of Metabolic Science, Addenbrookes Hospital, Cambridge, UK. [5]Department of Obstetrics and Gynecology, Medizinische Universität Graz, Graz, Austria. [6]Institut de Recerca de L'Hospital de la Santa Creu i Sant Pau, Barcelona, Spain. [7]CIBER Bioengineering, Biomaterials and Nanotechnology, Instituto de Salud Carlos III, Madrid, Spain. [8]Medical University of Vienna, Vienna City, Austria. [9]KU Leuven Department of Development and Regeneration: Pregnancy, Fetus and Neonate, Gynaecology and Obstetrics, University Hospitals Leuven, Leuven, Belgium. [10]Recherche en Santé Lawson SA, Bronschhofen, Switzerland. [11]University Hospital of Copenhagen - Rigshospitalet, Copenhagen, Denmark. [12]Akademia Medyczna im Karola Marcinkowskiego, Poznan, Poland. [13]BAP Health Outcomes Research SL, Oviedo, Spain. [14]Universita Degli Studi di Padova, Padova, Italy. [15]Università di Pisa, Pisa, Italy. [16]National University of Ireland, Galway, Ireland. [17]Odense University Hospital, Odense, Denmark. [18]Department of Medical Psychology, EMGO+ Institute for Health and Care Research, VU University Medical Centre, Amsterdam, The Netherlands. [19]Department of Medical Psychology, Academic Medical Centre, Amsterdam, The Netherlands.

References

1. Han S, Middleton P, Crowther CA. Exercise for pregnant women for preventing gestational diabetes mellitus. Cochrane Database Syst Rev. 2012;7, CD009021.
2. Goodwin A, Astbury J, McMeeken J. Body image and psychological well-being in pregnancy. A comparison of exercisers and non-exercisers. Aust N Z J Obstet Gynaecol. 2000;40:442–7.
3. Artal R. Exercise: the alternative therapeutic intervention for gestational diabetes. Clin Obstet Gynecol. 2003;46:479–87.
4. Dye TD, Knox KL, Artal R, Aubry RH, Wojtowycz MA. Physical activity, obesity, and diabetes in pregnancy. Am J Epidemiol. 1997;146:961–5.

5. Claesson IM, Klein S, Sydsjo G, Josefsson A. Physical activity and psychological well-being in obese pregnant and postpartum women attending a weight-gain restriction programme. Midwifery. 2014;30:11–6.
6. Downs DS, DiNallo JM, Kirner TL. Determinants of pregnancy and postpartum depression: prospective influences of depressive symptoms, body image satisfaction, and exercise behavior. Ann Behav Med. 2008;36:54–63.
7. Demissie Z, Siega-Riz AM, Evenson KR, Herring AH, Dole N, Gaynes BN. Physical activity and depressive symptoms among pregnant women: the PIN3 study. Arch Womens Ment Health. 2011;14:145–57.
8. Poudevigne MS, O'Connor PJ. Physical activity and mood during pregnancy. Med Sci Sports Exerc. 2005;37:1374–80.
9. Artal R, O'Toole M. Guidelines of the American College of Obstetricians and Gynecologists for exercise during pregnancy and the postpartum period. Br J Sports Med. 2003;37:6–12.
10. Petersen AM, Leet TL, Brownson RC. Correlates of physical activity among pregnant women in the United States. Med Sci Sports Exerc. 2005;37:1748–53.
11. Althuizen E, van Poppel MN, Seidell JC, van Mechelen W. Correlates of absolute and excessive weight gain during pregnancy. J Womens Health (Larchmt). 2009;18:1559–66.
12. Amezcua-Prieto C, Olmedo-Requena R, Jimenez-Mejias E, Hurtado-Sanchez F, Mozas-Moreno J, Lardelli-Claret P, et al. Changes in leisure time physical activity during pregnancy compared to the prior year. Matern Child Health J. 2013;17:632–8.
13. Kulie T, Slattengren A, Redmer J, Counts H, Eglash A, Schrager S. Obesity and women's health: an evidence-based review. J Am Board Fam Med. 2011;24:75–85.
14. Heslehurst N, Simpson H, Ells LJ, Rankin J, Wilkinson J, Lang R, et al. The impact of maternal BMI status on pregnancy outcomes with immediate short-term obstetric resource implications: a meta-analysis. Obes Rev. 2008;9:635–83.
15. Stuebe AM, Oken E, Gillman MW. Associations of diet and physical activity during pregnancy with risk for excessive gestational weight gain. Am J Obstet Gynecol. 2009;201:58.
16. Tobias DK, Zhang C, van Dam RM, Bowers K, Hu FB. Physical activity before and during pregnancy and risk of gestational diabetes mellitus: a meta-analysis. Diabetes Care. 2011;34:223–9.
17. Weir Z, Bush J, Robson SC, McParlin C, Rankin J, Bell R. Physical activity in pregnancy: a qualitative study of the beliefs of overweight and obese pregnant women. BMC Pregnancy Childbirth. 2010;10:18.
18. Poudevigne MS, O'Connor PJ. A review of physical activity patterns in pregnant women and their relationship to psychological health. Sports Med. 2006;36:19–38.
19. van Gool CH, Kempen GI, Bosma H, van Boxtel MP, Jolles J, van Eijk JT. Associations between lifestyle and depressed mood: longitudinal results from the Maastricht aging study. Am J Public Health. 2007;97:887–94.
20. Penedo FJ, Dahn JR. Exercise and well-being: a review of mental and physical health benefits associated with physical activity. Curr Opin Psychiatry. 2005;18:189–93.
21. Cooney GM, Dwan K, Greig CA, Lawlor DA, Rimer J, Waugh FR, et al. Exercise for depression. Cochrane Database Syst Rev. 2013;9, CD004366.
22. Williams A, Reilly T, Campbell I, Sutherst J. Investigation of changes in responses to exercise and in mood during pregnancy. Ergonomics. 1988;31:1539–49.
23. Da Costa D, Rippen N, Dritsa M, Ring A. Self-reported leisure-time physical activity during pregnancy and relationship to psychological well-being. J Psychosom Obstet Gynaecol. 2003;24:111–9.
24. Amador N, Juarez JM, Guizar JM, Linares B. Quality of life in obese pregnant women: a longitudinal study. Am J Obstet Gynecol. 2008;198:203–5.
25. Molyneaux E, Poston L, Ashurst-Williams S, Howard LM. Obesity and mental disorders during pregnancy and postpartum: a systematic review and meta-analysis. Obstet Gynecol. 2014;123:857–67.
26. Furber CM, McGowan L. A qualitative study of the experiences of women who are obese and pregnant in the UK. Midwifery. 2011;27:437–44.
27. Rohrer JE, Rohland BM. Psychosocial risk factors for obesity among women in a family planning clinic. BMC Fam Pract. 2004;5:20.
28. Green JM, Kafetsios K, Statham HE, Snowdon CM. Factor structure, validity and reliability of the Cambridge Worry Scale in a pregnant population. J Health Psychol. 2003;8:753–64.
29. Field T, Diego M, Hernandez-Reif M. Prenatal depression effects and interventions: a review. Infant Behav Dev. 2010;33:409–18.
30. Alder J, Fink N, Bitzer J, Hosli I, Holzgreve W. Depression and anxiety during pregnancy: a risk factor for obstetric, fetal and neonatal outcome? A critical review of the literature. J Matern Fetal Neonatal Med. 2007;20:189–209.
31. Hegaard HK, Kjaergaard H, Damm PP, Petersson K, Dykes AK. Experiences of physical activity during pregnancy in Danish nulliparous women with a physically active life before pregnancy. A qualitative study. BMC Pregnancy Childbirth. 2010;10:33.
32. Jelsma JG, van Poppel MN, Galjaard S, Desoye G, Corcoy R, Devlieger R, et al. DALI: Vitamin D and lifestyle intervention for gestational diabetes mellitus (GDM) prevention: an European multicentre, randomised trial - study protocol. BMC Pregnancy Childbirth. 2013;13:142.
33. Metzger BE, Gabbe SG, Persson B, Buchanan TA, Catalano PA, Damm P, et al. International association of diabetes and pregnancy study groups recommendations on the diagnosis and classification of hyperglycemia in pregnancy. Diabetes Care. 2010;33:676–82.
34. Lee KY, Macfarlane DJ, Cerin E. Comparison of three models of actigraph accelerometers during free living and controlled laboratory conditions. Eur J Sport Sci. 2013;13:332–9.
35. Sasaki JE, John D, Freedson PS. Validation and comparison of ActiGraph activity monitors. J Sci Med Sport. 2011;14:411–6.
36. Kelly LA, McMillan DG, Anderson A, Fippinger M, Fillerup G, Rider J. Validity of actigraphs uniaxial and triaxial accelerometers for assessment of physical activity in adults in laboratory conditions. BMC Med Phys. 2013;13:5.
37. Trost SG, McIver KL, Pate RR. Conducting accelerometer-based activity assessments in field-based research. Med Sci Sports Exerc. 2005;37:S531–43.
38. Evenson KR, Terry Jr JW. Assessment of differing definitions of accelerometer nonwear time. Res Q Exerc Sport. 2009;80:355–62.
39. Freedson PS, Melanson E, Sirard J. Calibration of the Computer Science and Applications, Inc. accelerometer. Med Sci Sports Exerc. 1998;30:777–81.
40. McParlin C, Robson SC, Tennant PW, Besson H, Rankin J, Adamson AJ, et al. Objectively measured physical activity during pregnancy: a study in obese and overweight women. BMC Pregnancy Childbirth. 2010;10:76.
41. Ainsworth BE, Haskell WL, Herrmann SD, Meckes N, Bassett Jr DR, Tudor-Locke C, et al. Compendium of physical activities: a second update of codes and MET values. Med Sci Sports Exerc. 2011;2011(43):1575–81.
42. Esliger DW, Copeland JL, Barnes JD, Tremblay MS. Standardizing and optimizing the use of accelerometer data for free-living physical activity monitoring. J Phys Act Health. 2005;3:366–83.
43. Lowe B, Spitzer RL, Grafe K, Kroenke K, Quenter A, Zipfel S, et al. Comparative validity of three screening questionnaires for DSM-IV depressive disorders and physicians' diagnoses. J Affect Disord. 2004;78:131–40.
44. Hajos TR, Pouwer F, Skovlund SE, Den Oudsten BL, Geelhoed-Duijvestijn PH, Tack CJ, et al. Psychometric and screening properties of the WHO-5 well-being index in adult outpatients with Type 1 or Type 2 diabetes mellitus. Diabet Med. 2013;30:e63–9.
45. Schwarzer R, Lippke S, Luszczynska A. Mechanisms of health behavior change in persons with chronic illness or disability: the Health Action Process Approach (HAPA). Rehabil Psychol. 2011;56:161–70.
46. McNamee R. Confounding and confounders. Occup Environ Med. 2003;60:227–34.
47. Plasqui G, Bonomi AG, Westerterp KR. Daily physical activity assessment with accelerometers: new insights and validation studies. Obes Rev. 2013;14:451–62.
48. Claesson IM, Josefsson A, Sydsjo G. Prevalence of anxiety and depressive symptoms among obese pregnant and postpartum women: an intervention study. BMC Public Health. 2010;10:766.
49. Cox JL, Holden JM, Sagovsky R. Detection of postnatal depression. Development of the 10-item Edinburgh Postnatal Depression Scale. Br J Psychiatry. 1987;150:782–6.
50. Pottinger AM, Trotman-Edwards H, Younger N. Detecting depression during pregnancy and associated lifestyle practices and concerns among women in a hospital-based obstetric clinic in Jamaica. Gen Hosp Psychiatry. 2009;31:254–61.
51. Foxcroft KF, Rowlands IJ, Byrne NM, McIntyre HD, Callaway LK. Exercise in obese pregnant women: the role of social factors, lifestyle and pregnancy symptoms. BMC Pregnancy Childbirth. 2011;11:4.

17

Psychological antecedents of excess gestational weight gain

Mufiza Zia Kapadia[1], Anca Gaston[2], Sherry Van Blyderveen[3], Louis Schmidt[4], Joseph Beyene[5], Helen McDonald[6] and Sarah D McDonald[7*]

Abstract

Background: Excess gestational weight gain (GWG), which has reached epidemic proportions, is associated with adverse outcomes during pregnancy and postpartum obesity in women and children. Psychological variables represent potentially modifiable factors. Moreover, previous systematic reviews on GWG interventions have called for the need for a clearer understanding of psychological factors affecting GWG. Hence, a systematic review was conducted to summarize the relation between psychological factors and GWG.

Methods: Eight databases were searched, and the guidelines on Preferred Reporting Items for Systematic Reviews and Meta-Analyses were followed. Methodological quality of the included studies was assessed using a modified Newcastle-Ottawa scale. Two assessors independently reviewed titles, abstracts and full articles, extracted data and assessed quality.

Results: A total of 6198 titles and abstracts were reviewed of which 90 full text articles were retrieved. Thirty-five studies (25 cohort, eight cross-sectional and two case–control) met the inclusion criteria, assessing 26 different psychological constructs in affect, cognitions and personality. Negative affective states such as depression, anxiety and stress were not related to excess GWG. Among weight-related and dietary-related cognitions, risk factors for excess GWG included concern about weight gain, negative body image and attitude towards weight gain, inaccurate perceptions regarding weight, higher than recommended target weight gain, less knowledge about weight gain, higher levels of cognitive dietary restraint, and perceived barriers to healthy eating. Protective factors included an internal locus of control for weight gain, lower than recommended target weight gain and higher self-efficacy for healthy eating. Only one study examined the relation between personality and excess GWG.

Conclusion: In this systematic review, a number of cognitive factors were identified that were associated with excess GWG. To address excess GWG, more high quality, adequately powered studies are required examining cognitions, motivation and personality factors.

Keywords: Psychological factors, Pregnancy, Weight gain, Systematic review

Background

Excess gestational weight gain (GWG) i.e., weight gain above that recommended Institute of Medicine (IOM) guidelines [1] occurs in half or more of women in many populations [2-6]. Excess GWG significantly increases the risks of serious maternal pregnancy complications such as gestational diabetes mellitus, gestational hypertension and caesarean section [1]. Excess GWG is also associated with an increased risk of obesity in mothers during the postpartum [7,8]. Some, but not all women who are overweight or obese have excess GWG [9]. Neonates born to women who have excess GWG are at risk of being born large for gestational age [10,11]. Being born large increases risks to the infants' health, both immediately after birth, (including seizure, hypoglycemia, polycythemia, and meconium aspiration [11]) and in the long term (including adiposity [12]). Thus, a cycle of obesity can be transmitted across generations.

* Correspondence: mcdonals@mcmaster.ca
[7]Division of Maternal-Fetal Medicine, Departments of Obstetrics & Gynecology, Radiology, and Clinical Epidemiology & Biostatistics, McMaster University, 1280 Main Street West, room 3N52B, Hamilton, Ontario L8S 4K1, Canada

To combat the immediate and long-term adverse outcomes associated with excess GWG, guidelines on GWG were published in 1990 by the US Institute of Medicine (IOM) [13], and updated in 2009 [1]. These guidelines were also adopted by other countries such as Canada and Finland [14]. Given that a high proportion of women gain above the recommendations, achieving a better understanding of factors related to excess GWG is a public health priority.

In contrast to biological or demographic determinants of excess GWG such as age, parity, ethnicity, or socioeconomic status, psychological variables represent potentially modifiable factors during pregnancy. Moreover, previous systematic reviews on GWG interventions have called for the need for a clearer understanding of psychological factors affecting weight gain. For example, Gardner highlighted a need to measure psychological mechanisms underpinning behavior change [15]. Kramer and colleagues suggested that whereas dietary modifications during pregnancy lowered GWG [16], interventions that focused on increasing physical activity through aerobic exercise were ineffective in reducing GWG [17]. These conclusions suggest that dietary modifications are critical in a pathway of behavioral modifications to GWG. These findings are further supported by systematic reviews of clinical trials that suggest that physical activity plus dietary interventions [18,19] are most effective in reducing GWG. One of those systematic reviews [18] found no effect on GWG with supervised physical activity *alone*. These findings further strengthen the key role of dietary interventions in reducing total GWG [20]. Skouteris and colleagues recommended that it was important to focus on the *antecedents* of psychological behavior which have previously not been targeted in interventions [21]. The authors particularly noted that psychological factors such as *affect* (feelings and emotional reactions to an occurrence [22-24]), and *cognitive factors* (thoughts and beliefs about the occurrence [22-24]) such as body image concerns, self-efficacy about making behavioral changes, and motivation might impede behavioral changes, and should therefore be targeted along with behavioral changes. Outside of pregnancy, another systematic review found one broad element of the Five Factor Model of personality, conscientiousness, was important. Moreover, this study suggested the need for future studies to examine lower level personality facets in relation to obesity prevention and treatment strategies [25]. A recent large cohort of young adults found that the effect sizes of various personality traits were on par with other well-established health risk factors such as socioeconomic status and smoking at predicting poor health in midlife [26]. Other research demonstrated that the magnitude of the effect of personality traits on mortality was similar to that of socioeconomic status [27]. Personality's role in preventive health care was deemed so pivotal that the American Psychological Association issued a recent Press Release entitled "Personality May be Key Risk Factor in Preventive Health Care" [28].

To date, there appears to be no systematic review that has addressed the relation between these psychological antecedents of pregnancy behavior and excess GWG. As a result, little is known about the psychological protective and risk factors associated with excess GWG. Hence, the aim of this systematic review was to provide a summary of the available evidence examining psychological antecedents of excess GWG, investigating three broad psychological domains, namely, *affect, cognitions* (related to dietary behavior, weight gain, or physical activity) and *personality.*

Methods

A systematic review of the literature was carried out in accordance with PRISMA (Preferred Reporting Items for Systematic Reviews and Meta-Analyses) [29] and Cochrane Handbook for Systematic Reviews of Interventions [30]. Separate, specific electronic searches were created with the aid of experienced reference librarians specializing in health sciences and psychology and conducted in the following databases from their inception (dates included wherever available in the databases) until May 3, 2013: Medline (1946 to 21 Jan 2015), EMBASE (1974 to 21 Jan 2015), PsychINFO (1806 to 21 Jan 2015), Cochrane Register, CINHAL, Web of Knowledge, Sociological Abstract, and Dissertation and Thesis (see Supporting information in Additional file 1 for the search strategies developed in the eight databases). Since it was a systematic review and did not directly involve human subjects, ethical approval was not required.

Study inclusion criteria

Study design

The following study designs were included: randomised controlled trials, cross-sectional studies, case–control studies and cohort studies. Reviews, editorials and opinion articles were excluded, since they did not contain primary data. Studies published as abstracts only (e.g., conference proceedings) were excluded, since their quality could not be adequately assessed. Duplicate or secondary publications on the same exposure in the same population were excluded to avoid multiple publication bias. There were no language restrictions.

Participants

Studies were restricted to women who were pregnant with a singleton or if recently postpartum, had already delivered a singleton.

Independent variables (exposures)

Studies were included if one or more of the psychological constructs, falling under the broad headings of *affect, cognitions* (related to dietary behavior, weight gain, or physical activity) or *personality* were assessed as exposure variables (Table 1). (However, examination of constructs related to physical activity are labeled 'post hoc' for transparency' sake, as a secondary objective, since they were added after the the initial development of the objectives and search strategy.) Studies that focused on the association between psychiatric disorders and GWG were excluded: We excluded studies that focused on a psychiatric diagnosis such as Major Depressive Disorder or a formal diagnosis of anxiety disorder, defined according to psychiatric criteria. We did this in two ways: Firstly, the Medical Subject Headings (MeSH) terms we used were designed to identify less severe forms of depression and anxiety, i.e. depressive and anxiety states of "mild to moderate" intensity. These terms we selected were in contrast to major depression or major anxiety. Secondly, when we screened the articles, we excluded ones focusing on major depression or anxiety.

Table 1 Psychological concepts covered in systematic review of psychological antecedents of excess gestational weight gain[$]

Psychological construct	Themes[$$]
1. Affect	Stress
	Distress
	Adaptation/coping behavior
	Depression
	Anxiety
	Mood/Affect
	Emotions/Feelings
2. Cognitions	
Related to weight gain	Self-esteem
	Self-efficacy
	Locus of control
	Body image
	Attitude
	Motivation
Related to dietary behavior	Eating attitudes
	Feeding behavior
	Knowledge
Personality	Personality traits related to Five Factor Model and Eysenck's personality model
	Resilience
	Impulsivity

[$]Search strategies related to these psychological constructs are provided in supporting information Additional file 1.
[$$]Studies were excluded if they measured a psychiatric disorder.

Outcome measures

Primary outcomes Studies were included if they had one or more of the following categorical outcomes of interest: total GWG in excess of the guidelines (i.e., weight gain above the recommended Institute of Medicine (IOM) guideline of 1990 [13] or 2009 [1]; rate of GWG (mean range of weight gain per week) above the IOM guidelines; or high adequacy ratio of GWG (expressed as the ratio of observed/expected total weight gain) above the IOM guidelines. *Secondary outcome:* Studies which defined GWG as a continuous outcome (as total GWG, either with or without reference a pre-pregnancy BMI) were included as secondary outcomes.

Study selection process

Two reviewers independently assessed the titles and abstracts of all identified citations (MZK and AG). Full-text articles were retrieved if either reviewer considered the citation potentially relevant with a low threshold for retrieval. The bibliographies of studies included for full-text review were also checked for additional relevant references. Inter-reviewer agreement for decision for full text review was assessed using an un-weighted kappa statistic. The final set of studies which was included in the systematic review was determined by consensus (between MZK and AG) with any disagreements resolved by the third reviewer (SDM).

Assessment of risk of bias

The methodological quality of the studies was assessed using a modified version of the Newcastle-Ottawa Scale [31]. The Newcastle-Ottawa Scale is comprised of three categories: 'Selection,' 'Comparability,' and 'Outcome' for cohort studies, and 'Selection,' 'Comparability,' and 'Exposure' for case control studies. Within the category of 'Selection,' one item was excluded for cohort studies and one item was excluded for case–control studies, namely 'Demonstration that outcome of interest was not present at start of study' and 'Definition of controls: no history of disease (endpoint),' respectively. These items were not relevant in the context of the present systematic review since our outcome of interest, GWG, could not have been present at the time of recruitment. To ensure the proper ascertainment of psychological constructs, the use of validated psychological scales was deemed to be important, hence the regular Newcastle-Ottawa Scale scoring items 'ascertainment of exposure' under the category of 'Selection' in cohort studies and 'Exposure' in case–control cohort studies were replaced with the following items: '≥50% of the tool(s) are stated /known validated' or '≥50% of the tool(s) are validated, but modified.' One point was awarded for ascertainment of exposure resulting in a maximum score of three points for 'Selection.'

With respect to criteria related to 'Comparability,' it was decided *a priori* that studies would receive one point if they controlled for pre-pregnancy BMI, as this is a key determinant of excess GWG [1]. Studies were given an additional point if they controlled for one or more of the following five potential confounders: age, parity, income, education or race. In evaluating the outcome, to be awarded points we required: that weight be measured objectively not self-reported, that there be sufficient duration of follow-up (we required that total GWG be evaluated at 37 weeks or beyond , the time frame which is considered 'term') and that there be complete or near complete (>90%) follow-up. In total, our modified Newcastle-Ottawa Scale awarded up to eight points. As there is no validation study that provides a cut off score for rating low quality studies, a cut off of less than 5 was used to consider a study as 'low quality' in this review. However, the studies were not excluded from the analysis in order to avoid publication bias based on their quality and because there is no validated NOS cut-off for excluding studies.

In addition, power was assessed by applying the general rule that regression models require a minimum of 10 events per predictor variable [32]. In cases where the number of variables entered into the model could not be determined, the study was categorized as 'unable to determine power.' For studies that performed only univariate analyses, a Bonferroni correction for multiple comparisons was applied, by dividing the *p*-value (α) of the test by the number of comparisons made in the study [33]. If the *p*-value for any given comparison was greater than the newly calculated *p*-value, then the study was classified as under-powered.

Thus, overall study quality was assessed through both the modified Newcastle-Ottawa Scale and the aforementioned power assessment, and is presented in the results. For exposures that were examined by five or more studies, we planned to assess publication bias with a funnel plot.

Data abstraction

To ensure consistency, an electronic data abstraction form was developed and subsequently piloted by three reviewers (MZK, AG, SDM) on one study [34]. For the remaining studies, two reviewers (MZK and AG) independently abstracted all available data. The following information was extracted from the included studies: date of publication, design, years the study was conducted, setting, population, inclusion/exclusion criteria, study outcomes, psychological scales/instruments, the timing of assessment of psychological exposure during gestation, and the results. Inconsistencies were checked and resolved through the consensus process described above.

Data synthesis

Data were not pooled for several reasons: Firstly, even when multiple studies examining the same exposure were available, different scales or, in some cases modified versions of the same scale, were often used. Secondly, some of the studies did not present an effect estimate, exact *p*-value, or sufficient data for it to be calculated, and instead only reported the presence and direction of an association. Thirdly, it was decided *a priori* that when available the results of a multivariate analysis would be preferentially reported. Lastly, some studies only reported effect estimates for a few items within a scale, or for subscales, and the effect estimates were not comparable across different studies.

Forest plots were generated in Revman 5.2 (Copenhagen, Denmark) to visually represent the magnitude and direction of the association of each exposure with the primary outcome. However, the pooled effect estimates were not reported in the forest plots due to the heterogeneity of the data. Instead two additional methods were used to visually represent our findings, which we have termed a pinwheel and a web plot. For the pinwheel, the center was divided into three main psychological constructs outlined in Table 1, namely affect, cognitions and personality and direction of association were shown through color coded boxes, each box representing an individual study.

Results

Our initial searches of the eight databases yielded 6198 records (Figure 1). After removal of duplicates (n = 1853), 4345 studies remained and were assessed based on titles and abstracts. Based on our screening criteria, 86 papers were selected for full-text review. Four additional papers were found through perusal of reference lists of full text of the included studies. A total of 35 studies [2,9,34-66] met inclusion criteria. The un-weighted κ for initial agreements on full study inclusion between two reviewers was 0.973. Twenty seven studies [2,9,35-38,40-43,45,46,48-59,61-63] reported our primary outcome of interest i.e., excess GWG as a categorical outcome.

Study characteristics

Baseline information on 25 cohort studies, eight cross-sectional studies and two case–control studies are presented in Tables 2 and 3. None of the included papers were in the format of RCTs (although a few secondary analyses of RCTs were included, the data in these instances were in the format of cohort studies). The majority of studies were from the United States (n = 26) and the remaining studies were from the United Kingdom [38], Canada [54,61], Australia [42,62,64], Japan [47], China [65] and Iran [35]. All of the included studies were in English. A total of 18,828 women were included, and study sizes ranged from 46 to 4528 participants. Study

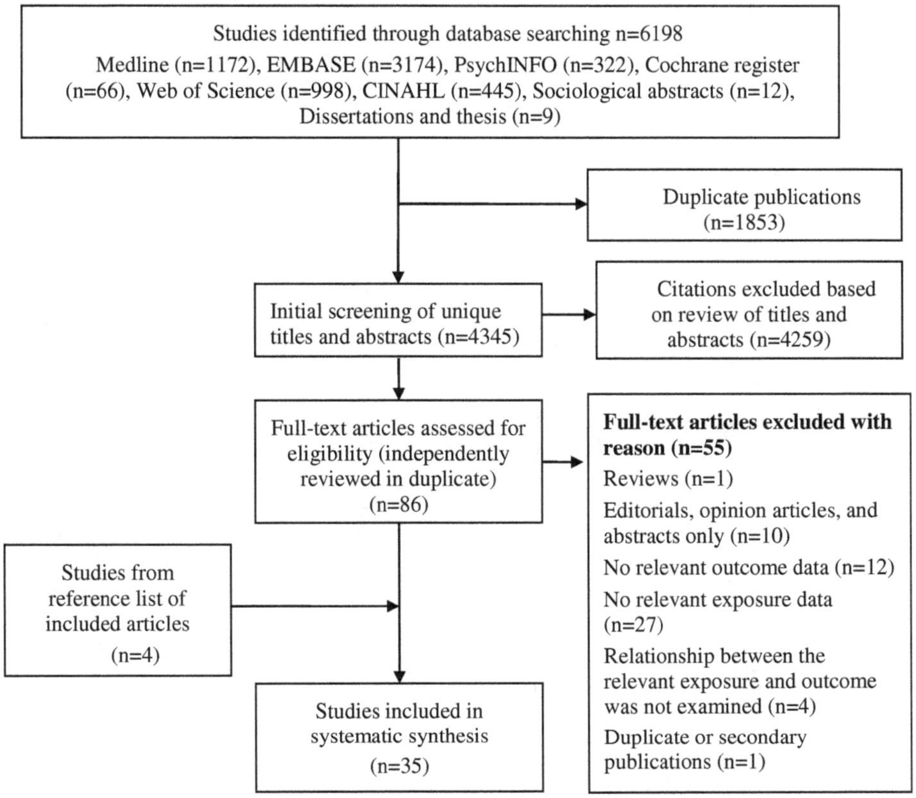

Figure 1 Flow diagram of study selection process in systematic review of psychological antecedents of excess gestational weight gain.

populations included women from most often drawn from the general population, although a few focused on specific populations (particular ethnic groups:2 studies, adolescents: 2 studies and low income populations:2 studies). There were several publications from the same cohort but they examined different psychological exposures with excess GWG: four studies examined the Pregnancy, Infection and Nutrition (PIN) cohort [2,43,46,48], two studies examined Rochester Study of Adolescent Pregnancy cohort [45,52] and two studies examined data collected as part of the ongoing Pregnancy Risk Assessment Monitoring System (PRAMS) [56,58]. The timing of assessments of exposure varied widely between the studies. Most studies assessed exposures in second trimester [2,34,36,38,39,41,42, 45-50,52-55,59,60,62,64,66], however, some studies assessed exposures in third trimester [9,35,37,40,43,44,61,62,65] or retrospectively during the immediate postpartum period [51,56-58]. The psychological scales used in the ascertainment of exposure are described in Additional file 1: Table S1.

Quality assessment

Cohort studies

A detailed breakdown of the quality evaluation of the 29 included studies [2,9,34,36,37,39,41-50,52-55,57-60,62-66] is provided in supplementary information Additional file 1: Table S2. Four studies [44,50,54,58] had a score less than five. Women were generally representative of an average pregnant population in the community. In nine studies [37,41,44,47,54,58,59,63,65], fewer than half of the scales for the ascertainment of exposure were validated. The non-exposed cohort was almost always drawn from the same population. Follow-up was generally adequate in duration. Twenty-one studies [2,34-44,47,48,50,51,53-58, 62,64-66] had a loss of 10% or greater at follow-up (or an unclear proportion), although the follow-up ranged from 48% to 95%. Eight studies were assessed as underpowered [36,42,50,52-54,57,59], and in two, the power could not be determined [2,62].

Case–control and cross-sectional studies

Detailed breakdown of quality evaluation of the six included studies [35,38,40,51,56,61] according to the modified Newcastle-Ottawa Scale for case–control studies is provided in supplementary information Additional file 1: Table S3. Two studies [38,40] had a score less than five. Only one study did not adjust for important confounders [38]. Five studies did not provide sufficient details about the response rate [35,40,51,56,61]. Two studies were underpowered [38,40].

Table 2 Characteristics of included cohort studies in systematic review of psychological antecedents of excess gestational weight gain

Author, year (*years study span*)	Sample size	Setting	Population
Allison 2012 [34] *(NR)*	105	University-based hospital in USA for women on community-based health insurance	African-American English speaking women, who were ≥ 18 years with a pre-gravid BMI of ≥25 kg/m^2, had a singleton pregnancy; no pre-existing diabetes mellitus or autoimmune disorder, or regular use of steroid treatment
Brawarsky 2005 [9] *(NR)*	1100	Project WISH (Women and Infants Starting Healthy) cohort participants received prenatal care and planned to deliver at participating hospitals in San-Francisco, USA	Women who had a singleton, full-term birth (>37 weeks), identified their race as white, 'black', Latina, or Asian, and had complete pregnancy weight gain information, including a weight measured within four weeks of delivery
Chasan-Taber 2008 [36] *(2000–2003)*	770	Latina Gestational Diabetes Mellitus (GDM) cohort study based in public obstetrics/gynecology clinic and midwifery practice of a large tertiary care facility in Western Massachusetts, USA	Women who were Hispanic, 16–40 years old, <24 weeks, had a singleton pregnancy; no history of type 2 diabetes, hypertension or heart disease, chronic renal disease; treatment with medications thought to influence glucose tolerance adversely
Cogswell 1999 [37] *(1993)*	1661	Identified through a consumer mail panel (of 500, 000 households), representative of USA population in terms of geographic region, annual income, population density, household size and age	Women who had a singleton pregnancy, and were expecting to deliver within 3 months
Copper 1995 [39] *(1985–1988)*	1000	Data obtained from a prospective study of risk factors for fetal growth restriction that included pregnant women who delivered at the University of Alabama hospital, USA	Multiparous women, who had a live singleton birth at full term, predominantly 'black', and medically indigent; last available weight was within 2 weeks before delivery; oversampled women with one or more risk factors for Fetal Growth Restriction, including, but not limited to, smoking, a history of an low birth weight infant, and small stature
Herring 2008 [41] *(1999–2002)*	1537	Women recruited from project Viva having their first prenatal visit in one of eight urban and suburban obstetric clinics associated with multispecialty group practice in eastern Massachusetts, USA	Women with a fluency in English, <22 weeks, with a singleton; excluded: underweight women
Hill 2013 [42] *(NR)*	104	Participants recruited from Australian pregnancy online forum and in pregnancy and parenting magazines distributed at state and national level	Pregnant women >18 years and between 10 and 16 weeks
Laraia 2013 [43] *(2001–2005)*	1041 for univariate, 922 for multivariate	Pregnancy, Infection and Nutrition (PIN3) prospective cohort study recruited through the University of North Carolina Hospital and private physician obstetrics clinics in USA	Women ≥16 years, English speaking, planning to continue care or deliver at the study site and having a singleton pregnancy
Loris 1985 [44] *(1979–1982)*	46	Teen obstetric clinic of the University of Carolina Davis Medical Centre, USA	Teenagers delivering a singleton
McAnarney 1992 [45] *(1986–1989)*	116	Participants recruited from Rochester Study of Adolescent Pregnancy in New York, USA	Participants of a cohort of poor, 'black', 12 to 19 years
Mehta 2011 [46] *(2001–2005)*	1192	Pregnancy, Infection and Nutrition (PIN) cohort study delivering at the University of North Carolina Hospital, USA	Participants of a cohort who were >16 years, spoke English, were ≤20 weeks on their second prenatal visit, were planning to continue care or deliver at the study site, had access to a phone for telephone interviews, and were having singleton pregnancies
Mehta-Lee 2013 [63] *(2008–2010)*	775	Secondary analysis of data collected for two randomized-controlled trials of routine provider, primary care based breastfeeding promotion interventions in the Bronx, New York United States	English or Spanish speaking women >18 years, 1st or 2nd trimester of a singleton pregnancy without known risk factors for premature birth, medical contraindications to breastfeed, or infant conditions that prevent breastfeeding. Inclusion criteria for this study: medical record data for height, self-reported pre-pregnancy weight or a pregnancy weight <22 weeks, and a weight > 12 weeks later; exclusion: underweight

Table 2 Characteristics of included cohort studies in systematic review of psychological antecedents of excess gestational weight gain *(Continued)*

McPhie 2015 [62] *(NR)*	183	Participants were recruited via advertising on online mother, child and baby forums, in parenting magazines, at baby and children's markets, and at obstetrician clinic waiting rooms in Geelong/Melbourne in the state of Vicotria, Australia	Women over the age of 18 years
Morling 2003 [47] *(NR)*	56 American women; 94 Japanese women	American women recruited from four obstetric clinics in the city of Schenectady, New York; Japanese women were recruited from the Centre of Obstetrics at the Central Hospital of Ethime	Women who were middle class, recruited during second trimester
Mumford 2008 [48] *(2001 to 2005)*	1223	PIN cohort study participant recruited from both public and private prenatal clinics at the University of North Carolina Hospital, USA	Participants who were ≥16 years, spoke English, ≤20 weeks on their second prenatal visit, planning to continue care or deliver at the study site and had a singleton pregnancy
Olson 2003 [49] *(NR)*	622	Women registered for prenatal care in a hospital and primary care clinic system serving a 10 county area of Upstate New York, USA	Women who entered prenatal care < third trimester, were ≥ 18 years at the time of delivery, planned to deliver within the local hospital and keep the baby, were healthy and mentally competent and gave birth to live singleton infants
Pomerleau[$]2000 [50] *(NR)*	68	Participants from studies at the Nicotine Research Laboratory, recruited from the general community in Michigan, USA	Women who had a first-born child age ≤10 years, singleton pregnancy, delivered at ≥ 37 weeks, smoked at least five cigarettes/day prior to first pregnancy, were smokers at the time of their first pregnancy (regardless of whether they quit during pregnancy or of their current smoking status); participants with a wide range of weight concerns and oversampled those who scored high on measures of dieting and bingeing severity
Steven-Simon 1993 [53] *(1986–1989)*	99	Participants were enrolled in the Colorado Adolescent maternity program at the University Hospital, USA	Participants who were 13 to 18 year old from diverse ethnic backgrounds
Steven-Simon 1995 [52] *(1986–1989)*	122	Participants of Rochester study of Adolescent pregnancy in New York, USA	Participants who were poor, 'black' and 12 to 19 years
Strychar[$] 2000 [54] *(NR)*	115	Prenatal clinics at 3 university teaching hospitals in Montreal, Canada	Primiparous women with singleton pregnancies, ≥ 19 years; excluded: high-risk pregnancies, gestational diabetes, edema, preeclampsia, 'black' women and women of Asiatic and Hispanic origin
Sui 2013 [64] *(2010–2012)*	442	Prospective cohort study nested within the LIMIT (LIMITing weight gain in overweight an dobese women during pregnancy to improve health outcomes) randomized trial, evaluating the effect of an antenatal dietary and lifestyle intervention for women who are overweight or obese; public maternity hospitals in South Australian metropolitan area	Women with BMI >25 kg/m2 were recruited with a live singleton pregnancy form 10–20 weeks' gestation at the time of their 1st antenatal appointment
Tovar 2012 [55] *(2006–2011)*	952	Proyecto Buena Salud Cohort based in the public obstetrics and gynecology clinic and midwifery practice at a large tertiary care facility in Western Massachusetts, USA	Hispanic 16 to 40 year old women of Puerto Rican or Dominican Republic heritage (Caribbean Islanders), who were either themselves, or one of their a parent, or at least 2 of their grandparents born in the Caribbean Islands; women who had a full-term, live singleton birth; excluded: women with current use of medications that could influence glucose tolerance, history of diagnosis of diabetes prior to pregnancy, hypertension, heart disease or chronic renal disease
van der Wijden 2014 [66] *(2005–2006)*	161	Pregnant women from eight midwifery practices in The Netherlands were invited to participate in a randomized control trial on the New Life(style) intervention program consisting of five individual counselling session by one of two trained counsellors with the aim of preventing excess GWG. (Secondary analysis)	Women were eligible if <14 weeks pregnant (1st ongoing pregnancy) and fluent in Dutch. Exclusion criteria for current study: pre-pregnancy BMI or objectively measured pregnancy weight gain could not be established, or if >/=2 items per scale missing in the Dutch Eating Behaviour Questionnaire or >/=3 items on other scales.

Table 2 Characteristics of included cohort studies in systematic review of psychological antecedents of excess gestational weight gain *(Continued)*

Walker[$]2002 [57] *(NR)*	305	Austin New Mothers Study cohort who completed the post-delivery panel in USA	White, African-American, and Hispanic low income women who could read and speak in English, were ≥ 18 years, had full term delivery (between 37 and 42 weeks based on medical records), singleton birth, no medical risks such as diabetes or hypertension during pregnancy, parity of ≤3, and who had Medicaid coverage for prenatal care
Webb 2009 [2] *(2001–2005)*	1605	PIN cohort study conducted in central North Carolina, USA	Women who were >16 years, had a singleton pregnancy, were <20 weeks at their second prenatal visit, had a live birth, and had GWG data
Wells 2006 [58] *(2000–2002)*	4528	Data from the Centre for Disease Control and Prevention's Pregnancy Risk Assessment Monitoring System (PRAMS) for Colorado, USA	Women with live births, were ≥ 15 years
Wright[$] 2013 [59] *(NR)*	101	Participants from Pennsylvania, USA. Details about the study setting not reported	Low income, English or Spanish speaking women who delivered a single live infant
Zhu 2013 [65] *(2008)*	1800	Women at Hefei Maternal and Child Health Hospital, Hefei, China	Women >32 weeks (retrospectively assessed stress in 1st and 2nd trimesters), singleton gestations. Exclusion criteria: >35 years, medically indicated preterm birth, birth defects, stillbirth, assisted reproductive technology, mental disorders, complications of pregnancy including diabetes, hypertension, heart failure, thyroid disease, intrahepatic cholestasis of pregnancy, moderate or severe anemia, history of abnormal pregnancy outcome including premature birth, spontaneous abortion, fetal death, stillbirth, birth defect, neonatal death
Zuckerman 1989 [60] *(1984–1987)*	1014	Prenatal clinic at Boston City Hospital, USA	Women who had the ability to communicate in English or Spanish, who gave informed consent

Note. [$]Cross-sectional study; however, treated similar to a cohort study by authors; NR: Not Reported; GWG: Gestational Weight Gain.

Table 3 Characteristics of included case–control and cross-sectional studies in systematic review of psychological antecedents of excess gestational weight gain

Author, year ***(Years study span)***	**Sample size**	**Setting**	**Population**
Bagheri 2013 [35] *(2010)*	362	Women referred for prenatal care to a large women's hospital in the south of Tehran, Iran	Fifteen to forty-six year-old pregnant women who were referred for prenatal care in a women's hospital; >34 weeks and had a singleton pregnancy; cases were defined as pregnant women who gained weight in excess of Institute of Medicine guidelines and controls as women who gained weight within the guidelines; excluded: pregnant women with abnormal fetuses and those who received hormonal treatment during pregnancy or had diabetes, hypertension, thyroid or, renal chronic diseases
Conway[$] 1999 [38] *(1995–1996)*	62	A large London hospital in United Kingdom	Caucasian women, who were expecting their first or second singleton baby, >18 years and free from known medical conditions which might affect nutrition or fetal outcomes
Dipietro[$] 2003 [40] *(NR)*	130	Obstetric clinic in Baltimore, USA	Women with low risk, normal, singleton pregnancies, delivered at term, and with no history of smoking; predominantly well-educated, middle class women
McDonald[$] 2013 [61] *(2012)*	330	Seven obstetrical and two midwifery clinics in southwestern Ontario, Canada	Women who had had at least one prenatal visit, could read English sufficiently well to complete the survey, and had a live singleton pregnancy
Sangi-haghpeykar[$] 2013 [51] *(2011)*	282	Women delivering at a general hospital in Houston, USA	Women who were Hispanic, recruited immediately post-partum before leaving the hospital
Walker 2009 [56] *(2000–2003)*	1988	Pregnancy Risk Assessment Monitoring System (PRAMS) study data in New Mexico, USA	Hispanic mothers, ≥ 18 years, who had a singleton live birth during their most recent pregnancy, and had a full term (≤37 weeks) delivery

[$]Cross-sectional study; however, treated similar to a case–control study by authors; NR: Not Reported; GWG: Gestational Weight Gain.

There was insufficient information available in the included studies to construct funnel plots to assess publication bias.

Psychological factors and excess GWG

Results are shown for the three main psychological constructs (affect, cognitions related to weight gain, and cognitions related to dietary behavior) pertaining to our primary outcome, excess GWG (Figure 2, Tables 4, 5, 6 and 7, and Additional file 1: Figures S1,S2 and S3 and summarized in the section below.

Affect and excess GWG

Overall, affective states were not found to be related to excess GWG (Figure 2, Table 4, and Additional file 1: Figure S1). Only one of the six studies examining depression [45], found a significant association and this was between a severe measure of depression 'suicidal thoughts and attempts' and excess GWG (among 'black'

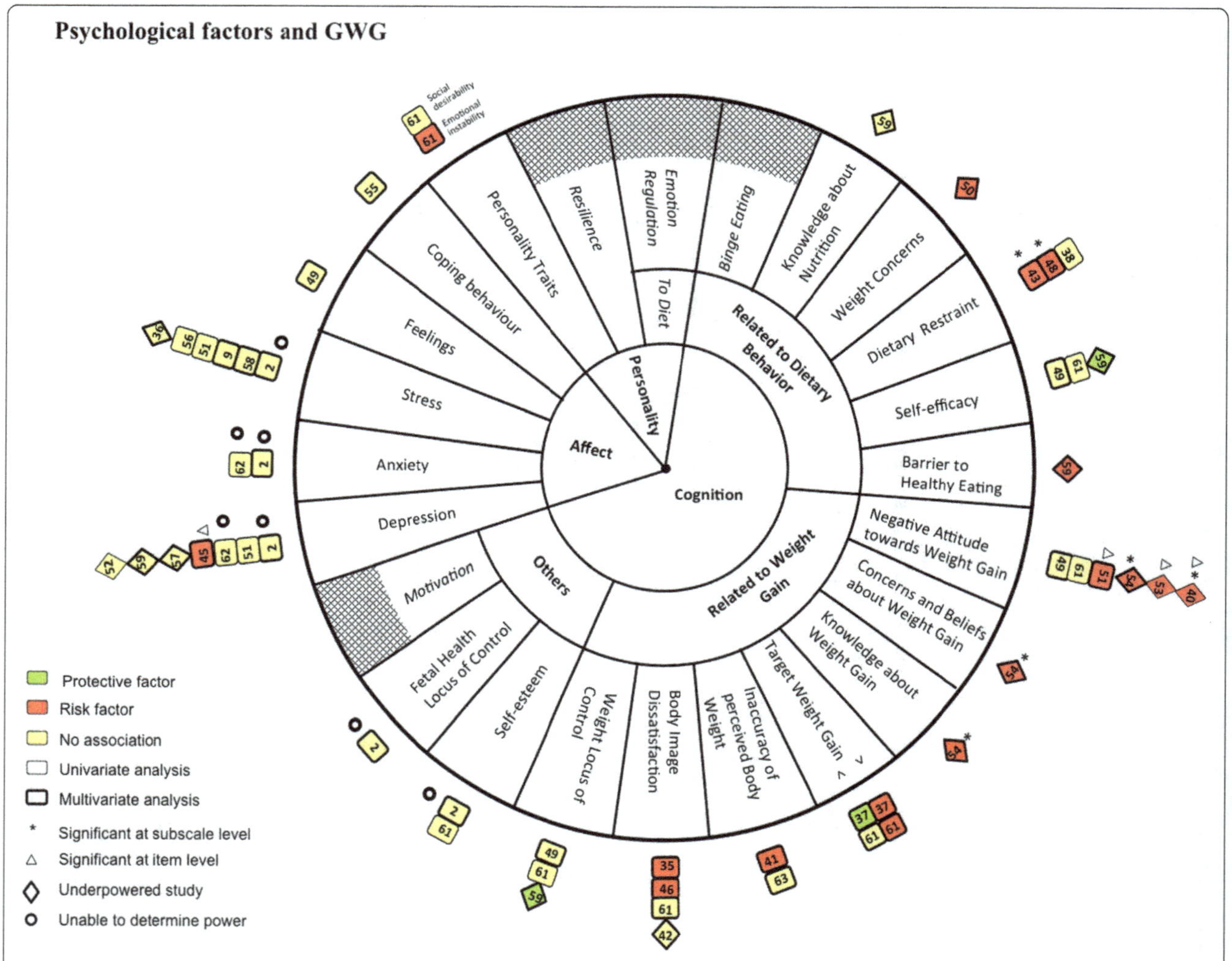

Figure 2 Diagrammatic representation (pinwheel) of relation between affect, cognition and personality and excess gestational weight gain in systematic review of psychological antecedents of excess gestational weight gain. The results of the systematic review on the relation of affect, cognitions and personality with excess GWG are depicted in Figure 2. The major domains are positioned in the innermost circle. In the next circle, cognition is further divided into three sub-domains. These sub-domains are further divided to represent the individual exposures investigated. Boxes (□) have been used to represent adequately powered studies and diamonds (◇) represent underpowered studies. The number within the boxes and diamonds corresponds to each study's reference as listed in Tables 4, 5, 6 and 7. Boxes and diamonds are further coded as follows: Studies which performed multivariate analysis are shown with a thick border; studies which performed univariate analysis are shown with a thin border; Green = significant negative association (protective factor), red = significant positive association (risk factor) and yellow = non-significant association. Adjacent to the boxes and diamonds, symbols represent the following: O = studies for which we were unable to determine power. * = significant only at subscale level of an exposure scale and △ = significant only at item level of an exposure scale. Exposures which were not investigated by any of the studies included in this systematic review are shown using crosshatching (▩). >: Greater than recommended target weight gain; <: Less than recommended target weight gain.

Table 4 Summary table of the relationship of affect and excess gestational weight gain during pregnancy in systematic review of psychological antecedents of excess gestational weight gain

Author, Year (Study reference number)*	Scale used**, Validation	Outcome	Crude (unadjusted) results	Adjusted results	Confounders adjusted for	Summary of results
Exposure: Depression						
McAnarney 1992 [45]	Centre for Epidemiological Studies-Depression Scale (CES-D), validated	Rate of weight gain categorized as slow, average and rapid	Mean (SD) CES-D in each weight gain category: 22 (±9); 20 (±7); 24 (±8) ($p < 0.05$)	OR (95% CI) of rapid weight gain:	Covariates used but not reported	Only 1 item was significant on multivariate analysis ➔
			Item: Suicidal thoughts and attempts	Item: 'Suicidal thoughts and attempts' 5.0 (1.28 to 19.57)		
			Proportion within each weight gain category 13%; 4.6%; 19.4% ($p < 0.05$)			
McPhie 2015 [62]	Depression, Anxiety, and Stress Scale-21 (DASS-21), validated	Excess GWG	In 1st trimester, mild depression in 8.5% of those who gained in excess and 8.9% who gained within guidelines (for moderate depression, 2.8% and 0.9%, respectively); mild anxiety in 9.9% and 11.6%, respectively (for moderate anxiety, 7.0% and 0.9%, respectively)	NA	NA	NS on univariate analysis
Sangi-Haghpeykar 2013 [51]	Patient Health Questionnaire (PHQ), validated	Excess GWG	Proportion with GWG categories: 9%, 9% (p-value NS)	NA	NA	NS on univariate analysis; variable not entered in the multivariate study
Steven-Simon 1995 [52]	CES-D, validated		Effect estimate not reported; (p-value NS)	NA	NA	NS on univariate analysis Multivariate analysis was not done
Walker 2002 [57]	CES-D, validated	Excess GWG	Correlation co-efficient (p-value): r = 0.02 (p-value NS)	β (SE): 0.0 (0.1)	Pre-pregnancy BMI, age, parity, ethnicity, newborn gender, maternal height, food habits	NS on univariate or multivariate analyses
Webb 2009 [2]	CES-D, validated	Excess GWG; Adequacy Ratio	RR (95% CI): **CES-D score (<20 weeks)** Low 1.0 (Reference); Moderate 1.06 (1.0 to 1.2); High 1.03 (0.9 to 1.1) **CES-D score (24–29 weeks)** Low 1.0 (Reference); Moderate 1.08 (1.0 to 1.2); High 1.12 (1.0 to 1.1)	RR (95% CI): **CES-D score (<20 weeks)** Low 1.0 (Reference); Moderate 1.01 (0.9 to 1.1); High 0.98 (0.9 to 1.1) (p = 0.91) **CES-D score (24–29 weeks)** Low 1.0 (Reference); Moderate 1.02 (0.9 to 1.1); High 1.02 (0.9 to 1.1) (p = 0.76)	Pre-gravid BMI, other socio-demographic, dietary and physical activity covariates	NS on univariate or multivariate analyses; Adequacy ratio outcome was significant only on univariate analysis

Table 4 Summary table of the relationship of affect and excess gestational weight gain during pregnancy in systematic review of psychological antecedents of excess gestational weight gain *(Continued)*

Wright 2013 [59]	Edinburgh Postnatal Depression Scale (EPDS), validated	Excess GWG [$;] GWG (continuous)[$$];	β (95% CI): 0.88 (0.1 to 1.7)	Effect estimate not reported for excess GWG β (95% CI) for secondary outcome: 0.3 (−1.0 to 1.5)	Pre-pregnancy BMI, age, race	Results were reported to be similar to secondary outcome but estimates were not reported, hence considered non-significant on univariate or multivariate analysis
Exposure: Anxiety						
McPhie 2015 [62]	Depression, Anxiety, and Stress Scale-21 (DASS-21), validated	Excess GWG	In 1st trimester, mild anxiety in 9.9% of those who gained in excess and 11.6% who gained within guidelines, respectively (for moderate anxiety, 7.0% and 0.9%, respectively)	NA	NA	NS on univariate analysis
Webb 2009 [2]	State and Trait Anxiety Inventory (STAI), validated	Excess GWG; Adequacy Ratio	RR (95% CI): **STAI-T (<20 weeks)** Low 1.0 (Reference); Moderate 1.04 (1.0 to 1.1); High 0.98 (0.9 to 1.1) **STAI-S (<20 weeks)** Low 1.0 (Reference); Moderate 0.94 (0.9 to 1.0); High 0.94 (0.9 to 1.0) **STAI-S (24–29 weeks)** Low 1.0 (Reference); Moderate 1.00 (0.9 to 1.1); High 0.95 (0.9 to 1.0)	RR (95% CI): **STAI-T (<20 weeks)** Low 1.0 (Reference); Moderate 1.02 (1.0 to 1.1); High 1.01 (1.0 to 1.1) **STAI-S (<20 weeks)** Low 1.0 (Reference); Moderate 1.06 (1.0 to 1.1); High 1.00 (0.9 to 1.1) **STAI-S (24 to29 weeks)** Low 1.0 (Reference); Moderate 1.01 (0.9 to 1.1); High 0.99 (0.9 to 1.1)	Pre-gravid BMI, other socio-demographic, dietary and physical activity covariates	NS on univariate or multivariate analyses; adequacy ratio was also NS on univariate or multivariate analyses
Exposure: Stress						
Brawarsky 2005 [9]	Perceived Stress Scale-PSS (short form), validated	Excess GWG	Proportion within GWG categories: Stress categorised as: Yes: 46.4%, 32.2% No: 55.4%, 32.2%	NA	NA	NS on univariate or multivariate analyses
Chasan-Taber 2008 [36]	Perceived Stress Scale-PSS (short form), validated	Excess GWG	Proportion within GWG categories: 0-2: 51.5%, 25.0%; 3-5: 39.5%, 38.4%; 6-8: 43.4%, 34.4%;	OR (95% CI): Maternal stress categorised as: 0-2: 1.0 (Reference); 3-5: 0.5 (0.3 to 0.9); 6-8: 0.6 (0.4 to 1.1);	Pre-pregnancy BMI, parity, age, generation in USA, prenatal care, caloric intake, household activity	NS on univariate or multivariate analyses

Table 4 Summary table of the relationship of affect and excess gestational weight gain during pregnancy in systematic review of psychological antecedents of excess gestational weight gain *(Continued)*

			≥9: 51.3%, 28.6%; (p for trend = .75 and .82, respectively)	≥9: 0.9 (0.5 to 1.6); Missing: 1.1 (0.4 to 3.2)		
Chasan-Taber 2008 [36]	PRAMS standard questions – based on modified Life Event Inventory, validated	Excess GWG	Proportions within GWG categories: Number of life events categorised as: None: 46.4%, 33.6%; 1: 46.0%, 35.4% 2: 50.0%, 28.8; ≥3: 42.6%, 31.1% (p for trend = .51 and .37 respectively)	NA	NA	NS on univariate analysis; variable not entered in a multivariate model
Sangi-haghpeykar 2013 [51]	Prenatal Psychosocial Profile Hassles Scale, validated	Excess GWG [$] and [$$]	Mean (±SD): 13.7 (±2.8), 14.4 (±4.0)	NA	NA	NS on univariate analysis; Variable not entered in the multivariate model
Walker 2009 [56]	PRAMS standard questions – based on modified Life Event Inventory, validated (18 items were used)	Excess GWG	Proportions within GWG categories: Maternal stress categorised as: None: 20.93%, 18.48% 1-2: 38.76%, 40.65%; 3-5: 32.11%, 31.49%; 6-18: 8.20%, 9.39%	NA	NA	NS on univariate analysis; Variable not entered in the multivariate model
Webb 2009 [2]	Perceived Stress Scale (PSS), validated	Excess GWG	RR (95% CI): **PSS 17–22 weeks** Low 1.0 (Reference); Moderate 0.99 (0.9 to 1.0); High 1.03 (1.0 to 1.1) ; **PSS 27–30 weeks** Low 1.0 (Reference); Moderate 1.04 (1.0 to 1.1); High 1.07 (1.0 to 1.2)	RR (95% CI): **PSS 17–22 weeks** Low 1.0 (Reference); Moderate 0.99 (0.9 to 1.0); High 0.99 (0.9 to 1.1) **PSS 27–30 weeks** Low 1.0 (Reference); Moderate 1.01 (1.0 to 1.1); High 1.01 (1.0 to 1.1)	Pre-gravid BMI, other socio-demographic, dietary and physical activity covariates	NS on univariate or multivariate analyses; NS results for adequacy ratio outcome
Wells 2006 [58]	PRAMS standard question – based on	Excess GWG	Proportions within GWG categories:	OR (95% CI):		NS on univariate level or multivariate analyses

Table 4 Summary table of the relationship of affect and excess gestational weight gain during pregnancy in systematic review of psychological antecedents of excess gestational weight gain *(Continued)*

	modified Life Event Inventory, validated (13 items were used)		Maternal stress categorised as: 0 Stressors: 41.3%, 36.4%; 1-2 Stressors: 41.7%, 36.2%; 3 or more stressors: 39.9%, 32.5%	0 Stressor: 1.0 (Reference); 1-2 stressors: 1.03 (0.84 to 1.26); ≥3 stressors: 1.04 (0.82 to 1.32)		
Exposure: Feelings						
Olson 2003 [49]	Investigator developed series of statement on Feelings about motherhood, Not validated	Excess GWG $$	Proportion of exposure within Excess GWG category: Low 43.8%; Medium 37.1% High 41.9%	NA	NA	NS on univariate analysis; variable not entered in a multivariate model
Exposure: Coping behavior						
Tovar 2012 [55]	Psychological Acculturation Scale, validated	Excess GWG $	Proportions within GWG categories: Low acculturation 49.3%, 30.6%; Medium acculturation 42.2%, 31.1%; High acculturation 47%, 31.5% (p = 0.4)	OR (95% CI): Continuous acculturation score 1.0 (0.8 to 1.3)	Pre-pregnancy weight, age, parity, perceived stress, gestational age and physical activity	NS on univariate or multivariate analysis; NS association with other weight gain outcomes (rate of weight gain, weight gain as continuous)

*Study reference number correspond to those cited in a pinwheel and web plot; **Scale details can be found in Additional file 1: Table S1; $2009 IOM GWG guidelines; $$ GWG measured in pounds (lb); →Positive association (Risk factor); ← Negative association (Protective factor); BMI: Body Mass Index; CES-D: Centre for Epidemiological Studies-Depression Scale; GWG: Gestational Weight Gain; NA: Not Applicable; NR: Not Reported; NS: Not Significant; PHQ: Patient Health Questionnaire; PRAMS: Pregnancy Risk Assessment Monitoring System; PSS: Perceived Stress Scale; STAI-S: State and Trait Anxiety Inventory-State; STAI-T: State and Trait Anxiety Inventory-Trait.

Table 5 Summary table of the relationship between cognitions related to weight gain and excess gestational weight gain in systematic review of psychological antecedents of excess gestational weight gain

Author, year (Study reference number)*	Scale used**, Validation	Outcomes	Crude(unadjusted) results	Adjusted results	Confounders adjusted for	Summary of results
Exposure: Negative attitude towards weight gain						
DiPietro 2003 [40]	Pregnancy and Weight Gain Attitude Scale, validated	Excess GWG	Proportions within GWG categories (p-value): **Individual items:** -Embarrassed about weight 28%, 8% (p <0.05) -Worried will get fat 43%, 37% (p-value NS) Feel unattractive 28%, 14% (p-value NS) -Embarrassed when nurse weight me 21%, 21% (p-value NS) -Cannot wear what is in style 18%, 27% (p-value NS) **Subscales:** Negative pregnancy body image r = 0.28 (p < 0.001) Pregnancy experience scale r = 0.20 (p < 0.001)	NA	Pre-pregnancy BMI	Only 1 item and two sub-scales were significant on univariate analyses →
McDonald 2013 [61]	Pregnancy and Weight Gain Attitude Scale, validated (Attitude towards weight gain scale)	Excess GWG	Mean (SD) in those gaining above 17.4 (3.4) vs within 17.9 (2.8); OR 0.95 (0.86 to 1.05)	NA	NA	NS on univariate therefore not included in multivariate
Olson 2003 [49]	Pregnancy and Weight Gain Attitude Scale, validated	Excess GWG $$ ($$$modified 1990 Institute of Medicine guidelines)	Effect estimate not reported; (p-value NS)	NA	NA	NS on univariate analysis Variable not entered in the multivariate model
Sangi-haghpeykar 2013 [51]	Pregnancy and Weight Gain Attitude Scale, validated	Excess GWG $	Proportions within GWG categories (p-value): **Individual items** -Worried will get fat: 28%, 15% (p <0.05)	OR (95% CI) -Embarrassed when nurse weighed me: 4.61 (1.18 to 29.80)	Pre-pregnancy BMI, USA born, unmarried	Only a few items were significant on univariate or multivariate analyses →

Table 5 Summary table of the relationship between cognitions related to weight gain and excess gestational weight gain in systematic review of psychological antecedents of excess gestational weight gain *(Continued)*

			-Embarrassed when nurse weighed me: 14%, 3% (p <0.05) -Don't care how much I gain: 23%, 9% (p <0.05)	-Don't care how much I gain: 3.80 (1.47 to 11.36)		
Stevens-Simon 1993 [53]	Pregnancy and Weight Gain Attitude Scale, validated	Rate of weight gain categorised into slow (<0.23 kg/wk), average (0.23 – 0.4 kg/wk), rapid (>0.4 kg/wk)	Correlation co-efficient (p-value): Total scale score r = 0.12 (p <0.14) **Mean (± SD) attitude score among three outcome categories** 3.4(±0.6), 3.5(±0.5), 3.5(±0.6) (p >0.05) **Individual items** (Correlation co-efficient not reported): -Liked wearing maternity clothes: (p <0.05) -Felt unattractive: (p <0.05) -Embarrassed when nurse weighed me: (p <0.05) -Cannot wear what is in style: (p <0.05)	NA	NA	Only a few items were significant on univariate analyses ➔ Multivariate analysis was not done
Strychar 2000 [54]	Investigator developed, Not validated	Excess GWG	NR	**Sub-scale** – less favourable attitude towards weight gain led to excess weight gain Effect estimate not reported (p <0.05	Pre-pregnancy BMI, age, marital status, education, smoking, and alcohol	Only a sub-scale was significant on multivariate analysis ➔
Exposure: Concerns and beliefs about weight gain						
Strychar 2000 [54]	Investigator developed, Not validated	Excess GWG	NR	**Sub-scale:** Perceived concern about their weight – more concerned leads to excess weight gain Effect estimate not reported; (p <0.05)	Pre-pregnancy BMI, age, marital status, education, smoking, and alcohol	Only a sub-scale, namely, 'perceived concern' was significant on multivariate analysis ➔
Exposure: Knowledge about weight gain						
Strychar 2000 [54]		Excess GWG	NR			

Table 5 Summary table of the relationship between cognitions related to weight gain and excess gestational weight gain in systematic review of psychological antecedents of excess gestational weight gain *(Continued)*

	Investigator developed, Not validated			**Sub-scale:** Importance of not gaining an excess amount of weight– Less knowledge leads to excess weight gain Effect estimate not reported; (p <0.05)	Pre-pregnancy BMI, age, marital status, education, smoking, and alcohol	Only a sub-scale, namely, ' importance of not gaining an excess amount of weight' was significant on multivariate analysis ➔
Exposure: Target weight gain						
Cogswell, 1999 [37]	Investigator developed single item; Not validated	Excess GWG	NR	OR (95% CI) Target weight gain categories <Recommended 0.4 (0.2 to 0.6) Recommended 1.0 (Reference) >Recommended 6.1 (4.1 to 8.9)	Pre-pregnancy BMI, maternal height, age, race, education, marital status, parity, prenatal care, WIC participants,, income	Significant on multivariate analysis ➔ (> recommended) ← (< recommended)
McDonald 2013 [61]	Investigator developed single item; Investigator developed, not validated	Excess GWG	OR (95% CI)	OR (95% CI)	Pre-pregnancy BMI group, first birth, planned	Planned gain above the guidelines Significant on both univariate and multivariate analysis
			Planned gain above the guidelines 9.31 (3.86 to 22.42), planned gain below 0.78 (0.33 to 1.84)	Planned gain above the guidelines 11.18 (4.45 to 28.06); planned gain below 0.69 (0.26 to 1.80)	weight gain, daily soda or juice consumption, watching television before bedtime, locus of control to Eysenck's neurotic scale of emotional instability, and satisfaction with pre-pregnancy weight	➔ (> recommended) planned gain below NS on univariate or multivariate multivariate
Exposure: Inaccuracy of perceived body weight						
Herring 2008 [41]	Previously published single item adopted National Health and Nutrition Examination Survey, No reference to validation	Excess GWG	Proportion of Excess GWG within each exposure category: Normal weight, accurate assessor 47% Normal weight, over-assessor 57% Overweight, accurate assessor 62%	OR (95% CI): Normal weight, accurate assessor 1.0 (reference); Normal weight, over-assessor 2.0 (1.3 to 3.0);	Pre-pregnancy BMI, age, education, marital status, income, employment, ethnicity, parity, smoking, gestational length	Significant on univariate or multivariate analyses ➔

Table 5 Summary table of the relationship between cognitions related to weight gain and excess gestational weight gain in systematic review of psychological antecedents of excess gestational weight gain *(Continued)*

				Overweight accurate assessor 2.9 (2.2 to 3.9);		
			Overweight under-assessor 81% (p <0.05)	Overweight under-assessor 7.6 (3.4 to 17.0)		
Mehta-Lee 2013 [63]	Single item, Perceived weight status was defined as "accurate" or "inaccurate" based upon the level of concordance between BMI (derived from actual weight) and self reported overweight or obesity (no reference to validation)	Excess GWG	OR (95% CI): Inaccurate reporters 1.2 (0.8, 1.8);	OR (95% CI): Inaccurate reporters 1.1 (0.7, 1.7);	Stratified by BMI; adjusted for: WIC status, employment status, race, native born, smoking, parity and either pre-gestational or gestational diabetes	NS on univariate and on multivariate analyses
Exposure: Body image dissatisfaction						
Bagheri 2013 [35]	Body Image Assessment for Obesity (BIA-O), Validated	Excess (cases) vs. Adequate (controls) GWG	OR (95% CI): Heavier body size preference 0.54 (0.27 to 1.04) Thinner Body Size Preference 2.17 (1.17 – 4.02)	OR (95% CI): Heavier body size preference 0.44 (0.18 to 1.10) Thinner body size preference 3.12 (1.97 to 4.95)	Pre-pregnancy BMI, age, parity, social class, energy intake	Significant on univariate or multivariate analyses ➔
Hill 2013 [42]	Body Attitude Questionnaire (BAQ), Validated, modified	Excess GWG [$]	NR	Effect estimates were not reported; p-value NS	Pre-pregnancy BMI, age, parity, education level	NS on multivariate analysis
Mehta 2011 [46]	Body Image Assessment for Obesity (BIA-O), Validated	Excess GWG	RR (95% CI): Heavier body size preference 1.79 (0.52-9.58) Thinner body size preference 0.88 (0.82 to 0.94)	RR (95% CI): Thinner body size preference <16 years of education 1.11 (1.00 to 1.22) ≥16 years of education 0.92 (0.83 to 1.01)	Pre-pregnancy BMI	Significant on multivariate analysis ➔
McDonald 2013 [61]	Satisfaction with pre-pregnancy weight , not stated if validated or not	Excess GWG	OR (95% CI): Not or not at all satisfied vs. satisfied or very satisfied 0.25 (0.10 to 0.60)	NA	NA	Significant on univariate analysis NS on multivariate analysis
Exposure: Weight Locus of Control						
McDonald 2013 [61]		Excess GWG	OR (95% CI) 1.12 (1 to 1.26)	NA	NA	

Table 5 Summary table of the relationship between cognitions related to weight gain and excess gestational weight gain in systematic review of psychological antecedents of excess gestational weight gain *(Continued)*

	Locus of control score, validated					NS on univariate analysis; Variable not entered in the multivariate model
Olson 2003 [49]	Weight Locus of Control (WLOC), Validated	Excess GWG $^{\$\$}$	Effect estimate not reported; p-value NS	NA	NA	NS on univariate analysis; Variable not entered in the multivariate model
Wright 2013 [59]	Single item from Attitude towards weigh gain scale by Palmer, Validated, modified	Excess GWG;	Effect estimate not reported for Adequacy ratio	Effect estimate not reported for Excess GWG	Pre-pregnancy BMI, age, race	Results were reported to be similar to secondary outcome , hence considered significant on univariate or multivariate analysis ←
		GWG (continuous)$^{\$\$}$	β (95% CI) for secondary outcome:-11.6 (−21.4 to −1.9)	β (95% CI) for secondary outcome: −16.1 (−28.7 to −3.4)		

*Study reference number correspond to those cited in a pinwheel and web plot; **Scale details can be found in Additional file 1: Table S1; $^{\$}$2009 IOM GWG guidelines; $^{\$\$}$ GWG measured in pounds (lb); → Positive association (Risk factor); ← Negative association (Protective factor); $^{\$\$\$}$ For obese women, upper limit of recommended weight gain was set as same as that of the overweight women; BAQ: Body Attitude Questionnaire; BIA-O: Body Image Assessment for Obesity; BMI: Body Mass Index; GWG: Gestational Weight Gain; NA: Not Applicable; NR: Not Reported; NS: Not Significant;

Table 6 Summary table of the relationship of cognitions related to dietary behavior to excess gestational weight gain in systematic review of psychological antecedents of excess gestational weight gain

Author, year (Study reference number)*	Scale used**, Validation	Outcome(s)	Crude (unadjusted) results	Adjusted results	Confounders adjusted for	Summary of results
Exposure: Knowledge about nutrition						
Wright 2013 [59]	Investigator developed, Validated	Excess GWG;	β (95% CI):	Effect estimate not reported for excess GWG	Pre-Pregnancy BMI, age, race	Results were reported to be similar to secondary outcome but estimates were not reported. Hence considered NS on univariate or multivariate analyses
		GWG (continuous)$^{\$\$}$	−1.2 (−3.2 to 0.69)	β (95% CI) for secondary outcome: −0.14 (−2.8 to 2.5)		
Exposure: Weight concerns						
Pomerleau 2000 [50]	Dieting and Binge Eating Severity Scale (DBESS), Validated	Difference between actual and current maximum recommended weight gain (continuous)	Mean (± SD) excess GWG between two weight concern categories: Low Weight Concern ;=2.9 (±12.7); High Weight Concern 15.6 (±21.9) (p <0.01)	Effect estimates not reported ANOVA F-test statistics = 7.614 (p <0.01)	NR	Significant on multivariate analysis; weight gain (lb) as a continuous outcome also has a positive significant association with weight concern categories ➔
Cognitive dietary restraint						
Conway 1999 [38]	Revised Restraint Scale (RRS), Validated	Excess GWG	Proportions with GWG categories (p-value): Dietary Restraint (Full scale) 48%, 30% (p = 0.07); Weight Fluctuation subscale 46%, 31% (p = 0.054); Concern for dieting subscale 50%, 33% (p = 0.601)	NA	NA	NS on univariate analysis Multivariate analysis was not done
Laraia 2013 [43]	RRS, Validated	Excess GWG for univariate; Adequacy Ratio for univariate and multivariate	Proportion within GWG category: Low dietary Restraint Food secure 52.7%, 35.4%; Marginally food insecure 52.7%, 25.5% High dietary Restraint Food secure 71.5%, 16.8%; Marginally food insecure 74.0%, 11.0% Overall x^2(p-value) :57.3 (p <0.001)	β (95% CI): Interaction between Marginally Food Insecure and: High Restraint 0.53 (0.33 to 0.73) Dieters 0.50 (0.30 to 0.70) Weight Cyclers 0.54 (0.34 to 0.74)	Pre-pregnancy BMI, maternal race, age, income, education, marital status, parity, gestational age, smoking, physical activity in 1st trimester	Full scale was significant on univariate or multivariate analyses; subscales were significant on multivariate analysis ➔

Table 6 Summary table of the relationship of cognitions related to dietary behavior to excess gestational weight gain in systematic review of psychological antecedents of excess gestational weight gain *(Continued)*

Mumford 2008 [48]	RRS, Validated	Adequacy Ratio	NR	OR (95% CI): **Overall** Restrained eating 1.12 (0.94 to 1.31) Non-Restrained eating 0.95 (0.78 to 1.12) **Dieters vs. Non-Dieters** Underweight 0.94 (0.68 to 1.19); 1.02 (0.89 to 1.16); Normal Weight 1.50 (1.40 to 1.60); 1.31 (1.23 to 1.40); Overweight 1.97 (1.80 to 2.15); 1.79 (1.54 to 2.03); Obese 2.09 (1.98 to 2.21); 1.73 (1.53 to 1.93) **Cyclers vs. Non-Cyclers** Underweight 0.88 (0.66 to 1.11); 0.94 (0.77 to 1.11); Normal Weight 1.38 (1.25 to 1.52); 1.25 (1.12 to 1.37); Overweight 1.92 (1.72 to 2.12); 1.58 (1.35 to 1.80); Obese 2.11 (1.96 to 2.26); 1.73 (1.54 to 1.91)	Pre-pregnancy BMI, race, education, poverty, physical activity, weight gain attitude	Only subscales were significant on multivariate analyses ➔
Exposure: Self-efficacy						
McDonald 2013 [61]	Self-efficacy in achieving healthy weight, ii) towards controlling food Intake; iii) towards weight Management, not stated if validated	Excess GWG	OR (95% CI): 0.97 (0.92 to 1.02); ii) 0.91 (0.79 to 1.05); iii) 0.94 (0.86 to 1.03)	NA	NA	NS on univariate Analysis; not entered in the multivariate model

Table 6 Summary table of the relationship of cognitions related to dietary behavior to excess gestational weight gain in systematic review of psychological antecedents of excess gestational weight gain *(Continued)*

Olson 2003 [49]	Investigator Developed, Not validated	Excess GWG $^{\$\$}$	Effect estimate not reported (p-value NS)	NA	NA	NS on univariate analysis; variable not entered in the multivariate model
Wright 2013 [59]	Investigator developed, Not validated	Excess GWG; GWG (continuous)$^{\$\$}$	Effect estimate not reported for excess GWG β (95% CI) for secondary outcome: β (95% CI) -1.3 (−2.6 – 0.0)	Effect estimate not reported for excess GWG β (95% CI) for secondary outcome: −3.6 (−6.8 to −0.3)	Pre-pregnancy BMI, age, race	Results were reported to be similar to secondary outcome but Estimates were not reported, hence considered significant on univariate or multivariate analysis ←
Exposure: Barriers to healthy eating						
Wright 2013 [59]	Fowles' Barriers to Health Eating Scale (BHES), Validated	Adequacy ratio; Excess GWG $^{\$\$}$	β (95% CI): 0.12 (−0.6 to 0.8)	β (95% CI): 2.0 (0.3 to 3.7)	Pre-pregnancy BMI, age, race	Results were reported to be similar to secondary outcome but estimates were not reported, hence considered significant on multivariate analysis →

*Study reference number correspond to those cited in a pinwheel and web plot; **Scale details can be found in Additional file 1: Table S1; $^{\$}$2009 IOM GWG guidelines; $^{\$\$}$ GWG measured in pounds (lb); →Positive association (Risk factor); ← Negative association (Protective factor); ANOVA: Analysis of Variance; BMI: Body Mass Index; GWG: Gestational Weight Gain; NA: Not Applicable; NS: Not Significant; RRS: Revised Restraint Scale.

Table 7 Summary table of the relationship between personality and 'other' cognitions, and excess gestational weight gain, in systematic review of psychological antecedents of excess gestational weight gain

Author, year (Study reference number)*	Scale used**, Validation	Outcome(s)	Crude (unadjusted) results	Adjusted results	Confounders adjusted for	Summary of results
Exposure: Personality Traits						
McDonald 2013 [61]	Eysenck's Neurotic Scale of Emotional Instability (Personality trait), validated;	Excess GWG	OR 95% CI 1.24 (1.11 to 1.39) (per unit increase on scale)	OR 95% CI 1.26 (1.10 to 1.44) (per unit increase on scale)	pre-pregnancy BMI group, first birth, planned weight gain, daily soda or juice consumption, watching television before bedtime, locus of control to Eysenck's neurotic scale of emotional instability, and satisfaction with pre-pregnancy weight	Neurotic Scale of Emotional Instability Significant on univariate analysis and multivariate ➔ Lie Scale of Social Desirability NS on univariate; not included in multivariate
McDonald 2013 [61]	Eysenck's Lie Scale of Social Desirability (Personality trait), validated	Excess GWG	OR 95% CI 1.24 0.95 (0.84 to 1.08)	NA	NA	NS on univariate; Not entered into multivariate analyses
Exposure: 'Other' Cognitions (Fetal Health Locus of Control)						
Webb 2009 [2]	Fetal Health Locus of Control (FHLC), Validated	Excess GWG; Adequacy ratio	RR (95% CI): **FHLC-(Internality scale)** Low 1.07 (1.0 to 1.2) Moderate 1.03 (0.9 to 1.1) High 1.0 (Reference) **FHLC-(Powerful** **others scale)** Low 1.0 (Reference) Moderate 1.10 (1.0 to 1.2) High 1.05 (1.0 to 1.1) **FHLC-(Chances scale)** Low 1.0 (Reference) Moderate 1.07 (1.0 to 1.2) High 1.08 (1.0 to 1.2)	RR (95% CI): **FHLC–(Internality Scale)** Low 1.02 (1.0 to 1.1) Moderate 1.01 (0.9 to 1.1) High 1.0 (Reference) **FHLC-(Powerful** **others scale)** Low 1.0 (Reference) Moderate 1.00 (0.9 to 1.1) High 0.96 (0.9 to 1.0) **FHLC-(Chances scale)** Low 1.0 (Reference) Moderate 1.00 (0.9 to 1.1)	Pre-pregnancy BMI and other identified maternal socio-demographic, dietary and physical activity variables (exact variables not reported)	NS on univariate or multivariate analyses; similar results for adequacy ratio outcome

Table 7 Summary table of the relationship between personality and 'other' cognitions, and excess gestational weight gain, in systematic review of psychological antecedents of excess gestational weight gain *(Continued)*

				High 1.01 (0.9 to 1.1)		
Exposure: 'Other' Cognitions (Self-esteem)						
McDonald 2013 [61]	Robins Self-esteem scale, validated	Excess GWG	OR (95% CI) for "Not very true" vs. other in terms of positive self esteem 0.28 (0.04 to 2.19)	NA	NA	NS on univariate therefore not included in multivariate
Webb 2009 [2]	Self-esteem scale, Previously published, no reference to validation	Excess GWG; Adequacy Ratio	RR (95% CI)	RR (95% CI)	Pre-pregnancy BMI, other socio-demographic, dietary and physical activity covariates	NS on univariate or multivariate analyses; NS results for adequacy ratio outcome
			Low 1.01 (0.9 to 1.1);	Low 0.99 (0.9 to 1.1);		
			Moderate 1.03 (1.0 to 1.1);	Moderate 1.02 (0.9 to 1.1);		
			High 1.0 (Reference)	High 1.0 (Reference)		

*Study reference number corresponds to those cited in a pinwheel and web plot; **Scale details can be found in Additional file 1: Table S1; FHLC: Fetal Health Locus of Control; NA: Not Applicable. ➔ Positive association (Risk factor).

adolescents; OR 5.0; 95% CI 1.28 to 19.57). Only one [65] of seven studies found a negative association between stress and excess GWG [2,9,36,51,56,58], however this study retrospectively assessed first trimester stress when the participants were at least 32 weeks gestation There was no association between excess GWG and feelings about motherhood [49], psychological acculturation (as a measure of coping behavior) [55] or anxiety [2].

Cognitions related to weight gain and excess GWG

Variable associations were found between cognitions related to weight gain and excess GWG. Of the eight cognitions related to weight gain, most were investigated by single studies while three were examined by more than one study (Figure 2, Table 5, and Additional file 1: Figure S2). Target weight gain 'greater than recommended' increased the risk of excess GWG (OR 6.1; 95% CI 4.1 to 8.9), whereas target weight gain 'less than recommended' decreased the risk (OR 0.4; 95% CI 0.2 to 0.6) of excess GWG [37], and similar associations were also found in a cross-sectional study [61]. Inaccuracy of perceived prepregnancy body weight was a risk for excess GWG among both normal weight women (OR 2.0; 95% CI 1.3 to 3.0) and overweight women (OR 7.6; 95% CI 3.4 to 17.0) [41] but was not in another study [63]. Less knowledge about the 'importance of not gaining too much weight' and more 'perceived concern' about weight gain were risk factors for excess GWG [54]. A non-significant association was found between self-esteem and excess GWG in two studies [2,61] .

Two of four studies found an association between body image dissatisfaction (preference for thinner body size) and excess GWG; one [35] noted this in their whole population (OR 3.12; 95% CI 1.89 to 4.95), whereas it held true only in women with less than 16 years of education in the other (RR 1.11; 95% CI 1.00 to 1.22) [46]. Two other studies reported non-significant associations [42,61], potentially due to lack of statistical power, given that the examination of GWG as a continuous outcome was significantly associated with the attractiveness subscale in one of the studies [42].

Four of six studies reported that a negative attitude towards weight gain, at a subscale or individual item level, was associated with excess GWG [40,51,54] or a rapid rate of weight gain [53] although two of these studies examined the association only with univariate analysis [40,53], while two others reported a non-significant effect [49,61] .

Weight locus of control appeared as a protective factor in one study [59], but had a non-significant effect in the other two studies [49,61] .

Cognitions related to dietary behavior and excess GWG

Variable associations were found between cognitions related to dietary behavior and excess GWG. Positive associations were found in two studies examining weight concerns [50] and barriers to healthy eating [59] with excess GWG, but both studies were underpowered (Figure 2, Table 6, and Additional file 1: Figure S3). Knowledge about nutrition was not significantly associated with excess GWG [59]. Two studies found no association between self-efficacy and excess GWG [49,61], and a third reported a negative association [59].

One of three studies found a positive association between dietary restraint on the full scale as well as on the two sub-scales of dietary restraint, namely dieters and weight cyclers, with excess GWG [38,43,48]. Laraia [43] found a positive association between high dietary restraint (OR 1.65; 95% CI 1.35 to 2.01), dieting (OR 1.72; 95% CI 1.40 to 2.10) and weight cycling (OR 1.70; 95% CI 1.39 to 2.08) and excess GWG for marginally food insecure women only. A second study [48] found a significant association between the dieting and weight cycling sub-scales (although not the full scale) and the adequacy of weight gain ratio. A third study [38] found no association between dietary restraint and excess GWG but only performed univariate analyses.

Personality and excess GWG

The only study to examine personality found a positive association between higher emotional instability and excess GWG, but no association with the social desirability scale [61] (Figure 2 and Table 7).

'Other' psychological factors in cognitions and excess GWG

One study [2] found non-significant associations between three sub-scales of fetal health locus of control (i.e., internality, powerful others and chance) and excess GWG (Figure 2, Table 7, and Additional file 1: Figure S3). None of the included studies examined motivation in relation to excess GWG.

Psychological factors and weight gain as a secondary outcome

The findings pertaining to GWG as a secondary outcome were from a relatively small number of studies [34,39,44, 47,60,64-66], and showed generally inconclusive results (Additional file 1: Table S4).

Cognitions related to physical activity and excess GWG (post hoc objective)

None of the included studies examined cognition related to physical activity and excess GWG.

Discussion

This is the first systematic review to our knowledge to examine the relation between psychological predictors and excess GWG, a condition now affecting approximately half of all pregnant women in some populations.

Taken together, the available evidence from 35 studies indicates that excess GWG is not related to negative affective states (such as non-clinical depression or anxiety), but is related to a number of weight-related and dietary-related cognitions, while personality traits and motivations remain underexplored constructs in relation to GWG. Specifically, negative cognitions/attitudes or inaccurate perceptions about weight gain appear to act as risk factors for excess GWG in some instances, whereas positive cognitions/attitudes appear to play a protective role. Risk factors for excess GWG may include higher levels of dietary restraint, perceived barriers to healthy eating, negative attitude towards weight gain, negative body image, concern about weight gain, high target weight gain, inaccurate perceptions regarding one's own body weight, and less knowledge about weight gain. In contrast, protective factors include higher self-efficacy for healthy eating, lower than recommended target weight gain, and an internal locus of control with respect to weight gain. A number of these findings warrant further discussion. Overall, the evidence was more consistent in showing a lack of relation for affective states and excess GWG. However, many of the studies investigating cognitions related to weight gain were underpowered.

Affect and excess GWG

The available evidence on negative affective states, such as symptoms of depression, anxiety and stress, indicated that they are not directly related to excess GWG. These findings are in contrast to the evidence from the general population which clearly indicates that depression and anxiety are associated with weight [67-70] with a dose–response relation between depression and weight demonstrated in a meta-analysis of 15 longitudinal studies [67] and a similar graded relation between anxiety and weight gain [69,70]. Reasons for why a relation between negative affect and excess GWG may have failed to emerge in our systematic review include firstly, the mild degree of the affective symptoms experienced by the participants included in this systematic review. This was supported by the fact that one study in our systematic review did find an association between an item pertaining to severe symptoms of depression (i.e., history of suicidal thoughts or attempts) and excess GWG [45]. A second but related reason stems from our decision to exclude studies which focused on participants diagnosed with an eating disorder. Meta-analytic evidence indicates that negative affect is a risk factor for eating pathology [71]. However, a history of severe morbidities that impact weight gain such as anorexia and bulimia together constitute less than 1% of pregnant women [72]. A third reason may be the relatively short time frame of studies during pregnancy (i.e., often only a few months), compared to the longitudinal studies in non-pregnant populations which have examined the relation between affective symptoms and weight gain across several years [67,69,70]. A growing body of research has identified 'pregnancy-specific anxiety' as a particularly robust risk factor for a number of negative birth outcomes [73]. It is possible that the relation between excess GWG and affect may be different for women who enter pregnancy with more negative affect compared to those whose negative affect is pregnancy-specific.

The available evidence from six of seven included studies indicates that overall, perceived stress is not related to excess GWG [2,9,36,51,56,58]. This finding was robust, given that most of the scales had been validated for use during pregnancy, two studies were large and population-based, and four studies included women from diverse ethnic backgrounds. In contrast, among non-pregnant populations, a consistent body of evidence demonstrates that higher levels of stress are associated with increased weight gain [74-76], possibly due to activation of the HPA axis, with higher glucocorticoid levels leading to increased adiposity [77,78]. Pregnancy is also associated with increased HPA axis function beginning as early as the 11th week of gestation [79] and by the third trimester, blood cortisol levels are more than twofold higher among pregnant women compared to non-pregnant controls [79]. Hence there may be a 'ceiling effect' since levels of cortisol are higher during pregnancy regardless of the degree of stress. Hence, pregnancy-related changes in HPA axis function may dampen the relation between stress and weight gain seen in the general population.

Cognitions related to weight gain and excess GWG

In contrast to affective states, a number of significant findings were found among studies examining negative cognitions related to weight gain and excess GWG, including most studies on *negative* attitudes towards weight gain [40,51,53,54], and negative body image (i.e., 'thinner body size preference') [35,46]. Furthermore, women who inaccurately perceived their weight to be greater than it was, were more likely to gain excess weight [41] as were women who were more concerned about weight gain [54] or had less knowledge about weight gain during pregnancy [54]. Consistent with the above findings, research in non-pregnant women has also shown an association between BMI tertile and negative body image [80].

Conflicting results were found between weight locus of control and weight gain during pregnancy. Consistent with the literature among non-pregnant women, which suggests that women with an internal locus of control perform better in weight loss programs [81], one underpowered study found that having an internal locus of control was associated with a lower risk of excess GWG [59]. However, the other study did not find a significant effect between either an internal or external locus of control and GWG [49], hence more research is required.

A lower than recommended target weight gain was a protective factor for excess GWG while a higher than recommended target weight gain was a risk factor for excess GWG [37,61]. The latter factor is particularly concerning given that only 29% of pregnant women reported that they were counseled to gain a certain amount of weight, but only 12%, reported receiving a recommendation in accordance with the IOM guidelines [82]. Barriers to GWG counseling by the health providers, include insufficient training, concern about the sensitivity of the topic, and the perception that counseling is ineffective [83]. Although few women reported receiving accurate recommendations about GWG and the lack of knowledge associated with excess GWG are both concerning, it is reassuring that appropriate GWG targets are a protective factor, as the provision of such information is an easily modifiable factor. This is consistent with evidence that the provision of information regarding weight gain represents a key intervention strategy in preventing excess GWG [84].

Cognitions related to dietary behaviors and excess GWG

Although the existing evidence on cognitions related to dietary behaviors and excess GWG is limited, the available studies suggest that having higher dietary restraint, weight concerns and perceived barriers to healthy eating are all risk factors for excess GWG, while higher self-efficacy for healthy eating was a protective factor in one study [59]. Such findings are consistent with qualitative research which suggests that pregnant women regard themselves as less restrained in their eating behavior [85]. Furthermore, previous research has found that chronic dietary restraint eventually breaks down and results in impulsive eating, binge eating [86], although no studies were found investigating the association between impulsivity and GWG. Laraia [43] found that the association of restrained eating with excess GWG holds true only among women who experienced marginal food insecurity. Food insecurity appears to be associated with intake of low cost, high caloric food , which in turns is associated with weight gain [87].

The perception of barriers to healthy eating was associated with excess GWG [59], similar to the non-pregnant literature [88]. Although, no relation emerged between lack of knowledge about nutrition and weight gain among low income women [59], given that outside of pregnancy it has been perceived to be linked to weight loss in overweight and obese low income women [88], more studies are needed in a more varied pregnant population.

Self-efficacy regarding healthy eating, which in the general population is related to weight loss [89], was protective against excess GWG in one of three studies [59] but not in the others. Self-efficacy, a major domain associated with health behavior [90], may be especially important during pregnancy, a time of physiological challenges to the maintenance of health behaviors related to GWG (e.g. nausea and food cravings) [1,91]. In light of documented pregnancy-specific challenges and the modifiable nature of self-efficacy, future studies should explore whether targeting self-efficacy represents a viable intervention strategy for helping prevent excess GWG.

Personality and excess GWG

The single study [61] which examined the relation between excess GWG and personality and found that per unit increase on Eysenck's Neurotic Scale of Emotional Instability, the adjusted OR for excess gain was 1.26 (1.10 to 1.44). Hence, personality traits represent important areas for future research, given that outside of pregnancy a recent meta-analysis found that certain personality traits, such as conscientiousness (in an adjusted analysis) and higher openness to experience (in an unadjusted analysis), were related to a reduction in the risk of developing obesity [25], while weight fluctuation over time was predicted by personality traits such as neuroticism and impulsivity [92].

This is the first systematic review to our knowledge to examine the relation between psychological factors and excess GWG. Strengths include the comprehensiveness of the searches that were performed, using eight databases and variations on a wide selection of search terms, and the use of rigorous methodology in accordance with PRISMA (Preferred Reporting Items for Systematic Reviews and Meta-Analyses) [29]. There were a number of strengths in the methodology and design of the included studies. For example, the majority of studies investigating our primary outcomes obtained women's final pregnancy weight from medical records, rather than self-report. Most studies were longitudinal cohort designs, allowing for stronger conclusions to be drawn regarding the predictive utility of the constructs under review and most adjusted for pre-pregnancy BMI, a known confounder of GWG [1].

The challenges associated with the current systematic review stem primarily from the limitations inherent in the individual included studies. Firstly, by considering only the relation between each construct and GWG, studies failed to evaluate a likely interaction between various psychological constructs and its impact on weight gain. AbuSabha and Achterberg [90] suggest that evaluating such constructs individually might result in weak predictive abilities and contradictory results, and this appears to have been the case so far. Secondly, the methodological quality of the included studies was not consistently high and the results should be interpreted with caution due to poor quality of some of the included studies. For instance, a large number of studies did not report effect size and confidence intervals. Moreover, many of the included studies were underpowered, and underpowered studies contribute biased effect size estimates. Thirdly, studies failed to assess whether the timings of assessment of psychological constructs during gestation had an effect on the outcome. There is a need for more work on psychological predictors of GWG according to each trimester. Fourthly, publication bias [93] may be a limitation of this systematic review but could not be assessed even with a funnel plot. Only few constructs had a sufficient number of related studies, and when such was the case (e.g., with stress), the relevant studies did not always provide sufficient information to calculate effect estimates needed to produce funnel plot, hence, limiting our ability to draw definite conclusions regarding publication bias. Fifthly, all but one of the psychological constructs assessed were not pregnancy-specific. Lastly, the considerable heterogeneity in the scales used to assess each psychological construct and the failure of many studies to report comprehensive data precluded us from computing a pooled effect estimate with meta-analytic techniques.

Conclusion

This is the first systematic review to our knowledge to examine the relation between excess GWG and psychological antecedents, answering the call from other systematic reviews of generally non-successful interventions for preventing excess GWG to study the antecedents. Based on the studies included in this review, affective symptomatology was unrelated to excess GWG, except for severe symptoms of depression (i.e., suicidality). Negative cognitions/attitudes or inaccurate perceptions about weight gain emerged as risk factors for excess GWG whereas positive cognitions/attitudes appear to play a protective role. Specifically, risk factors for excess GWG include higher levels of cognitive dietary restraint, perceived barriers to healthy eating, negative attitude towards weight gain, negative body image, being concerned about weight gain, high target weight gain, inaccurate perceptions regarding one's own body weight, and less knowledgeable about weight gain. Although fewer factors were protective, some evidence emerged for the association between a reduced risk of excess GWG and higher self-efficacy for healthy eating, lower than recommended target weight gain, and an internal locus of control with respect to weight gain. Finally, we identified important areas for future study, as there was little available information on the association of excess GWG with personality traits and motivation. This study forms the basis of a better understanding of psychological factors, a critical first step in developing effective interventions to prevent the current epidemic of excess GWG and help prevent the resultant trans-generational cycle of obesity. Although pregnancy spans only a short period of time, but represents a potentially critical window influencing the mother's weight trajectory, and the fetus' in utero programming, there is a need for further investigation on psychological factors influencing GWG.

Additional files

Additional file 1: Supporting information: Final search strategies. Table S1. Description of psychological scales used in the included studies. **Table S2.** Quality assessment of included cohort studies using the modified Newcastle-Ottawa scale in systematic review of psychological antecedents of excess gestational weight gain. **0 S3.** Quality assessment of included case-control and cross-sectional studies using the modified Newcastle-Ottawa scale in systematic review of psychological antecedents of excess gestational weight gain. **Figure S1.** Forest plots showing relation of affect and excess gestational weight gain in systematic review of psychological antecedents of excess gestational weight. **Figure S2.** Forest plots showing relation of cognitions related to weight gain and other cognitions and excess gestational weight gain in systematic review of psychological antecedents of excess gestational weight gain. **Figure S3.** Forest plots showing relation of cognitions related to dietary behavior and excess gestational weight gain in systematic review of psychological antecedents of excess gestational weight gain. **Table S4.** Summary table of secondary outcomes and the relation of affect, cognition related to on dietary behavior or weight gain, in systematic review of psychological antecedents of excess gestational weight gain.

Competing interests

The authors declare that they have no competing interests.

Authors' contributions

MZK designed and performed the literature review, collected data from individual studies, participated in statistical analysis, data interpretation and was primary author of the manuscript. AG participated in study design, collected data from individual studies, participated in statistical analysis, data interpretation and contributed in writing the manuscript. JB participated in statistical analysis and interpretation. HM, SVB and LS contributed in the study design and data interpretation. SMD conceived the study, and supervised in its design, coordination, analysis, interpretation and writing the manuscript. All authors were involved in drafting or revising the manuscript, and approving the final version.

Acknowledgements

This work was supported by a Canadian Institute of Health Research (CIHR) grant number KRS124594. SDM is supported by a Canadian Institutes of Health Research (CIHR) New Investigator Salary Award. JB is supported John D. Cameron Chair in the Genetic Determinants of Chronic Disease at McMaster University. CIHR and McMaster University had no role in the conduct analyses, writing of the report, interpretation of data or decision to submit the manuscript.
We would like to thank Neera Bhatnager, B.Sc., M.L.I.S., Head of Systems, Coordinator of Research & Graduate Education Support, Health Sciences Library, McMaster University; and Marisa Surmacz, B.Sc., M.L.I.S., Research and Instructional Services Librarian, Allyn & Betty Taylor Library, University of Western Ontario for their assistance in developing the search strategies. We thank Olha Lustiv for her assistance with a number of administrative aspects of the study and Sabnam Mahmuda and Christina Park for their contribution in the creation of the figures for this manuscript.

Author details

[1]Department of Obstetrics and Gynecology, McMaster University, Hamilton, Canada. [2]School of Kinesiology, University of Western Ontario, London, Ontario, Canada. [3]New Leaf Psychology, Milton, Canada. [4]Department of Psychology, Neuroscience & Behavior, McMaster University, Hamilton, Canada. [5]Department Clinical Epidemiology and Biostatistics, McMaster

University, Hamilton, Canada. [6]Midwifery Education Program, Department of Family Medicine, McMaster University, Hamilton, Canada. [7]Division of Maternal-Fetal Medicine, Departments of Obstetrics & Gynecology, Radiology, and Clinical Epidemiology & Biostatistics, McMaster University, 1280 Main Street West, room 3N52B, Hamilton, Ontario L8S 4K1, Canada.

References

1. Rasmussen KM, Yaktine AL. Weight gain during pregnancy: reexamining the guidelines. Washington, D.C.: National Academies Press; 2009.
2. Webb JB, Siega-Riz AM, Dole N. Psychosocial determinants of adequacy of gestational weight gain. Obesity. 2009;17(2):300–9.
3. Chu SY, Callaghan WM, Bish CL, D'Angelo D. Gestational weight gain by body mass index among US women delivering live births, 2004–2005: fueling future obesity. Am J Obstet Gynecol. 2009;200(3):271. e1-7.
4. Li N, Liu E, Guo J, Pan L, Li B, Wang P, et al. The effect of gestational weight gain by body mass index on maternal and neonatal outcomes. J Obstet Gynaecol Can. 2009;31(1):28–35.
5. Kowal C, Kuk J, Tamim H. Characteristics of weight gain in pregnancy among Canadian women. Matern Child Health J. 2012;16(3):668–76.
6. Li N, Liu E, Guo J, Pan L, Li B, Wang P, et al. Maternal prepregnancy body mass index and gestational weight gain on pregnancy outcomes. PLoS One. 2013;8(12):e82310.
7. Amorim AR, Rossner S, Neovius M, Lourenco PM, Linne Y. Does excess pregnancy weight gain constitute a major risk for increasing long-term BMI? Obesity (Silver Spring). 2007;15(5):1278–86.
8. Mamun AA, Kinarivala M, O'Callaghan MJ, Williams GM, Najman JM, Callaway LK. Associations of excess weight gain during pregnancy with long-term maternal overweight and obesity: evidence from 21 y postpartum follow-up. Am J Clin Nutr. 2010;91(5):1336–41.
9. Brawarsky P, Stotland N, Jackson R, Fuentes-Afflick E, Escobar G, Rubashkin N, et al. Pre-pregnancy and pregnancy-related factors and the risk of excessive or inadequate gestational weight gain. Int J Gynecol Obstet. 2005;91(2):125–31.
10. Siega-Riz AM, Viswanathan M, Moos MK, Deierlein A, Mumford S, Knaack J, et al. A systematic review of outcomes of maternal weight gain according to the Institute of Medicine recommendations: birthweight, fetal growth, and postpartum weight retention. Am J Obstet Gynecol. 2009;201(4):339. e1-339.e14.
11. Stotland NE, Cheng YW, Hopkins LM, Caughey AB. Gestational weight gain and adverse neonatal outcome among term infants. Obstet Gynaecol. 2006;108(3, Part 1):635–43.
12. Oken E, Taveras EM, Kleinman KP, Rich-Edwards JW, Gillman MW. Gestational weight gain and child adiposity at age 3 years. Am J Obstet Gynecol. 2007;196(4):322. e1-322. e8.
13. Institute of Medicine. Nutrition During Pregnancy: Part I, Weight Gain: Part II, Nutrient Supplements: Summary. Washington, D.C.: National Academies Press; 1990.
14. Alavi N, Haley S, Chow K, McDonald SD. Comparison of national gestational weight gain guidelines and energy intake recommendations. Obes Rev. 2013;14(1):68–85.
15. Gardner B, Wardle J, Poston L, Croker H. Changing diet and physical activity to reduce gestational weight gain: a meta-analysis. Obes Rev. 2011;12(7):e602–20.
16. Kramer MS, Kakuma R. Energy and protein intake in pregnancy. Cochrane Database Syst Rev. 2003;(4):Cd000032.
17. Kramer, MS, McDonald, SW. Aerobic exercise for women during pregnancy. Cochrane Database Syst Rev. 2006;(3):Cd000180.
18. Choi J, Fukuoka Y, Lee JH. The effects of physical activity and physical activity plus diet interventions on body weight in overweight or obese women who are pregnant or in postpartum: A systematic review and meta-analysis of randomized controlled trials. Prev Med. 2013;56(6):351–64.
19. Streuling I, Beyerlein A, von Kries R. Can gestational weight gain be modified by increasing physical activity and diet counseling? A meta-analysis of interventional trials. Am J Clin Nutr. 2010;92(4):678–87.
20. Tanentsapf I, Heitmann B, Adegboye A. Systematic review of clinical trials on dietary interventions to prevent excessive weight gain during pregnancy among normal weight, overweight and obese women. BMC Pregnancy Childbirth. 2011;11(1):81.
21. Skouteris H, Hartley-Clark L, McCabe M, Milgrom J, Kent B, Herring SJ, et al. Preventing excessive gestational weight gain: a systematic review of interventions. Obes Rev. 2010;11(11):757–68.
22. Duncan S, Barrett LF. Affect is a form of cognition: A neurobiological analysis. Cogn Emot. 2007;21(6):1184–211.
23. Farley SD, Stasson MF. Relative influences of affect and cognition on behavior: are feelings or beliefs more related to blood donation intentions? Exp Psychol. 2003;50(1):55–62.
24. Eagly AH, Chaiken S. The psychology of attitudes. Orlando, FL, US: Harcourt Brace Jovanovich College Publishers. xxii; 1993. p. 794.
25. Jokela M, Hintsanen M, Hakulinen C, Batty GD, Nabi H, Singh-Manoux A, et al. Association of personality with the development and persistence of obesity: a meta-analysis based on individual-participant data. Obes Rev. 2013;14(4):315–23.
26. Israel S, Moffitt TE, Belsky DW, Hancox RJ, Poulton R, Roberts B, et al. Translating personality psychology to help personalize preventive medicine for young adult patients. J Pers Soc Psychol. 2014;106(3):484–98.
27. Roberts BW, Kuncel NR, Shiner R, Caspi A, Goldberg LR. The power of personality- The comparative validity of personality traits, socioeconomic status, and cognitive ability for predicting important life outcomes. Perspect Psychol Sci. 2007;2(4):313–45.
28. American Psychological Association. Personality May be Key Risk Factor in Preventive Health Care. 2014. [cited 2015 30 Jan]; Available from: http://www.apa.org/news/press/releases/2014/03/personality-health.aspx.
29. Moher D, Liberati A, Tetzlaff J, Altman DG. Preferred reporting items for systematic reviews and meta-analyses: the PRISMA statement. BMJ. 2009;339:b2535.
30. Higgins JP, Green S. Collaboration, *Cochrane handbook for systematic reviews of interventions*. Vol. 5. 2008: Wiley Online Library. Available from: www.cochrane-handbook.org.
31. Wells GA, Shea B, O'Connell D, Peterson J, Welch V, Losos M, et al. The Newcastle-Ottawa Scale (NOS) for assessing the quality of nonrandomized studies in meta-analyses. 2013. Available from: http://www.ohri.ca/programs/clinical_epidemiology/oxford.asp.
32. Peduzzi P, Concato J, Kemper E, Holford TR, Feinstein AR. A simulation study of the number of events per variable in logistic regression analysis. J Clin Epidemiol. 1996;49(12):1373–9.
33. Miller RG. Simultaneous statistical inference. New York: Springer-Verlag; 1981.
34. Allison KC, Wrotniak BH, Pare E, Sarwer DB. Psychosocial Characteristics and Gestational Weight Change among Overweight, African American Pregnant Women. Obstet Gynecol Int. 2012;2012:878607.
35. Bagheri M, Dorosty A, Sadrzadeh-Yeganeh H, Eshraghian M, Amiri E, Khamoush-Cheshm N. Pre-pregnancy Body Size Dissatisfaction and Excessive Gestational Weight Gain. Matern Child Health J. 2013;17(4):699–707.
36. Chasan-Taber L, Schmidt MD, Pekow P, Sternfeld B, Solomon CG, Markenson G. Predictors of Excessive and Inadequate Gestational Weight Gain in Hispanic Women. Obesity. 2008;16(7):1657–66.
37. Cogswell ME, Scanlon KS, Fein SB, Schieve LA. Medically Advised, Mother's Personal Target, and Actual Weight Gain During Pregnancy. Obstet Gynecol. 1999;94(4):616–22.
38. Conway R, Reddy S, Davies J. Dietary restraint and weight gain during pregnancy. Eur J Clin Nutr. 1999;53(11):849–53.
39. Copper RL, DuBard MB, Goldenberg RL, Oweis AI. The relationship of maternal attitude toward weight gain to weight gain during pregnancy and low birth weight. Obstet Gynecol. 1995;85(4):590–5.
40. Dipietro JA, Millet S, Costigan KA, Gurewitsch E, Caulfield LE. Psychosocial influences on weight gain attitudes and behaviors during pregnancy. J Am Diet Assoc. 2003;103(10):1314–9.
41. Herring SJ, Oken E, Haines J, Rich-Edwards JW, Rifas-Shiman SL, Kleinman Sc DK. Misperceived pre-pregnancy body weight status predicts excessive gestational weight gain: findings from a US cohort study. BMC Pregnancy Childbirth. 2008;8:54.
42. Hill B, Skouteris H, McCabe M, Fuller-Tyszkiewicz M. Body image and gestational weight gain: a prospective study. J Midwifery Womens Health. 2013;58(2):189–94.
43. Laraia B, Epel E, Siega-Riz AM. Food insecurity with past experience of restrained eating is a recipe for increased gestational weight gain. Appetite. 2013;65:178–84.
44. Loris P, Dewey KG, Poirier-Brode K. Weight gain and dietary intake of pregnant teenagers. J Am Diet Assoc. 1985;85(10):1296–305.

45. McAnarney ER, Stevens-Simon C. Determinants of weight gain in pregnant adolescents. J Am Diet Assoc. 1992;92(11):1348–51 (Note: authors' order is reversed in Pubmed).
46. Mehta U, Siega-Riz A, Herring A. Effect of Body Image on Pregnancy Weight Gain. Matern Child Health J. 2011;15(3):324–32.
47. Morling B, Kitayama S, Miyamoto Y. American and Japanese women use different coping strategies during normal pregnancy. Pers Soc Psychol Bull. 2003;29(12):1533–46.
48. Mumford SL, Siega-Riz AM, Herring A, Evenson KR. Dietary restraint and gestational weight gain. J Am Diet Assoc. 2008;108(10):1646–53.
49. Olson CM, Strawderman MS. Modifiable behavioral factors in a biopsychosocial model predict inadequate and excessive gestational weight gain. J Am Diet Assoc. 2003;103(1):48–54.
50. Pomerleau CS, Brouwer RJ, Jones LT. Weight concerns in women smokers during pregnancy and postpartum. Addict Behav. 2000;25(5):759–67.
51. Sangi-Haghpeykar H, Lam K, Raine SP. Gestational weight gain among hispanic women. Maternal and Child Health Journal. 2013;(Pagination): p. No Pagination Specified.
52. Stevens-Simon C, McAnarney ER. Change in depressive symptoms during pregnancy: Relationship to birth outcome. Adolesc Pediatr Gynecol. 1995;8(1):29–33.
53. Stevens-Simon C, Nakashima I, Andrews D. Weight gain attitudes among pregnant adolescents. J Adolesc Health. 1993;14(5):369–72.
54. Strychar IM, Chabot C, Champagne F, Ghadirian P, Leduc L, Lemonnier MC, et al. Psychosocial and lifestyle factors associated with insufficient and excessive maternal weight gain duping pregnancy. J Am Diet Assoc. 2000;100(3):353–6.
55. Tovar A, Chasan-Taber L, Bermudez OI, Hyatt RR, Must A. Acculturation and gestational weight gain in a predominantly puerto rican population. BMC Pregnancy Childbirth. 2012;12:133.
56. Walker LO, Hoke MM, Brown A. Risk Factors for Excessive or Inadequate Gestational Weight Gain Among Hispanic Women in a U.S.-Mexico Border State. J Obstet Gynecol Neonatal Nurs. 2009;38(4):418–29.
57. Walker LO, Kim M. Psychosocial thriving during late pregnancy: relationship to ethnicity, gestational weight gain, and birth weight. J Obstet Gynecol Neonatal Nurs. 2002;31(3):263–74.
58. Wells CS, Schwalberg R, Noonan G, Gabor V. Factors influencing inadequate and excessive weight gain in pregnancy: Colorado, 2000–2002. Matern Child Health J. 2006;10(1):55–62.
59. Wright C, Bilder D, DeBlasis T, Mogul M, Rubin D, Shea JA. Psychosocial factors associated with gestational weight gain in a low-income cohort. J Health Care Poor Underserved. 2013;24(1):332–43.
60. Zuckerman B, Amaro H, Bauchner H, Cabral H. Depressive symptoms during pregnancy: relationship to poor health behaviors. Am J Obstet Gynecol. 1989;160(5 Pt 1):1107–11.
61. McDonald SD, Park CK, Timm V, Schmidt L, Neupane B, Beyene J. What psychological, physical, lifestyle, and knowledge factors are associated with excess or inadequate weight gain during pregnancy? A cross-sectional survey. J Obstet Gynaecol Can. 2013;35(12):1071–82.
62. McPhie S, Skouteris H, Fuller-Tyszkiewicz M, Hill B, Jacka F, O'Neil A. Relationships between mental health symptoms and body mass index in women with and without excessive weight gain during pregnancy. Midwifery. 2015;31(1):138–46.
63. Mehta-Lee SS, Lischewski Goel JL, Xu L, Brittner MR, Bernstein PS, Bonuck KA. Perception of weight status and its impact on gestational weight gain in an urban population. Maternal & Child Health Journal. 2013;17(10):1931–9.
64. Sui Z, Turnbull D, Dodd J. Effect of body image on gestational weight gain in overweight and obese women. Women Birth. 2013;26(4):267–72.
65. Zhu P, Huang W, Hao JH, Huang K, Jiang XM, Tao FB. Time-specific effect of prenatal stressful life events on gestational weight gain. Int J Gynaecol Obstet. 2013;122(3):207–11.
66. van der Wijden CL, Steinbach S, van der Ploeg HP, van Mechelen W, van Poppel MNM. A longitudinal study on the relationship between eating style and gestational weight gain. Appetite. 2014;83:304–8.
67. Luppino FS, de Wit LM, Bouvy PF, Stijnen T, Cuijpers P, Penninx BWJH. Overweight, obesity, and depression: a systematic review and meta-analysis of longitudinal studies. Arch Gen Psychiatry. 2010;67(3):220.
68. Blaine B. Does Depression Cause Obesity?: A Meta-analysis of Longitudinal Studies of Depression and Weight Control. J Health Psychol. 2008;13(8):1190–7.
69. Rofey DL, Kolko RP, Iosif AM, Silk JS, Bost JE, Feng W. A longitudinal study of childhood depression and anxiety in relation to weight gain. Child Psychiatry Hum Dev. 2009;40(4):517–26.
70. Zhao G, Ford ES, Dhingra S, Li C, Strine TW, Mokdad AH. Depression and anxiety among US adults: associations with body mass index. Int J Obes (Lond). 2009;33(2):257–66.
71. Stice E. Risk and maintenance factors for eating pathology: a meta-analytic review. Psychol Bull. 2002;128(5):825–48.
72. Swann RA, Von Holle A, Torgersen L, Gendall K, Reichborn-Kjennerud T, Bulik CM. Attitudes Toward Weight Gain During Pregnancy: Results from the Norwegian Mother and Child Cohort Study (MoBa). Int J Eat Disord. 2009;42(5):394–401.
73. Dunkel Schetter C, Tanner L. Anxiety, depression and stress in pregnancy: implications for mothers, children, research, and practice. Curr Opin Psychiatry. 2012;25(2):141–8.
74. Block JP, He Y, Zaslavsky AM, Ding L, Ayanian JZ. Psychosocial stress and change in weight among US adults. Am J Epidemiol. 2009;170(2):181–92.
75. Overgaard D, Gamborg M, Gyntelberg F, Heitmann BL. Psychological workload and weight gain among women with and without familial obesity. Obesity. 2006;14(3):458–63.
76. Serlachius A, Hamer M, Wardle J. Stress and weight change in university students in the United Kingdom. Physiol Behav. 2007;92(4):548–53.
77. Vicennati V, Pasqui F, Cavazza C, Pagotto U, Pasquali R. Stress-related development of obesity and cortisol in women. Obesity. 2009;17(9):1678–83.
78. Adam TC, Epel ES. Stress, eating and the reward system. Physiol Behav. 2007;91(4):449–58.
79. Lindsay JR, Nieman LK. The hypothalamic-pituitary-adrenal axis in pregnancy: challenges in disease detection and treatment. Endocr Rev. 2005;26(6):775–99.
80. Riley NM, Bild DE, Cooper L, Schreiner P, Smith DE, Sorlie P, et al. Relation of self-image to body size and weight loss attempts in black women: the CARDIA study. Coronary Artery Risk Development in Young Adults. Am J Epidemiol. 1998;148(11):1062–8.
81. Adolfsson B, Andersson I, Elofsson S, Rossner S, Unden AL. Locus of control and weight reduction. Patient Educ Couns. 2005;56(1):55–61.
82. McDonald SD, Pullenayegum E, Taylor VH, Lutsiv O, Bracken K, Good C, et al. Despite 2009 guidelines, few women report being counseled correctly about weight gain during pregnancy. Am J Obstet Gynecol. 2011;205(4):333. e1-333.e6.
83. Stotland NE, Gilbert P, Bogetz A, Harper CC, Abrams B, Gerbert B. Preventing excessive weight gain in pregnancy: how do prenatal care providers approach counseling? J Womens Health. 2010;19(4):807–14.
84. Hill B, Skouteris H, Fuller-Tyszkiewicz M. Interventions designed to limit gestational weight gain: a systematic review of theory and meta-analysis of intervention components. Obes Rev. 2013;14(6):435–50.
85. Clark M, Ogden J. The impact of pregnancy on eating behaviour and aspects of weight concern. Int J Obes Relat Metab Disord. 1999;23(1):18–24.
86. Polivy J, Herman CP. Dieting and binging: a causal analysis. Am Psychol. 1985;40(2):193.
87. Drewnowski A, Specter S. Poverty and obesity: the role of energy density and energy costs. Am J Clin Nutr. 2004;79(1):6–16.
88. Andajani-Sutjahjo S, Ball K, Warren N, Inglis V, Crawford D. Perceived personal, social and environmental barriers to weight maintenance among young women: a community survey. Int J Behav Nutr Phys Act. 2004;1(1):15.
89. Van Buren DJ, Sinton MM. Psychological aspects of weight loss and weight maintenance. J Am Diet Assoc. 2009;109(12):1994–6.
90. AbuSabha R, Achterberg C. Review of self-efficacy and locus of control for nutrition-and health-related behavior. J Am Diet Assoc. 1997;97(10):1122–32.
91. Tuffery O, Scriven A. Factors influencing antenatal and postnatal diets of primigravid women. J R Soc Promot Health. 2005;125(5):227–31.
92. Sutin AR, Ferrucci L, Zonderman AB, Terracciano A. Personality and obesity across the adult life span. J Pers Soc Psychol. 2011;101:579–92.
93. Rosenthal R. Meta-analytic procedures for social research. Vol. 6. Newbury Park: SAGE Publications, Inc; 1991.

18

Maternal obesity and fetal deaths: results from the Brazilian cross-sectional demographic health survey, 2006

Mariana Santos Felisbino-Mendes[1], Fernanda Penido Matozinhos[1], J Jaime Miranda[2], Eduardo Villamor[3] and Gustavo Velasquez-Melendez[1*]

Abstract

Background: Obesity is highly related to negative reproductive health outcomes, but its relationship with spontaneous abortion and stillbirth remains to be understood, especially in transitioning economies. This study aimed to examine the relationship between obesity and spontaneous abortions and stillbirths in a representative sample of the Brazilian population.

Methods: Cross-sectional study using secondary data of Brazilian women of reproductive age (15–45 years old) from the National Demographic and Health Survey in 2006. Obesity was measured by body mass index (BMI), waist circumference (WC) and waist-to-height ratio (WHR). Logistic regression modeling of the survey data was used to evaluate the relationship between obesity and the study outcomes.

Results: The three obesity markers used were found to be strongly and positively associated with spontaneous abortion and stillbirth occurrence. In the adjusted models, there was strong evidence that for each unit increase in BMI (OR = 1.05; 95%CI: 1.02-1.08) and WHR (OR = 1.32; 95%CI: 1.03-1.69), the odds of having a spontaneous abortion was higher. In addition, compared to those of optimal weight, obese women were more likely to have negative outcomes. Maternal age, parity, skin color, educational level and household income were important covariates for adjustment. A sensitivity analysis among women who had only one pregnancy was also performed and showed similar results.

Conclusion: Obesity is potentially associated with an increased risk of spontaneous abortion and stillbirth in a representative sample of the Brazilian population. These findings are in accordance with previous studies and thus reinforce the need for obstetric care providers to counsel obese reproductive-age women regarding the risks, complications and importance of weight loss and weight control prior to pregnancy.

Keywords: Spontaneous abortion, Stillbirth, Obesity, Body mass index, Waist circumference

Background

Obesity is increasing worldwide and has significant health-related consequences, including increased mortality [1,2]. Obesity is a growing problem, particularly among women, who have a combined prevalence of overweight and obesity of over 20% [3-5].

This increase is also observed in middle-income countries, such as Brazil, a country that is rapidly transitioning with an emerging economy. For instance, national surveys in the last 34 years have shown a continuous increase in overweight and obesity prevalence among Brazilian men and women. Most up-to-date estimates show that overweight and obesity levels are approximately 50% and 15%, respectively [6]. In reproductive-age women, the prevalence of obesity is approximately 17%.

Being overweight is a significant handicap in women undergoing infertility treatment, and women are often encouraged to lose weight before treatment [2,7]. Additionally,

* Correspondence: guveme@ufmg.br
[1]Department of Maternal and Child Nursing and Public Health, Escola de Enfermagem, Universidade Federal de Minas Gerais (UFMG), Av. Alfredo Balena, 190 - Bairro Santa Efigênia, 30130-100, Belo Horizonte, MG, Brasil
Full list of author information is available at the end of the article

maternal obesity is associated with various risks in pregnancy and to offspring [7]. It leads to changes in maternal metabolism, and some studies have also associated obesity with abortion, late fetal death and infertility risk [2,8,9]. Moreover, consequences of maternal obesity may extend beyond fetal life into childhood and adulthood, when the fetus becomes a viable and live birth [2,10,11]. This relationship has been consistently shown in studies in high-income countries, but poorly explored in low and middle-income nations, such as Brazil [12-14], where obesity is a rapidly growing problem for public health.

Most of the previous research regarding the association between obesity and reproductive outcomes only used body mass index (BMI) as an obesity marker. On the other hand, waist circumference (WC), a more direct measure of the abdominal accumulation of fat [15], and waist-to-height ratio (WHR), a more practical index for screening the risk of obesity-related disorders that could be applied uniformly to all ethnicities and ages [16], are also important and reliable obesity indexes [16-18]. This study aimed to examine the potential relationship between obesity and the occurrence of spontaneous abortion and stillbirths in a representative sample of the Brazilian female population.

Methods

Data sources, study population and sample size

The data for this study came from the 2006–2007 Brazilian National Demographic and Health Survey (DHS), which is a nationally representative cross-sectional study carried out in 2006 by the Ministry of Health designed to evaluate maternal and child health. Data collection was performed through home interviews and exams of non-institutionalized women at reproductive age (15 to 49 years). Detailed sampling plans, data collection information and data quality assurance are available in the DHS 2006 survey final reports at http://bvsms.saude.gov.br/bvs/pnds/index.php.

The DHS 2006 sample was stratified by urban and rural areas and by geographic region: Northeast, Southeast, North, Mid-West and South. The sample was composed of 14,617 households with 56,365 women; 15,575 of them were of reproductive age and 6,833 had reported at least one pregnancy after 2001. From this number, 109 women were excluded due to twin births or absence of data regarding the event (birth or death). Thus, from the 6,724 women available for the study, 11.6% (SE 0.7) declared fetal deaths. Of these deaths, 70.2% (SE 3.0) were spontaneous abortions and 11.4% (SE 1.9) were stillbirths. Other types of deaths, such as ectopic pregnancy and induced abortion, were not considered in this study (18.4%; SE 2.6) (n = 109). Pregnant women were also excluded from the sample (n = 433). The total sample subpopulation was 6,182 (Figure 1).

Outcome, exposure of interest and confounders

The endpoint for our study was fetal deaths, derived from the pregnancies that occurred from 2001 until the time of the interview. This general outcome included spontaneous abortions (≤ 20 weeks of gestational age) and stillbirths (> 20 weeks of pregnancy). Both of them were self-reported and binary (1 = abortion/stillbirth, 0 = otherwise).

Obesity was the exposure of interest, and it was ascertained through three different indicators: WC, WHR and BMI. The waist circumference categories were determined as follows: normal (< 80 cm), overweight (80–87.9 cm) and obesity (≥ 88 cm). WHR was calculated dividing the women's WC by their height, both measured in centimeters, and the categories were defined by quartiles of distribution, where the first quartile consisted of the lowest values and the fourth consisted of the highest. Height and weight were used to calculate BMI according to the formula weight/height^2, and the women were classified into the following categories: undernutrition (< 18.5 kg/m^2), eutrophic (18.5-24.9 kg/m^2), overweight (25.0-29.9 kg/m^2), obesity class I (30.0-34.9 kg/m^2) and obesity class II-III (≥ 35.0 kg/m^2). All indexes were analyzed as continuous and categorical variables, and WC and BMI were classified according to conventional cut-off points [1,19].

The potential confounders were considered according to the conceptual model (Figure 2) [20,21], and important adjustments were made when related to the outcome and the exposure of interest, such as maternal age group (15–19; 20–24; 25–29; 30–34; 35–39; ≥ 40), educational level in years (illiteracy; 1–4; 5–8; 9–11; 12 or more years), skin color as a proxy for race and socioeconomic status (white, brown, black, others), parity (0–1; 2–3; ≥ 4 children) marital status (single; married or cohabitating; widowed; divorced), occupation (yes or no), smoking status (yes or no), and quartiles of household income (1st quartile: 0–270, 2nd quartile: 271–500, 3rd quartile: 501–972 and 4th quartile: ≥ 973; in 2006–2007, approximately US$ 0.47 dollars per Brazilian *real*) and area of residence (urban/rural).

Analysis

Analyses were performed with STATA version 12.0 (Stata Corp., College Station, TX, USA), using survey commands, to account for the complex sample survey data composition: strata, clusters and weights. Instead of excluding participants, we conducted an unconditional subpopulation analysis [22], restricting the estimate to a subpopulation of interest. This type of performance is highly recommended when analyzing complex designed data because it is a more appropriate approach to variance estimates [22]. Out of a total sample of 6,724 participants, our subpopulation included 6,182 non-pregnant women with a history of pregnancy after 2001 to data collection

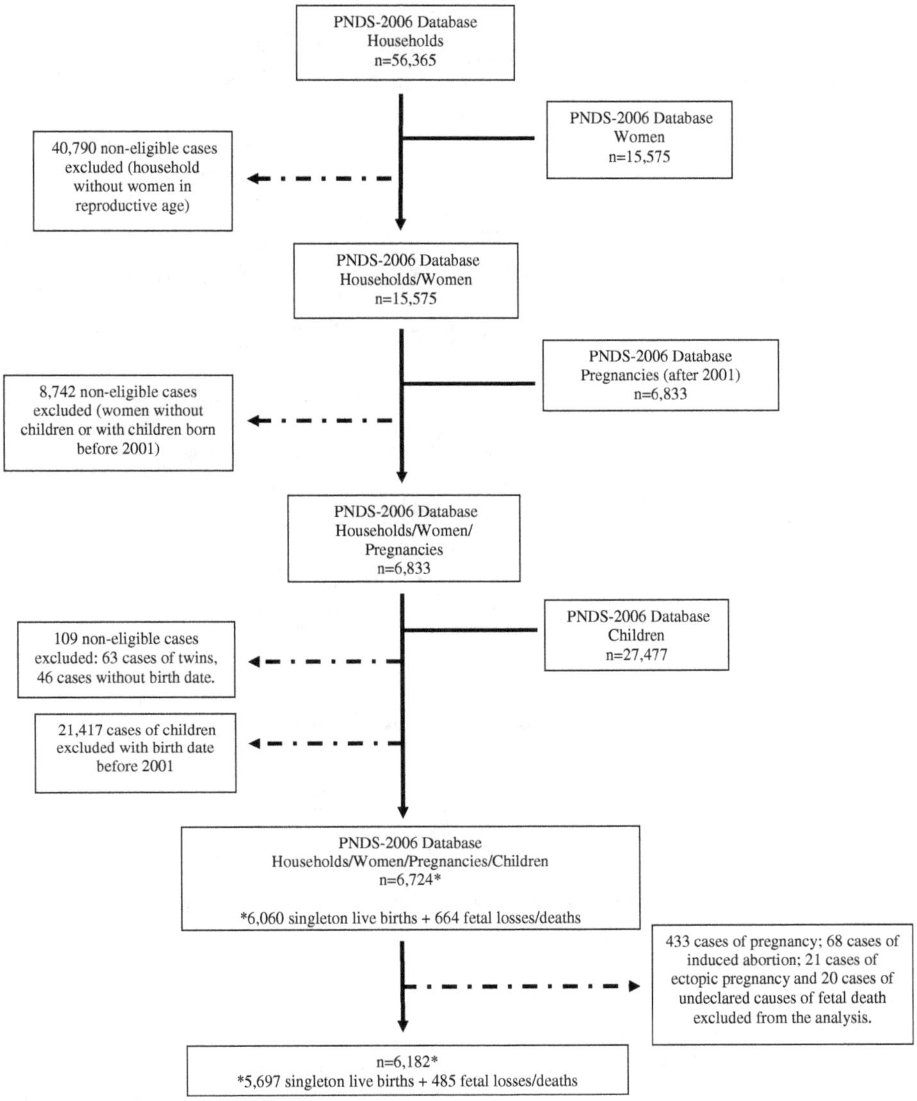

Figure 1 Study population flowchart.

(single live births or incomplete pregnancies) (Figure 1). Thus, we treated the exclusion conditions as category 0 of the subpopulation indicator and the population of interest as category 1 [22].

Proportions and standard errors (SE) were estimated by descriptive analysis. We also estimated unadjusted and adjusted odds ratios (OR) and 95% confidence intervals (95% CI) for all outcomes according to obesity markers. The logistic regression models were adjusted by maternal age group, parity, skin color, household income, maternal education and maternal smoking status. Wald design-based chi-square and goodness of fit tests were also performed to evaluate the fitted models [23].

Finally, we conducted a sensitivity analysis that consisted of the same performance but restricted to the women who reported only one pregnancy at the time of the interview. This analysis consisted in an effort to attenuate potential effect of changes, usually increases, in obesity indicators in multiparous women.

Ethical review

Our study used de-identified data. The DHS was conducted following standard ethical guidelines established by Helsinki Declaration and was approved by the Ethical Committee Council of the State Health Secretary of Sao Paulo.

Results

Sociodemographic characteristics

We examined the distribution of demographic and socioeconomic characteristics in the total population and according to the reproductive health outcomes studied (Table 1). The majority of women in the sample analyzed were < 40 years old (93%), living in urban areas (80%)

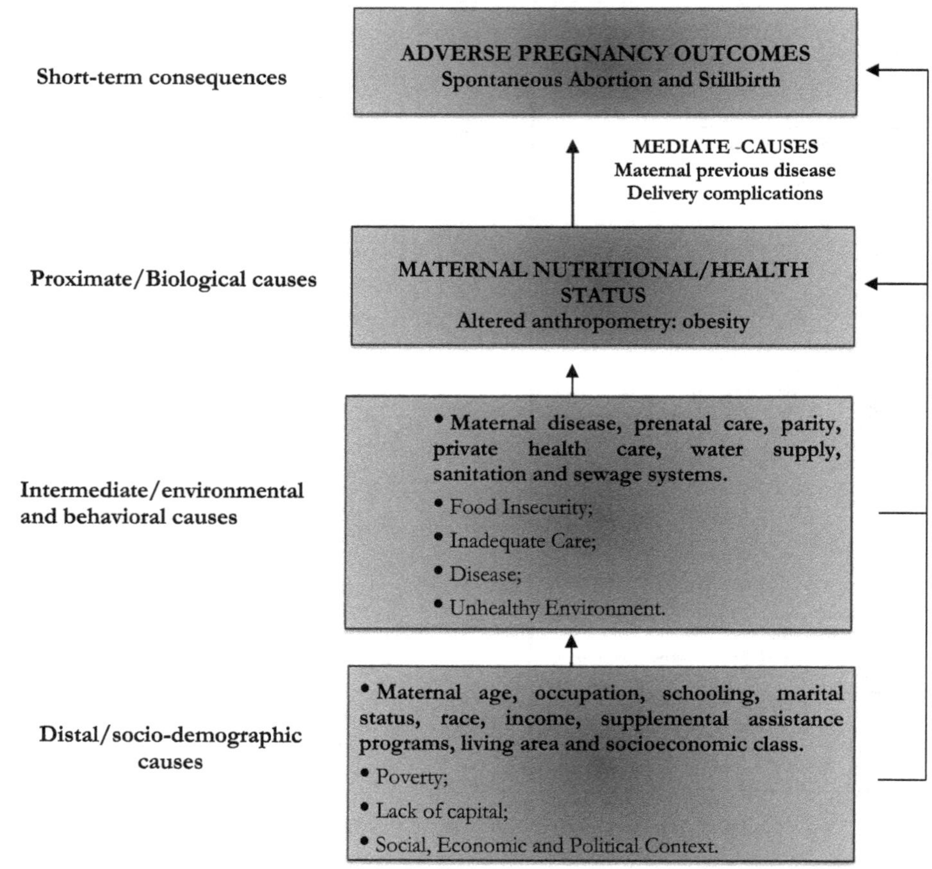

Figure 2 Framework of the relationship between the causes of maternal obesity and the fetal consequences. Adapted from Black et al., 2008 and Mosley & Chen, 1984.

and had a higher educational level with 9 or more years of education (43%). Of all participants, 51% had 2 or 3 children and approximately 85% of the women were married.

Prevalence of abortion and stillbirths

Women of advanced age had a higher proportion of abortions and stillbirths. Stillbirths were more frequent at either very young or very old ages. The proportion of abortions also increased with maternal education, but an inverse relationship was observed for stillbirths. Furthermore, total fetal deaths were more frequent among women with a marital status of single, women who reported 0–1 children and women whose skin color was declared black and brown (Table 1).

The proportion of abortions and stillbirths were higher among overweight and obese women (Table 2). The proportion of fetal deaths was also higher in abdominally obese women (10.2%) and in women with the highest values of WHR (4th quartile, 10.9%). The unadjusted association between any index of obesity and total deaths was significant (Table 2). In these preliminary models, women with higher BMI values (≥ 35 Kg/m^2) presented an almost twofold higher odds of abortion (OR = 1.96; 95%CI: 1.16-3.30) compared to those with lower values of this anthropometric marker. This relationship was not found for abdominal obesity (WC) or higher values of WHR, only after controlling for confounders.

Association between obesity markers and outcomes

Women with WC values equal to or greater than 88 cm were also more likely to report a stillbirth (OR = 2.61; 95%CI: 1.13-6.04) when compared to those with lower and median values for these measures ($p < 0.05$). The same pattern was observed for those who had WHR values in the 4th quartile of the distribution ($p < 0.05$). These associations remained unchanged after adjusting for maternal age group, parity, skin color, educational level, smoking status and household income (Table 3). Adjusted OR and 95% confidence intervals for the associations between obesity markers and the reproductive outcomes showed that all anthropometric indexes positively associated with the total deaths. There was strong evidence that for each unit increase in BMI (OR = 1.05; 95%CI: 1.02-1.08) and WHR (OR = 1.32; 95%CI: 1.03-1.69), the odds of having a spontaneous abortion was higher. We

Table 1 Demographic and socioeconomic characteristic distribution in the total study population and according to reproductive outcome – DHS/2006, Brazil

Characteristics	Total population		Spontaneous abortion	Stillbirth	All deaths[a]
	n[b]	% ± (SE)	% ± (SE)	% ± (SE)	% ± (SE)
Age					
15-19	448	8.8 (0.8)	8.4 (1.7)	2.4 (1.3)	10.6 (2.1)
20-24	1726	30.3 (1.2)	6.9 (1.2)	1.2 (0.5)	7.9 (1.2)
25-29	1733	25.4 (1.0)	5.6 (0.9)	1.4 (0.4)	6.9 (1.0)
30-34	1215	17.7 (1.0)	7.4 (1.3)	0.7 (0.3)	8.1 (1.3)
35-39	678	11.1 (0.8)	11.1 (2.4)	1.7 (0.9)	12.6 (2.5)
≥ 40	382	6.8 (0.7)	15.1 (3.2)	3.2 (2.0)	17.9 (3.5)
Area of residence					
Urban	4063	79.6 (1.6)	8.1 (0.8)	1.2 (0.3)	9.0 (1.2)
Rural	2119	20.5 (1.6)	6.8 (1.2)	2.4 (0.7)	9.2 (0.8)
Schooling (years)					
0	205	2.7 (0.4)	2.9 (2.0)	6.5 (4.2)	9.2 (4.4)
1-4	1424	19.0 (1.3)	6.0 (1.2)	1.7 (0.7)	7.6 (1.3)
5-8	2215	35.7 (1.4)	7.9 (1.0)	1.5 (0.4)	9.3 (1.1)
9-11	1911	35.4 (1.5)	8.1 (1.1)	0.7 (0.2)	8.7 (1.1)
12+	380	7.2 (0.8)	11.9 (2.7)	1.9 (1.4)	13.6 (3.1)
Skin color					
White	2093	33.9 (1.4)	6.9 (0.9)	1.3 (0.5)	8.1 (1.0)
Brown	3068	49.5 (1.6)	7.4 (1.0)	1.8 (0.4)	9.1 (1.0)
Black	620	11.0 (1.1)	11.5 (2.1)	0.9 (0.5)	12.3 (2.1)
Other	329	5.6 (0.7)	10.7 (3.3)	0.1 (0.1)	10.8 (3.3)
Parity					
0-1	1944	38.3 (1.4)	12.8 (1.4)	1.9 (0.5)	14.5 (1.4)
2-3	3070	51.2 (1.4)	4.9 (0.7)	1.1 (0.4)	6.0 (0.7)
≥ 4	1168	10.5 (0.6)	3.8 (1.1)	1.0 (0.4)	4.8 (1.1)
Marital status					
Single	337	5.5 (0.8)	9.0 (2.9)	2.4 (1.2)	11.1 (3.0)
Married	5157	85.2 (1.1)	7.8 (0.7)	1.5 (0.3)	9.1 (0.8)
Widowed	38	0.6 (0.2)	3.1 (2.6)	0.6 (0.6)	3.6 (2.8)
Divorced	646	8.7 (0.8)	8.0 (1.7)	0.4 (0.2)	8.3 (1.7)
Smoking Status					
Yes	1,000	16.3 (1.0)	10.2 (1.8)	1.8 (0.9)	11.8 (1.8)
No	5,182	86.7 (1.0)	7.4 (0.7)	1.4 (0.3)	8.6 (0.7)
Income[c]					
1st Quartile (0–270)	1325	22.0 (1.4)	6.1 (1.0)	2.2 (0.8)	8.2 (1.2)
2nd Quartile (271–500)	1521	26.4 (1.6)	6.4 (1.1)	2.2 (0.7)	8.5 (1.1)
3rd Quartile (501–972)	1187	21.6 (1.1)	8.3 (1.4)	1.3 (0.6)	9.5 (1.5)
4th Quartile (≥ 973)	1406	30.0 (1.7)	10.3 (1.7)	0.5 (0.3)	10.8 (1.7)

[a]Abortions and Stillbirths [b]n = real sample values. [c]Value in reais (in 2006–07, US$ 0.47 per real). *SE* Standard Error.

also observed that abdominal obesity (WC ≥ 88 cm) was strongly associated with stillbirths (OR = 2.91; 95%CI: 1.32-6.44), while global obesity (BMI ≥ 35 Kg/m^2) was highly predictive of abortion occurrence (OR = 2.49; 95% CI: 1.45-4.26). We observed no association between overweight women and fetal deaths.

Table 2 Proportions (SE) and unadjusted OR (95% CI) of spontaneous abortions and stillbirths according to maternal anthropometry – Brazil, DHS/2006

Maternal anthropometry	n	Spontaneous abortions		Stillbirths		Total deaths	
		% ± (SE)	Unadjusted OR (95%CI)	% ± (SE)	Unadjusted OR (95%CI)	% ± (SE)	Unadjusted OR (95%CI)
Maternal BMI (Kg/m²)							
Underweight (<18.5)	251	4.5 (1.7)	0.55 (0.25-1.22)	0.1 (0.1)	0.08 (0.01-0.63)*	4.6 (1.7)	0.49 (0.22-1.06)
Normal (18.5-24.9)	3,302	7.8 (0.8)	1.00	1.2 (0.3)	1.00	9.0 (0.8)	1.00
Overweight (25-29.9)	1,645	7.4 (1.3)	0.94 (0.63-1.41)	1.4 (0.5)	1.10 (0.44-2.79)	8.6 (1.3)	0.96 (0.67-1.56)
Obese 1 (≥ 30 -34.99)	625	6.6 (1.6)	0.84 (0.49-1.44)	2.2 (0.9)	1.83 (0.72-4.67)	8.7 (1.8)	0.97 (0.60-1.56)
Obese 2–3 (≥ 35)	359	14.3 (3.1)	1.96 (1.16-3.30)*	3.4 (2.4)	2.81 (0.60-13.22)	17.1 (2.8)	2.10 (1.36-3.25)*
Maternal BMI (per 1 Kg/m²)	**6,182**	-	1.03 (1.00-1.07)	-	1.07 (1.00-1.14)*	-	1.04 (1.01-1.07)*
Maternal WC (cm)							
Normal (< 80)	2,782	7.4 (0.8)	1.00	0.9 (0.3)	1.00	8.3 (0.9)	1.00
Overweight (80–87.9)	1,457	7.9 (1.2)	1.06 (0.71-1.60)	1.3 (0.6)	1.41 (0.48-4.23)	9.1 (1.3)	1.10 (0.75-1.60)
Obese (≥ 88)	1,758	8.2 (1.3)	1.10 (0.74-1.63)	2.4 (0.6)	2.61 (1.13-6.04)*	10.2 (1.3)	1.26 (0.90-1.75)
Maternal WC (per 1 cm)	**5,997**	-	1.01 (1.00-1.03)	-	1.03 (1.00-1.06)	-	1.02 (1.00-1.03)*
Maternal WHR							
1st quartile	1,494	6.6 (1.0)	1.00	0.8 (0.4)	1.00	7.4 (1.0)	1.00
2nd quartile	1,495	8.1 (1.3)	1.25 (0.78-1.98)	0.9 (0.4)	1.09 (0.30-3.92)	8.9 (1.3)	1.23 (0.80-1.90)
3rd quartile	1,490	8.0 (1.2)	1.23 (0.79-1.93)	1.3 (0.5)	1.53 (0.48-4.88)	9.2 (1.3)	1.27 (0.84-1.93)
4th quartile	1,494	8.4 (1.5)	1.30 (0.80-2.12)	2.8 (0.8)	3.42 (1.15-10.13)*	10.9 (1.5)	1.55 (1.02-2.35)*
Maternal WHR (per 0.1)	**5,973**	-	1.19 (0.94-1.51)	-	1.78 (1.13-2.81)*	-	1.29 (1.06-1.55)*

*$p < 0.05$; *BMI* Body Mass Index, *WC* Waist Circumference, *WHR* Waist-to-Height Ratio, *OR* Odds Ratio, *SE* Standard Error, *95%CI* 95% Confidence Interval.

Sensitivity analysis

Furthermore, a sensitivity analysis (data not shown) was performed and consisted of evaluating all these relationships, but only among women who declared only one pregnancy. The results showed the same direction of the associations found for the entire population. Obese women with a BMI ≥ 35 Kg/m^2 were found to have a greater chance of abortion, even after adjustment. Abdominally obese women had greater odds of stillbirth. Thus, for each unit increase in BMI, WC and WHR, the odds of total death were also increased. These associations remained significant even after adjusting for maternal age group, skin color, educational level, smoking status and household income, and confirmed the associations found for the whole population, regardless of the number of pregnancies.

Discussion

Main findings

In this study, obesity was associated with greater odds of spontaneous abortion and stillbirth among Brazilian women of reproductive age. This association was observed using different anthropometric markers of obesity (BMI, WC and WHR). The gain of each BMI unit increased the odds of spontaneous abortion and total deaths by approximately 5%. Women with higher BMI values (≥ 35.0 Kg/m^2) had the highest chance of total death, and this obesity index was shown to be a more important predictor of abortion. Moreover, a WC ≥ 88 cm was a better predictor of the occurrence of stillbirths, with an almost 3-times greater chance compared with the baseline of optimal-waist circumference women (WC < 80 cm). WHR also presented a positive association with fetal outcomes. For each increase of 0.1 units of this ratio, women presented 32% and 65% increased odds of abortion and stillbirth, respectively. These results were adjusted for maternal age group, parity, skin color, household income, educational level and smoking status, which did not attenuate the associations found.

Results in the context of other studies

These findings are consistent with those found in high-income countries [24-26] and low-income countries [12-14], although the majority of the studies focus on stillbirths and death after the child is born.

Anthropometric measures of obesity could contribute to fetal deaths. Similar studies have shown that obesity relates to the occurrence of adverse pregnancy outcomes, but most of these studies focused on maternal outcomes. We advanced these observations by considering fetal outcomes in the context of an emerging economy. Findings from a study that evaluated the risk of

Table 3 Adjusted OR (95% CI) of spontaneous abortions and stillbirths according to maternal anthropometry – Brazil, DHS/2006

Maternal anthropometry	Spontaneous abortions	Stillbirths	Total deaths
	Adjusted[a] OR (95%CI)	Adjusted[a] OR (95%CI)	Adjusted[a] OR (95%CI)
Maternal BMI (Kg/m^2)			
Underweight (<18.5)	0.44 (0.19-1.02)	0.06 (0.01-0.48)*	0.37 (0.16-0.83)
Normal (18.5-24.9)	1.00	1.00	1.00
Overweight (25–29.9)	1.02 (0.64-1.64)	1.07 (0.43-2.67)	1.04 (0.68-1.59)
Obese 1 (≥ 30 -34.99)	1.14 (0.63-2.05)	2.16 (0.82-5.73)	1.29 (0.76-2.17)
Obese 2–3 (≥ 35)	2.49 (1.45-4.26)*	2.51 (0.46-13.74)	2.54 (1.49-4.31)*
Maternal BMI (per 1 Kg/m^2)	1.05 (1.01-1.08)*	1.06 (1.00-1.13)	1.05 (1.02-1.08)*
Maternal WC (cm)			
Normal (< 80)	1.00	1.00	1.00
Overweight (80–87.9)	0.91 (0.58-1.43)	1.32 (0.48-3.67)	0.96 (0.64-1.46)
Obese (≥ 88)	1.30 (0.80-2.10)	2.91 (1.32-6.44)*	1.51 (1.00-2.31)
Maternal WC (per 1 cm)	1.02 (1.00-1.03)*	1.03 (1.00-1.06)	1.02 (1.01-1.04)*
Maternal WHR			
1st quartile	1.00	1.00	1.00
2nd quartile	0.98 (0.59-1.64)	0.89 (0.25-3.21)	0.97 (0.61-1.54)
3rd quartile	1.18 (0.73-1.92)	1.40 (0.48-4.12)	1.21 (0.78-1.89)
4th quartile	1.51 (0.89-2.59)	3.17 (1.17-8.56)*	1.75 (1.09-2.81)*
Maternal WHR (per 0.1)	1.32 (1.03-1.69)*	1.65 (1.06-2.57)*	1.39 (1.12-1.73)*

Notes: [a]Adjusted for maternal age group, parity, skin color, household income, maternal education and maternal smoking status. *BMI* Body Mass Index, *WC* Waist Circumference, *WHR* Waist-to-Height Ratio, *OR* Odds Ratio, *SE* Standard Error, *95%CI* 95% Confidence Interval; *$p < 0.05$.

spontaneous abortion in 1,644 pregnant, obese women from a United Kingdom hospital facility compared to a control group of 3,288 women with normal BMI suggests an increased risk of abortion and recurrent early abortions in obese women [27].

Beyond population-based studies, obesity also impacts heavily on the clinical setting and the individual's well-being. In addition to responding poorly to fertility treatments, obese women also have an increased risk of infertility [7]. Systematic reviews have shown that women who were overweight and obese had significantly lower clinical pregnancy and live birth rates (RR = 0.90 and 0.84), respectively. Obese women showed a higher abortion rate when compared to non-obese women (OR = 1.31, 95% CI 1.18 – 1.46) [28,29].

In addition to abortion, studies have also investigated the relationship of obesity leading to late fetal deaths. The results of one study that investigated the effect of obesity on pregnancy outcomes suggested that among nulliparous women in Sweden, the odds ratio for late fetal death was increased among women with a higher BMI compared with lean women (≤ 19.9 Kg/m^2) [30]. This study also observed an increased risk among women with normal BMI levels (OR = 2.2; 95%CI: 1.2-4.1), overweight women (OR = 3.2; 95%CI: 1.6-6.2), and obese women (OR = 4.3; 95%CI: 2.0-9.3) [30]. Thus, among parous Swedish women, only obese women had a significant increase in the risk of late fetal death (OR = 2.0; 95%CI: 1.2-3.3) [30]. Similar results have been shown in Danish obese women, who presented a more than two-fold risk of stillbirth (OR = 2.8; 95% CI: 1.5-5.3) (BMI ≥ 30 Kg/m^2) compared to normal BMI women [31]. Additionally, adjusted estimates showed a 63% greater likelihood of stillbirth among Swedish women who gained three or more BMI units between pregnancies when compared to those who changed less than one unit [24]. These authors also found that slight changes in BMI considerably increased the risk of adverse pregnancy outcomes. These studies corroborate our results, although we found WC to be related more to the occurrence of stillbirths than to BMI. Experimental data on obesity and abortion also provide support for our hypothesis [32,33].

Limitations

The cross-sectional design of the DHS 2006 data limits our causal inference because it was difficult to determine temporality for the association of obesity and fetal deaths. To avoid the possibility of reverse causation, the ideal measurement should occur before pregnancy or during the first trimester. This absence of data is a serious limitation of our study, and only prospective primary data collection would resolve the issue. As previously reported, longitudinal data on this matter with nationally representative data are scarce, especially in low- and middle-income countries [26]. In an attempt to overcome this limitation, we performed an analysis with only primiparous women. This subset consisted of approximately a third of the entire study population and hindered possible weight gain after having several pregnancies. The results from this analysis remained unchanged and showed the same direction of the associations found in the analysis with the entire population, even after adjusting for the same confounders. We recognize that women could gain weight for some reasons other than multiple pregnancies, and this lack of temporal information indicates that our results should be interpreted carefully. Another way to overcome this limitation could be to evaluate whether changes in BMI after birth differed between women who lost their babies and those who did not [14]; however, because of the lack of exact data of the outcome (abortion or stillbirth), we could not perform this evaluation. Even so, our observations align in direction and magnitude with those previously reported in other high-income settings, indicating that this bias might not heavily affect our estimates. Additionally, there is also the possibility of residual confounding by unmeasured diseases and other conditions that may be associated with adverse pregnancy outcomes.

We should also note that the outcomes were self-reported. Although it is uncommon for a woman to forget such an event, directly measuring the occurrence of abortions and stillbirths would be the ideal assessment.

Biological plausibility and implications

Despite these limitations, our findings are also consistent with those of similar studies, and plausible mechanisms that explain the link between obesity and fetal death have been proposed. This link may be directly related to obesity or to obesity-associated conditions, such as gestational diabetes and hypertensive disorders. Obesity is known to affect gonadal function, inhibiting ovarian follicle development throughout secreted adipokines that stimulate the hypothalamus. The adipokines also regulate embryo development in the early stages of cellular division, which, among other specific mechanisms, might justify the low reproduction performance in overweight and obese women [8]. Therefore, these changes could also explain harmful consequences to the child or even the unviability of the fetus. Additionally, previous studies have shown reproductive problems in obese women, such as proinflammatory cytokine accumulation, which could harm fetal membranes [34]; deregulation of metabolic, vascular and inflammatory pathways [10]; and hyperlipidemia, which reduces prostacyclin secretion and enhances peroxidase production, resulting in vasoconstriction and platelet aggregation [35]. We believe that some of these pathways offer plausible routes that provide reasonable explanations for the miscarriage and late fetal death observed in obese women.

The differential association of the two measures of obesity (BMI and WC) with early and late fetal deaths, respectively, is uncertain. This uncertainty might arise because WC is a more proximate measure of fat accumulation in the abdominal region, indicating a more deleterious form of obesity, a condition that is highly associated with inflammation, insulin resistance and the future development of diabetes [36]. Although very speculative, these events may have different triggers, and stillbirths are more closely related to a pre-diabetes condition while abortions are more closely related to the direct effects of obesity on reproductive function.

In public health terms, the findings of our study demonstrate the need for obstetric care providers to counsel obese reproductive-aged women regarding the risks, complications and importance of weight loss and weight control prior to pregnancy. In Brazil, non-communicable diseases have become the most important health problem. Brazil's Unified Health System (SUS) provides primary health care based on Family Health Programme teams. Improvements in access to integral care towards the prevention of chronic diseases have been observed since its implementation and continuous expansion. Specific programs, such as smoking cessation, diabetes screening, and the distribution of low cost, generic and even free medications, have already been implemented. Despite these advances, critical aspects of the chronic care model of this program still remain, such as pressure for the incorporation of high complexity care rather than making good use of cost-effective technologies, and the absence of legislative and regulatory norms. Other health professionals, such as nutritionists, physical educators, psychologists, and psychiatrists, should support primary health care teams [37]. This initiative could promote physical activity and dietary modifications as a strategy to improve weight control and to avoid postpartum weight retention, consequently preventing maternal obesity. Thus, lifestyle changes could result in significant improvement in women's reproductive function. From the standpoint of primary prevention, adverse pregnancy outcomes related to obesity may be preventable, and the identification of obesity in these women is a cost-effective prevention strategy because BMI calculation only requires simple measures, such as weight and height, along with the waist circumference, for the identification of abdominal obesity.

Conclusions

In summary, we analyzed data from a large national demographic survey in Brazil with an emphasis on spontaneous abortions, stillbirths and total fetal death outcomes of participating women. Our results provide important epidemiological information in the direction of a potential positive relationship between markers of obesity and the risk of spontaneous abortion and stillbirth occurrence in a representative sample of the Brazilian population. Our study also used the WC and WHR ratio as an obesity index, and we believe that this use reinforces the importance of the results found. Moreover, our findings provide further justification for the development of effective strategies to reverse the trends toward a higher prevalence of maternal overweight and obesity.

Abbreviations

95% CI: 95% Confidence interval; BMI: Body mass index; DHS: Demographic and health survey; OR: Odds ratio; RR: Risk ratio; SE: Standard error; WC: Waist circumference; WHR: Waist-to-height ratio.

Competing interests

The authors declare that they have no competing interests.

Authors' contributions

MSFM participated in the conception, design, analysis and interpretation of data, and drafted the manuscript. FMP participated in the conception, design and data analysis, and helped to draft the manuscript. JJM helped to draft the manuscript and critically revised it for important intellectual content. EV participated in analysis and interpretation of data and critically revised it for important intellectual content. GVM conceived of the study, and participated in its design, interpretation of data, coordination, and critically revised it for important intellectual content. All authors read and approved the final manuscript.

Acknowledgements

MSFM received PhD scholarship from FAPEMIG and would also like to thank the Coordenação de Aperfeiçoamento de Pessoal de Nível Superior – CAPES, Brazil, for a scholarship that supported a fellowship at the University of Michigan, USA. JJM is with CRONICAS Centre of Excellence in Chronic Diseases at Universidad Peruana Cayetano Heredia, which is funded by the National Heart, Lung and Blood Institute, National Institutes of Health, Department of Health and Human Services, under contract No. HHSN268200900033C. GVM is a research fellow from the Brazilian National Council for Scientific and Technological Development (CNPq) and FAPEMIG. GVM also acknowledge the support from Pró-Reitoria de Pesquisa of Universidade Federal de Minas Gerais.

Author details

[1]Department of Maternal and Child Nursing and Public Health, Escola de Enfermagem, Universidade Federal de Minas Gerais (UFMG), Av. Alfredo Balena, 190 - Bairro Santa Efigênia, 30130-100, Belo Horizonte, MG, Brasil. [2]CRONICAS Center of Excellence in Chronic Diseases, and Department of Medicine, School of Medicine, Universidad Peruana Cayetano Heredia, Lima, Peru. [3]Department of Epidemiology, School of Public Health, University of Michigan, Ann Arbor, MI, USA.

References

1. World Health Organization: **Obesity: preventing and managing the global epidemic. Report of a WHO consultation.** *World Health Organ Tech Rep Ser* 2000, **894:**1–253.
2. Sirimi N, Goulis DG: **Obesity in pregnancy.** *Hormones* 2010, **9:**299–306.
3. Mendez MA, Monteiro CA, Popkin BM: **Overweight exceeds underweight among women in most developing countries.** *Am J Clin Nutr* 2005, **81:**714–721.
4. Balarajan Y, Villamor E: **Nationally representative surveys show recent increases in the prevalence of overweight and obesity among women of reproductive age in Bangladesh, Nepal, and India.** *J Nutr* 2009, **139:**2139–2144.
5. Hillemeier MM, Weisman CS, Chuang C, Downs DS, McCall-Hosenfeld J, Camacho F: **Transition to overweight or obesity among women of reproductive age.** *J Womens Health (Larchmt)* 2011, **20:**703–710.
6. INSTITUTO BRASILEIRO DE GEOGRAFIA E ESTATÍSTICA/IBGE: *Pesquisa de orçamentos familiares 2008–2009: análise da disponibilidade domiciliar de alimentos e do estado nutricional no Brasil.* Rio de Janeiro: IBGE; 2010.
7. Yu CKH, Teoh TG, Robinson S: **Obesity in pregnancy.** *RCOG* 2006, **113:**1117–1125.
8. Metwally M, Li TC, Ledger WL: **The impact of obesity on female reproductive function.** *Obes Rev* 2007, **8:**515–523.
9. Guelincky I, Devlieger R, Beckers K, Vansant G: **Maternal obesity: pregnancy complications, gestational weigh gain and nutrition.** *Obes Rev* 2008, **9:**140–150.
10. Ramsay JE, Ferrell WR, Crawford L, Wallace AM, Greer IA, Sattar N: **Maternal obesity is associated with dysregulation of metabolic, vascular, and inflammatory pathways.** *JCEM* 2002, **87:**4231–4237.
11. Sen S, Carpenter AH, Hochstadt J, Huddleston JY, Kustanovich V, Reynolds A, Robert A: **Nutrition, weight gain and eating behavior in pregnancy: a review of experimental evidence for long-term effects on the risk of obesity in offspring.** *Physiol Behav* 2012, **107:**138–145.
12. Subramanian SV, Ackerson LK, Smith GD, John NA: **Association of maternal height with child mortality, anthropometric failure, and anemia in India.** *JAM* 2009, **301:**1691–1701.
13. Ozaltin E, Hill K, Subramanian SV: **Association of maternal stature with offspring mortality, underweight, and stunting in low- to middle-income countries.** *JAMA* 2010, **303:**1507–1516.
14. Cresswell JA, Campbell OMR, De Silva MJ, Filippi V: **Effect of maternal obesity on neonatal death in Sub-Saharan Africa: multivariable analysis of 27 national datasets.** *Lancet* 2012, **380:**1325–1330.
15. Beck CC, Lopes AS, Pitanga FJG: **Anthropometric indexes of overweight and obesity as predictors of lipid changes in adolescents.** *Rev Paul Pediatr* 2011, **29:**46–53.
16. Hsieh SD, Muto T: *Waist-to-height ratio is the best anthropometric index for screening the risk of obesity-related disorders*, Asian Perspectives and Evidence on Health Promotion and Education. Tokyo: Springer; 2011:358–363.
17. Misra A, Wasir JS, Vikram NK: **Waist circumference criteria for the diagnosis of abdominal obesity are not applicable uniformly to all populations and ethnic groups.** *Nutrition* 2005, **21:**969–976.
18. Brenner DR, Tepylo K, Eny KM, Cahill LE, El-Sohemy A: **Comparison of body mass index and waist circumference as predictors of cardiometabolic health in a population of young Canadian adults.** *Diabetol Metab Syndr* 2010, **2:**28.
19. World Health Organization: *Physical status: the use and interpretation of anthropometry.* Geneva: World Health Organization; 1995:36. Technical Report Series, 854.
20. Black RE, Allen LH, Bhutta ZA, Caulfield LE, de Onis M, Ezzati M, Mathers C, Rivera J: **Maternal and child undernutrition: global and regional exposures and health consequences.** *Lancet* 2008, **371:**243–260.
21. Mosley WH, Chen LC: **An analytical framework for the study of child survival in developing countries.** *Populat Dev Rev* 1984, **10:**25–45. Sup. Child Survival: Strategies for Research.
22. West BT, Berglund P, Heeringa SG: **A closer examination of subpopulation analysis of complex sample survey data.** *Stata J* 2008, **8:**520–531.
23. Heeringa SG, West BT, Berglund PA: *Applied survey data analysis.* Boca Raton: Chapman Hall/CRC Press; 2008.
24. Villamor E, Cnattingius S: **Interpregnancy weight change and risk of adverse pregnancy outcomes: a population-based study.** *Lancet* 2006, **368:**1164–1170.
25. Flenady V, Koopmans L, Middleton P, Froen JF, Smith GC, Gibbons K, Coory M, Gordon A, Ellwood D, McIntyre HD, Fretts R, Ezzati M: **Major risks for stillbirth in high-income countries: a systematic review and meta-analysis.** *Lancet* 2011, **377:**1331–1340.
26. Nohr EA: **Maternal obesity and neonatal mortality in an African setting.** *Lancet* 2012, **380:**1292–1293.
27. Lashen H, Fear K, Sturdee DW: **Obesity is associated with increased risk of first trimester and recurrent miscarriage: matched case control study.** *Hum Reprod* 2004, **19:**1644–1646.
28. Rittenberg V, Seshadri S, Sunkara SK, Sobaleva S, Oteng-Ntim E, El-Thouky T: **Effect of body mass index on IVF treatment outcome: an updated systematic review and meta-analysis.** *Reprod Biomed Online* 2011, **23:**421–439.

29. Boots C, Stephenson MD: **Does obesity increase the risk of miscarriage in spontaneous conception: a systematic review.** *Semin Reprod Med* 2011, **29**:507–513.
30. Cnattingius S, Berstrom R, Lipworth L, Kramer MS: **Prepregnancy weight and the risk of adverse pregnancy outcomes.** *N Engl J Med* 1998, **338**:147–152.
31. Kristensen J, Vestergaard M, Wisborg K, Kesmodel U, Secher NJ: **Pre-pregnancy weight and the risk of stillbirth and neonatal death.** *BJOG* 2005, **112**:403–408.
32. Hayes EK, Lechowicz A, Petrik JJ, Storozhuk Y, Paez-Parek S, Dai Q, Samjoo IA, Mansell M, Gruslin A, Holloway AC, Raha S: **Adverse fetal and neonatal outcomes associated with a life-long high fat diet: role of altered development of the placental vasculature.** *PLoS One* 2012, **7**:e33370.
33. Moran L, Tsagareli V, Norman R, Noakes M: **Diet and IVF pilot study: short-term weight loss improves pregnancy rates in overweight/obese women undertaking IVF.** *Aust N Z J Obstet Gynaecol* 2011, **51**:455–459.
34. Chen Z, Du J, Shao L, Zheng L, Wu M, Ai M, Zhang Y: **Prepregnancy body mass index, gestational weight gain, and pregnancy outcomes in China.** *Int J Gynecol Obstet* 2010, **109**:41–44.
35. Stone JL, Lockwood CJ, Berkowitz GS, Alvarez M, Lapinski R, Berkowitz RL: **Risk factors for severe preeclampsia.** *Obstet Gynecol* 1994, **83**:357–361.
36. Rocha VZ, Libby P: **Obesity, inflammation, and atherosclerosis.** *Nat Rev Cardiol* 2009, **6**:399–409.
37. Schmidt MI, Duncan BB, Silva GA, Menezes AM, Monteiro CA, Barreto SM, Chor D, Menezes PR: **Chronic non-communicable diseases in Brazil: burden and current challenges.** *Lancet* 2011, **377**:1949–1961.

19

Effect of maternal obesity with and without gestational diabetes on offspring subcutaneous and preperitoneal adipose tissue development from birth up to year-1

Kirsten Uebel[1,2], Karina Pusch[4], Kurt Gedrich[3], Karl-Theo M Schneider[5], Hans Hauner[2,4] and Bernhard L Bader[1,2,4*]

Abstract

Background: Maternal obesity and gestational diabetes mellitus (GDM) may independently influence offspring fat mass and metabolic disease susceptibility. In this pilot study, body composition and fat distribution in offspring from obese women with and without GDM and lean women were assessed within the 1st year of life, and maternal and newborn plasma factors were related to offspring adipose tissue distribution.

Methods: Serum and plasma samples from pregnant obese women with (n = 16) or without (n = 13) GDM and normoglycemic lean women (n = 15) at 3rd trimester and offspring cord plasma were used for analyzing lipid profiles, insulin and adipokine levels. At week-1 and 6, month-4 and year-1, offspring anthropometrics and skinfold thickness (SFT) were measured and abdominal subcutaneous (SCA) and preperitoneal adipose tissue (PPA) were determined by ultrasonography.

Results: Cord insulin was significantly increased in the GDM group, whereas levels of cord leptin, total and high molecular weight (HMW) adiponectin were similar between the groups. Neonates of the GDM group showed significantly higher SFT and fat mass until week-6 and significantly increased SCA at week-1 compared to the lean group that persisted as strong trend at week-6. Interestingly, PPA in neonates of the GDM group was significantly elevated at week-1 compared to both the lean and obese group. At month-4 and year-1, significant differences in adipose tissue growth between the groups were not observed. Multiple linear regression analyses revealed that cord insulin levels are independently related to neonatal PPA that showed significant relation to PPA development at year-1. Maternal fasted C-peptide and HMW adiponectin levels at 3rd trimester emerged to be determinants for PPA at week-1.

Conclusion: Maternal pregravid obesity combined with GDM leads to newborn hyperinsulinemia and increased offspring fat mass until week-6, whereas pregravid obesity without GDM does not. This strongly suggests the pivotal role of GDM in the adverse offspring outcome. Maternal C-peptide and HMW adiponectin levels in pregnancy emerge to be predictive for elevated PPA in newborns and might be indicative for the obesity risk at later life. Altogether, the findings from our pilot study warrant evaluation in long-term studies.

Keywords: Gestational diabetes mellitus, Maternal obesity, Fetal programming, Adiponectin, Insulin, C-peptide, Skinfold thickness, Ultrasonography, Subcutaneous adipose tissue, Preperitoneal adipose tissue

* Correspondence: bernhard.bader@tum.de
[1]PhD Graduate School 'Nutritional adaptation and epigenetic mechanisms', ZIEL - Research Center for Nutrition and Food Sciences, Technische Universität München, Freising-Weihenstephan, Germany
[2]Clinical Nutritional Medicine Unit, ZIEL - Research Center for Nutrition and Food Sciences, Technische Universität München, Freising-Weihenstephan, Germany
Full list of author information is available at the end of the article

Background

Emerging data suggest a permanent impact of the perinatal environment on the offspring risk for developing obesity, metabolic and cardiovascular diseases. The prevalence of obesity in US children and adolescents was 16.9% in 2009–2010 [1], while a German survey showed slightly lower rates [2]. Particularly worrying is the continuous increase in obesity prevalence within young women showing that more than 20.5% of US women at reproductive age were obese (BMI > 30 kg/m^2) in 2009 [3]. A similar trend was recently reported for the German population [4].

Pregravid obesity is, besides maternal age, ethnicity and family history of diabetes, also a major predictor for gestational diabetes mellitus (GDM) [5]. Importantly, maternal obesity and GDM are independent risk factors for fetal hyperinsulinemia, elevated weight and body fat at birth, suggesting that both GDM and pregravid obesity influence fetal development through similar mechanism [6-8]. Moreover, children born from obese and/or diabetic mothers are at higher risk for obesity and insulin resistance/type 2 diabetes from childhood periods [9-11] and adolescence [11,12] up to adulthood [13,14].

There is rising evidence from infants and adults that the distribution of fat depots is a stronger predictor for the metabolic and cardiovascular risk than the total amount of fat [15,16]. Notably, visceral fat has been associated with insulin resistance, decreased adiponectin and hypertriglyceridemia in children and adolescents [17]. Recently, ultrasonography was considered as a valid method for measuring infant abdominal fat distribution in clinical research [18,19]. Preperitoneal adipose tissue (PPA) assessed by ultrasonography has been proposed as a surrogate for visceral/intra-abdominal fat. However, there is missing information about metabolic markers, e.g. insulin, leptin and adiponectin, associated with the distribution of abdominal subcutaneous (SCA) adipose tissues and PPA in neonates and early infancy.

This pilot study comprised pregravid obese women with and without GDM and lean pregnant women, as well as their offspring. Maternal and umbilical cord plasma metabolic markers were determined and related to offspring anthropometrics and distribution of adipose tissues, skinfold thickness (SFT) and abdominal SCA and PPA, from birth/week-1 up to year-1 *post partum (pp).*

Methods

Study population

The study protocol of the *GesA*-Study (**Ges**tational diabetes mellitus and **a**diposity in early adipose tissue development) was approved by the Ethics Committee of the Technische Universität München (Ethics Committee Number: 2629/09) and was registered at the German clinical trials register (DRKS00004370). Singleton pregnant women were recruited at the Abteilung für Geburtshilfe und Perinatalmedizin der Frauenklinik, Klinikum rechts der Isar, Technische Universität München, Munich, Germany between week-33 and 36 of gestation. Written informed consent was obtained from participants before their first appointment. Exclusion criteria for pregnant women were preeclampsia, chronic hypertension and pregravid type 1 or type 2 diabetes. At delivery, participants were excluded if newborns were born preterm (< 37 weeks of gestation), small for gestational age (SGA) or with an APGAR < 5. The study group consisted of Caucasian pregnant women divided into three groups according to their self-reported pregravid BMI and the result of the oral glucose tolerance tests in the 2nd and 3rd trimester [normoglycemic lean (BMI 18.5-25 kg/m^2; n = 15), obese women without GDM (BMI > 30 kg/m^2; n = 13), and obese women with GDM (BMI > 30 kg/m^2; diet-controlled n = 7, insulin-treated n = 9)]. The diagnosis of GDM was defined according to the Hyperglycemia and Pregnancy Outcome (HAPO) criteria [20]: fasting glucose > 5.1 mmol/L (92 mg/dL), 1 h glucose > 10 mmol/L (180 mg/dL), 2 h glucose > 8.5 mmol/L (153 mg/dL). GDM was diagnosed if at least 1 of the threshholds was met or exceeded. Women, tested negatively in the OGTT in 2nd trimester, were retested in the 3rd trimester to confirm glucose tolerance and to re-evaluate their group allocation.

Biochemical analysis

Venous blood samples were obtained from fasted women between week-33 and 36 of gestation. Neonatal blood was collected immediately after delivery from umbilical cord vein. At Synlab (Munich, Germany), maternal and cord plasma glucose were assessed by the glucose oxidase method, and maternal and fetal serum lipid parameters (total, LDL and HDL cholesterol, triglycerides) were determined using established enzymatic methods (Roche Diagnostics, Mannheim, Germany). Fasted maternal plasma and cord plasma insulin as well as fasted maternal plasma C-peptide were analyzed using commercially available ELISAs (Dako, Glostrup, Denmark). Maternal insulin sensitivity was assessed according to the formula for the homeostasis model of assessment-insulin resistance: HOMA-IR-index = [Insulin (μU/mL) × Glucose (mmol/L)]/22.5. Maternal and cord plasma levels for leptin (R&D Systems, Minneapolis, USA), total adiponectin and HMW adiponectin (ALPCO, Salem, NH, USA) were determined by ELISA. The ratio of high molecular weight (HMW) to total adiponectin (S_A) was calculated for each plasma sample. All calculated intra- and interassay coefficients of variation (CV) were less than 10%.

Measurements of anthropometric parameters and adipose tissue distribution

Anthropometric data and SFT were assessed as originally described by Hauner et al. [21]. Briefly, birth weight, height and head circumference were obtained from the obstetric protocol. At visit week-6, month-4 and year-1 *pp*, the infant weight and height, head circumference, and waist circumference (only at year-1) were determined in the study center. Ponderal index (in kg/m^3) was calculated according to the measured variables.

SFT measurements were conducted by one well-trained researcher at 2–5 days *pp* in the obstetric clinic as well as at week-6, month-4 and year-1 *pp* at the study center. SFTs were determined in triplicate with a Holtain caliper (Holtain Ltd, Crosswell, Crymych, UK) at the infant's left body axis at the following four sites: triceps, biceps, subscapular and suprailiac. Total body fat was calculated via predictive SFT equation according to the method of Westrate and Deurenberg [22] and trunk-to total SFT (%) was evaluated by applying the equation (subscapular + suprailiac SFT)/(sum of 4 SFTs) × 100 [23].

Ultrasonographic imaging, as described originally by Holzhauer et al. [18] was performed by two researchers (including one pediatrician blinded to study group allocation) at week-1, week-6, month-4 and year-1. Briefly, abdominal SCA and PPA fat thicknesses were measured in sagittal planes as areas of 1-cm length just below the xiphoid process. Additionally, SCA was determined in axial planes as areas of 1-cm length in the middle of the xiphoid process and the navel directly above the linea alba. From each plane, three images were analyzed by one observer and 120 images were randomly controlled by a completely blinded second researcher. The inter-observer variability was calculated by interclass coefficient (ICC) and further validated by a Bland-Altman plot [24]. The ICC for the ultrasonographic analysis was 0.981 and the p-value < 0.001, indicating high correlation between independent assessments. In the Bland-Altman plot analysis, the mean of the differences (bias) between observers was −0.17 mm^2 and the *Limits of Agreement* were −0.65 mm^2 (mean −2 SD) and 0.31 mm^2 (mean +2 SD), excluding a systematic inter-observer bias (Additional file 1).

Statistical analysis

For all statistical analyses, IBM SPSS statistics software (version 20.0; IBM Corp.) was used. One-way ANOVA with Sidak's post hoc test was applied for group comparison of normally distributed variables and data are presented as means ± SD. In case of violation of the normality assumption, the Kruskal-Wallis test with Dunn's post hoc test was applied, and accordingly, data are presented as medians and interquartile ranges. The Fisher's Exact test was used for analyzing qualitative measurements. Comparative statistical evaluation of infant growth and fat development between the groups was performed by employing multiple linear regression models. The potential confounding factors offspring sex and pregnancy duration were taken into account when analyzing cord parameters and the covariate infant age at investigation was additionally applied for respective anthropometric and adipose tissue growth assessments. Generally, infant parameters at week-6, month-4 and year-1 were further adjusted for breastfeeding status.

Linear regression analyses were used to identify maternal parameters and cord insulin levels independently related to offspring adipose tissue distribution. If necessary, logarithmically transformed variables were applied to accomplish normality of residuals. Values for the unadjusted analyses are presented, whereas the indicated adjusted model considered the variables offspring sex, gestational duration, maternal pre-pregnancy BMI, area under the curve (AUC) $_{Glucose}$ (OGTT) and gestational weight gain. Applying adipose tissue markers at week-6, month-4 and year-1 as dependent variables, corresponding breastfeeding status was a further covariate. Spearman correlation analysis was used to determine the association of cord adiponectin levels with respective cord insulin levels and adipose tissue parameters at week-1, and respective partial correlations were applied including the covariables for infant sex, pregnancy duration, maternal pre-pregnancy BMI, AUC $_{Glucose}$ (OGTT) and gestational weight gain. All statistical tests were performed two-sided and a p-value < 0.05 was considered to indicate statistical significance.

Results

Maternal and fetal metabolic outcome

The main clinical and metabolic data of the study population are summarized in Table 1. Lean and obese participants with and without GDM did not significantly differ in parity or mode of delivery, but obese participants with GDM were slightly older at study entry, and pregnancy duration was shorter compared to obese subjects without GDM. Both obese groups had similar pregravid BMI and weight gain during pregnancy, whereas the glucose levels (fasted, 1 h, 2 h) upon OGTT were significantly higher in the obese GDM group than in the obese group without GDM. At baseline (week-33 to 36 of gestation), obese women with and without GDM had significantly increased levels of fasting insulin and C-peptide compared to lean subjects and showed increased insulin resistance estimated by HOMA-IR-index. HbA1c levels were similar between all groups. Plasma leptin levels of obese pregnant women were - irrespective of GDM - significantly higher, while HMW-total adiponectin ratios (S_A) were significantly lower compared to the lean group. Concerning the lipid profile, total cholesterol levels were significantly decreased in obese subjects, but HDL cholesterol and triglyceride levels were similar between study groups. Cord plasma insulin levels and HOMA-IR-index were significantly elevated in the obese group with GDM compared to the euglycemic

Table 1 Characterization of study participants

A Mother	Lean group	Obese group	Obese GDM group	P-value[1]
Number of women (n = 44)	15	13	16	
Age (year)	31.1 ± 3.1	28.5 ± 4.2	32.6 ± 4.8	0.040[c]
Primiparae (%) [n]	86.7 [13]	76.9 [10]	56.2 [9]	0.299
BMI (kg/m^2) before pregnancy	20.1 (19.5-22.0)	36.1 (32.2-38.3)	33.4 (31.1-36.1)	< 0.001[a,b]
Gestational weight gain (kg)	16.8 ± 4.4	11.6 ± 5.6	12.1 ± 5.8	0.022[a,b]
Parental history of diabetes (%) [n]	13.3 [2]	38.5 [5]	43.8 [7]	0.181
Duration of pregnancy (days)	278.2 ± 8.1	279.5 ± 8.2	271.3 ± 7.0	0.012[c]
Mode of delivery				
Spontaneous / cesarean section, n	9/6	6/7	6/10	0.483
75 g OGTT (mmol/L)				
Glucose fasted	4.22 (3.89-4.39)	4.33 (4.00-4.63)	5.11 (4.44-5.56)	< 0.001[b,c]
Glucose 1 h	7.41 ± 0.90	7.34 ± 1.42	10.85 ± 1.34	< 0.001[b,c]
Glucose 2 h	6.30 ± 0.96	6.49 ± 1.21	8.00 ± 1.57	< 0.001[b,c]
Area under curve (AUC) $_{Glucose}$	12.54 (11.90-13.24)	11.85 (11.65-14.10)	16.37 (16.04-18.13)	< 0.001[b,c]
Fasted plasma/serum parameters at 3rd trimester				
Gestational age (weeks)	33.9 ± 1.4	34.3 ± 1.7	34.1 ± 1.0	0.836
Glucose (mmol/L)	4.10 ± 0.32	4.19 ± 0.40	4.39 ± 0.28	0.161
Insulin (µU/mL)	5.66 (4.76-10.05)	11.54 (9.28-20.54)	13.99 (11.22-17.97)	0.002[a,b]
HOMA-IR-index	1.10 (0.86-1.79)	2.31 (1.98-4.15)	2.76 (2.08-3.63)	0.001[a,b]
C-peptide (ng/mL)	1.60 (1.42-2.23)	2.99 (2.05-3.51)	3.01 (2.64-3.14)	0.002[a,b]
HbA1c (%)	5.32 ± 0.31	5.45 ± 0.23	5.40 ± 0.28	0.474
Leptin (ng/mL)	9.30 (6.52-20.11)	46.03 (29.84-78.67)	42.24 (26.71-66.69)	< 0.001[a,b]
Total adiponectin (µg/mL)	4.98 ± 1.02	4.14 ± 1.78	3.81 ± 1.39	0.071
HMW adiponectin (µg/mL)	2.86 ± 0.82	2.06 ± 1.17	1.74 ± 0.91	0.008[b]
S_A	0.57 ± 0.1	0.48 ± 0.09	0.44 ± 0.07	< 0.001[a,b]
Total cholesterol (mmol/L)	7.49 ± 1.51	6.28 ± 0.96	6.60 ± 0.96	0.035[a]
LDL cholesterol (mmol/L)	4.86 ± 1.50	3.73 ± 0.87	3.92 ± 1.96	0.039
HDL cholesterol (mmol/L)	1.92 ± 0.49	1.73 ± 0.45	1.88 ± 0.28	0.524
Triglycerides (mmol/L)	2.53 ± 0.74	2.38 ± 0.57	2.76 ± 0.72	0.420

B Infant	Lean group	Obese group	Obese GDM group	P-value[1]	Adjusted p-value[2]
Offspring gender (male/female), n	8/7	8/5	13/3	0.275	
Umbilical cord plasma parameters					
Glucose (mmol/L)	4.46 ± 1.13	4.42 ± 1.03	4.60 ± 1.02	0.892	0.202
Insulin (µU/mL)	1.72 (1.08-5.14)	1.73 (1.33-3.97)	5.29 (4.21-8.33)	0.023[b,c]	0.014[b,c]
HOMA-IR-index	0.40 (0.22-1.23)	0.42 (0.23-0.74)	1.08 (0.81-1.52)	0.021[b,c]	0.009[b,c]
Leptin (ng/mL)	5.88 (2.15-9.70)	7.57 (4.56-16.65)	6.84 (4.76-11.58)	0.455	0.114
Total adiponectin (µg/mL)	20.68 ± 6.23	20.82 ± 8.56	22.03 ± 7.33	0.977	0.685
HMW adiponectin (µg/mL)	14.61 ± 5.15	14.28 ± 7.02	14.75 ± 5.80	0.860	0.884
S_A	0.70 ± 0.06	0.67 ± 0.06	0.65 ± 0.08	0.292	0.348
Total cholesterol (mmol/L)	1.71 (1.31-1.90)	1.53 (1.36-1.71)	1.55 (1.32-1.73)	0.718	0.886
LDL cholesterol (mmol/L)	0.54 (0.32-0.65)	0.52 (0.38-0.60)	0.47 (0.41-0.54)	0.905	0.271
HDL cholesterol (mmol/L)	0.72 (0.67-1.03)	0.62 (0.60-0.96)	0.72 (0.57-0.88)	0.691	0.724
Triglycerides (mmol/L)	0.35 (0.27-0.52)	0.35 (0.26-0.45)	0.40 (0.25-0.46)	0.959	0.847

Table 1 Characterization of study participants *(Continued)*

Breastfeeding status at week-6 (month-4), n				
Exclusively breastfed	10 (8)	7 (6)	6 (4)	0.257 (0.304)
Formula and breast milk	0 (2)	3 (0)	4 (4)	
Formula only	5 (5)	3 (6)	4 (6)	
Introduction of solid food (months)	5.0 (5.0-6.0)	5.0 (4.0-6.0)	5.0 (4.0-6.0)	0.411

HbA1c: hemoglobin A1c; HDL: high-density lipoprotein; HOMA-IR: homeostasis model assessment-insulin resistance; LDL: low-density lipoprotein; OGTT: oral glucose tolerance test; S_A: HMW-total adiponectin ratio.
Data are presented as mean ± SD; otherwise skewed variables are presented as median followed by interquartile range.
[1]One-way ANOVA with Sidak's post hoc test or nonparametric Kruskal-Wallis-test with Dunn's post hoc test.
[2]Statistical analyses for cord plasma parameters were performed by multiple linear regression models and p-values were adjusted for infant sex and pregnancy duration.
[a]p-value < 0.05 obese vs. lean group; [b]p-value < 0.05 obese GDM vs. lean group; [c]p-value < 0.05 obese GDM vs. obese group.

obese and lean group. In contrast, no significant differences were observed for cord plasma HMW and total adiponectin or S_A between all study groups. In addition, levels of LDL, HDL, and total cholesterol as well as triglycerides were similar in all groups. With regard to breastfeeding status at week-6 and month-4 and the introduction of solid food, no significant differences were observed between the study groups.

Infant anthropometrics, adipose tissue growth and distribution

Infant anthropometrics and adipose tissue development assessed by SFT measurement and ultrasonography from birth/week-1 to year-1 are shown in Tables 2 and 3, respectively. Anthropometric birth outcomes, namely weight, height, ponderal index and head circumference were similar for all groups. However, the sum of 4 SFT at week-1 was significantly higher in the obese GDM group than in the lean group after considering the potential confounders infant sex, pregnancy duration and age at investigation. Similarly, abdominal SCA was significantly elevated in the newborns of obese mothers with GDM compared to the lean group, whereas PPA was significantly increased compared to the normoglycemic lean and obese group. At week-6, only SFT and calculated fat mass were significantly higher in the obese group with GDM after considering indicated confounders. In contrast, SCA and PPA were not significantly larger in offspring of obese mothers with GDM at week-6. Notably, although the sum of all 4 SFT did not differ significantly between groups at year-1, the trunk-total SFT ratio was significantly higher in obese GDM offspring than in children of both euglycemic groups, indicating changes in adipose tissue distribution with increased trunk fat in these infants. With regard to further anthropometric and adipose tissue parameters at month-4 and year-1 and total weight and fat mass gain from birth to year-1, no significant differences were observed between the three groups (Tables 2 and 3).

Relation of cord plasma insulin to offspring fat distribution up to year-1

Linear regression analyses were used to explore the relation of cord plasma insulin to infant SFT, SCA and PPA at all ages investigated (Table 4). Thus, cord insulin levels were positively related to SFT at week-1 in the unadjusted analysis, however, in the adjusted model, the relationship did not remain significant ($p = 0.071$). After repeating the linear regressions with abdominal SCA and PPA at week-1, respectively, cord insulin levels also emerged as positive determinant for both adipose tissue markers in the unadjusted analysis (Table 4). This independent relationship still remained after adjusting for infant sex, pregnancy duration, maternal pre-pregnancy BMI, $AUC_{Glucose}$ (OGTT) and gestational weight gain. No significant relationships were found between cord insulin levels and fat distribution at week-6, month-4 and year-1 in the fully adjusted analyses (Table 4).

Relation of infant anthropometric parameters at birth/week-1 to respective year-1 measures

The influence of neonatal anthropometric parameters on corresponding primary endpoint parameters at year-1 were evaluated by linear regression. The adjusted analysis was further performed with the covariates infant sex, pregnancy duration, breastfeeding status at month-4, pre-pregnancy BMI, $AUC_{Glucose}$ (OGTT) and gestational weight gain (Table 5). Values for PPA at week-1 emerged as positive independent determinants of PPA at year-1 in both analyses. In contrast, no further significant relationships were observed between birth weight, ponderal index, SFT and SCA assessed at year-1 and respective parameters determined at birth/week-1.

Relation of maternal plasma C-peptide and adiponectin to offspring fat distribution up to year-1

Linear regression analyses were conducted to determine the relationship of maternal fasted C-peptide, HMW adiponectin levels and S_A at 3rd trimester with neonatal PPA at week-1 (Figure 1). For maternal C-peptide, a

Table 2 Anthropometric infant data from birth to year-1

	Lean group	Obese group	Obese GDM group	P-value[1]	Adjusted p-value[2]
Weight [g]					
Birth	3,449 ± 332 [15]	3,651 ± 285 [13]	3,617 ± 333 [16]	0.201	0.169
Week-6	4,701 ± 330 [15]	4,963 ± 635 [13]	5,285 ± 517 [12]	0.017[b]	0.170
Month-4	6,468 ± 522 [15]	6,929 ± 829 [11]	7,066 ± 732 [13]	0.071	0.211
Year-1	9,786 ± 915 [15]	10,356 ± 1273 [12]	10,392 ± 1212 [14]	0.286	0.549
Weight gain [g]					
Δ Week-6 - birth	1,265 (1,095-1,480) [15]	1,480 (775–1,690) [13]	1,550 (1,361-1,892) [12]	0.017[b]	0.394
Δ Month-4 - week-6	1,734 (1,390-2,100) [15]	2,070 (1,840-2,300) [11]	1,848 (1,460-2,100) [11]	0.112	0.042[a]
Δ Year-1 - month-4	3,318 ± 760 [15]	3,228 ± 801 [11]	3,329 ± 666 [13]	0.936	0.937
Δ Year-1 - birth	6,337 ± 996 [15]	6,665 ± 1,220 [12]	6,765 ± 1,102 [14]	0.554	0.722
Length [cm]					
Birth	51.8 ± 1.5 [15]	52.5 ± 1.4 [13]	52.3 ± 1.5 [16]	0.299	0.264
Week-6	55.6 ± 0.9 [15]	56.0 ± 1.8 [13]	56.4 ± 1.4 [12]	0.360	0.738
Month-4	63.3 ± 1.2 [15]	64.4 ± 2.0 [11]	63.7 ± 1.4 [13]	0.226	0.177
Year-1	76.5 ± 2.3 [15]	77.5 ± 2.6 [12]	76.7 ± 2.7 [14]	0.551	0.666
Ponderal index [g/cm^3]					
Birth	6.65 ± 0.54 [15]	6.95 ± 0.48 [13]	6.81 ± 0.51 [16]	0.291	0.287
Week-6	8.45 ± 0.55 [15]	8.86 ± 1.03 [13]	9.36 ± 0.75 [12]	0.018[b]	0.176
Month-4	10.21 ± 0.81 [15]	10.74 ± 1.06 [11]	11.04 ± 0.97 [13]	0.073	0.272
Year-1	12.80 ± 1.04 [15]	13.34 ± 1.38 [12]	13.52 ± 1.30 [14]	0.262	0.616
Head circumference [cm]					
Birth	34.0 (34.0-35.5) [15]	35.0 (34.5-36.5) [13]	35.5(34.0-36.0) [16]	0.072	0.410
Week-6	37.5 (37.0-38.8) [15]	38.3 (37.6-39.7) [13]	38.9 (37.7-40.0) [12]	0.023[b]	0.096
Month-4	41.1 ± 1.2 [15]	42.1 ± 1.7 [11]	42.0 ± 1.3 [13]	0.132	0.184
Year-1	45.6 ± 1.4 [15]	47.0 ± 1.6 [12]	47.1 ± 1.7 [14]	0.072	0.105
Waist circumference [cm]					
Year-1	45.1 ± 2.4 [15]	45.6 ± 4.0 [12]	45.7 ± 3.0 [14]	0.859	0.897

Data are presented as mean ± SD; otherwise skewed variables are presented as median followed by interquartile range, numbers in brackets represent number of infants included in the analysis.
[1]One-way ANOVA with Sidak's post hoc test or nonparametric Kruskal-Wallis-test with Dunn's post hoc test.
[2]Statistical analyses were performed by multiple linear regression models. P-values for parameters at week-1 were adjusted for infant sex, pregnancy duration and age at investigation. P-values at week-6, month-4 and year-1 were adjusted for infant sex, pregnancy duration, age at investigation and corresponding breastfeeding.
[a]P-value < 0.05 obese vs. lean group; [b]p-value < 0.05 obese GDM vs. lean group.

significantly positive relationship with infant PPA was found in the unadjusted analysis, and C-peptide remained an independent positive predictor after full adjustment for infant sex, pregnancy duration, pre-pregnancy BMI, OGTT-derived AUC $_{Glucose}$ and gestational weight gain. Decreasing levels of maternal HMW adiponectin and S_A were significantly related to higher offspring PPA at week-1 in the unadjusted analysis, whereas in the adjusted model, only maternal HMW adiponectin remained as negative determinant. Notably, no significant relationships were found for maternal C-peptide, HMW adiponectin or S_A with subcutaneous adipose tissues, namely SCA (Figure 1) and SFT (Additional file 2), at week-1. Indicated maternal parameters were no longer related to PPA at week-6, month-4 and year-1 in the fully adjusted analyses, however we found that maternal HMW adiponectin and S_A were significantly positively related to infant SCA only at month-4 (Additional file 2).

Discussion

Adipose tissue development within the 1st year in offspring born from obese and GDM mothers is poorly investigated. This study is the first reporting comparative longitudinally SFT assessment combined with complementary abdominal ultrasonography of SCA and PPA from birth to year-1 *pp* in offspring from obese mothers with and without GDM and normoglycemic lean mothers.

Our data show that offspring of obese GDM mothers have significantly higher cord insulin levels associated

Table 3 Infant adipose tissue growth assessed by skinfold thickness measurements and ultrasonography from week-1 to year-1

	Lean group	Obese group	Obese GDM group	P-value[1]	Adjusted p-value[2]
SFT [mm]					
Week-1	18.9 ± 3.1 [15]	20.3 ± 2.6 [13]	21.6 ± 2.4 [16]	0.031[a]	0.031[a]
Week-6	25.2 ± 3.7 [15]	26.1 ± 5.1 [13]	30.4 ± 3.4 [12]	0.007[a,b]	0.048[a]
Month-4	30.7 ± 6.6 [15]	31.2 ± 4.3 [11]	33.6 ± 4.8 [13]	0.336	0.258
Year-1	29.0 ± 4.3 [15]	30.3 ± 4.6 [12]	29.7 ± 4.8 [14]	0.749	0.536
Fat mass [g][3]					
Week-1	583 ± 139 [15]	660 ± 114 [13]	694 ± 117 [16]	0.051	0.042[a]
Week-6	1,008 ± 159 [15]	1,098 ± 285 [13]	1,307 ± 187 [12]	0.004[a,b]	0.048[a]
Month-4	1,581 ± 318 [15]	1,728 ± 327 [11]	1,847 ± 328 [13]	0.108	0.184
Year-1	2,260 ± 419 [15]	2,475 ± 536 [12]	2,444 ± 530 [14]	0.466	0.498
Trunk-total SFT ratio (%)[4]					
Week-1	47.4 ± 2.5 [15]	47.2 ± 3.3 [13]	48.1 ± 2.9 [16]	0.630	0.958
Week-6	48.4 ± 3.2 [15]	49.4 ± 3.4 [13]	49.1 ± 2.4 [12]	0.648	0.528
Month-4	49.0 ± 4.1 [15]	48.9 ± 2.4 [11]	49.6 ± 3.1 [13]	0.841	0.647
Year-1	45.1 ± 2.6 [15]	44.9 ± 2.6 [12]	48.5 ± 3.3 [14]	0.002[a,b]	0.035[a,b]
SCA (mm^2)[5]					
Week-1	12.7 (9.5-15.4) [12]	16.7 (14.0-19.9) [12]	17.7 (16.8-19.4) [12]	0.020[a]	0.014[a]
Week-6	24.0 ± 6.6 [15]	26.5 ± 10.7 [13]	34.6 ± 7.9 [12]	0.008[a,b]	0.058[a]
Month-4	41.3 ± 12.8 [15]	42.9 ± 9.4 [11]	45.6 ± 12.7 [13]	0.644	0.458
Year-1	24.6 (18.6-27.7) [15]	29.0 (26.8-36.2) [12]	34.2 (22.8-43.6) [14]	0.132	0.217
PPA (mm^2)[5]					
Week-1	5.6 (4.9-7.9) [12]	7.9 (6.3-9.3) [12]	10.0 (8.9-12.2) [12]	0.001[a]	0.001[a,b]
Week-6	10.0 ± 2.7 [15]	11.4 ± 3.6 [13]	13.9 ± 2.9 [12]	0.009[a]	0.183
Month-4	13.5 (9.7-14.1) [15]	16.9 (12.1-18.6) [11]	15.6 (11.5-18.0) [13]	0.221	0.525
Year-1	17.5 ± 4.9 [15]	22.3 ± 7.0 [12]	20.8 ± 6.7 [14]	0.130	0.368

PPA: preperitoneal adipose tissue; SCA: subcutaneous adipose tissue; SFT: sum of the 4 skinfold thickness measurements (biceps + triceps + subscapular + suprailiac).
Data are presented as mean ± SD; otherwise skewed variables are presented as median followed by interquartile range; numbers in brackets represent number of infants included in the analysis.
[1]One-way ANOVA with Sidak's post hoc test or nonparametric Kruskal-Wallis-test with Dunn's post hoc test.
[2]Statistical analyses were performed by multiple linear regression models. P-values for parameters at week-1 were adjusted for infant sex, pregnancy duration and age at investigation. P-values at week-6, month-4 and year-1 were adjusted for infant sex, pregnancy duration, age at investigation and corresponding breastfeeding status.
[a]P-value < 0.05 obese GDM vs. lean group; [b]p-value < 0.05 obese GDM vs. obese group.
[3]Fat mass was estimated from the sum of 4 SFTs by using the equations of Weststrate and Deurenberg [22].
[4]Trunk-total SFT ratio (%) was evaluated by applying the equation (subscapular + suprailiac SFT)/(sum of 4 SFTs) × 100 of Westrate et al. [23].
[5]SCA and PPA were measured as areas of 1-cm length according to the method of Holzhauer et al. [18]. SCA indicates mean area from axial + sagittal plane.

with higher fat mass than offspring of euglycemic lean and obese mothers. The major novel findings were that abdominal SCA and PPA in infants from obese women with GDM were significantly higher at week-1 and SFT was significantly elevated at week-1 and week-6 compared to offspring of lean mothers. Moreover, our analysis revealed that neonatal PPA is highly related to PPA development at year-1. Searching for maternal markers as predictors for offspring adipose tissue growth and obesity risk, we identified a significantly positive relationship for maternal C-peptide levels and a significantly inverse relationship for HMW adiponectin with infant PPA at week-1. However, these associations of maternal factors did not prolong afterwards in the first year of life.

Our data are compatible with the hypothesis proposed by Pedersen et al. [25] indicating that fetal hyperinsulinemia is an adaptive process resulting from elevated maternal glucose levels [6], and that fetal insulin is associated with neonatal fat mass and growth due to the role of insulin in adipogenesis and stimulation of insulin-like-growth factor 1 (IGF-1) production [6,26]. Moreover, the data are in line with two other studies that did not observe fetal hyperinsulinemia in pregnancies of euglycemic obese women [27,28]. In contrast, Catalano et al. [7] reported

Table 4 Regression of fat distribution parameters up to year-1 on cord plasma insulin levels

	Cord plasma insulin					
		Unadjusted analysis		Adjusted analysis		
	N	β	P-value	β	P-value	Adjusted model r^2
Week-1						
SFT	44	0.398	0.007	0.325	0.071	0.195; p = 0.026
SCA	36	0.464	0.004	0.390	0.039	0.310; p = 0.008
PPA	36	0.445	0.007	0.436	0.022	0.311; p = 0.008
Week-6						
SFT	40	0.294	0.065	0.292	0.146	0.122; p = 0.127
SCA	40	0.335	0.035	0.241	0.217	0.163; p = 0.074
PPA	40	0.307	0.054	0.287	0.119	0.268; p = 0.014
Month-4						
SFT	39	0.281	0.084	0.196	0.335	0.080; p = 0.215
SCA	39	0.175	0.287	0.056	0.794	−0.044; p = 0.615
PPA	39	0.146	0.368	0.011	0.961	−0.090; p = 0.799
Year-1						
SFT	41	−0.072	0.653	−0.017	0.937	−0.080; p = 0.769
SCA	41	0.027	0.866	0.085	0.680	−0.034; p = 0.585
PPA	41	0.062	0.698	0.198	0.290	0.137; p = 0.099

β: standardized regression coefficient; PPA: preperitoneal adipose tissue; r^2: coefficient of determination; SCA: subcutaneous adipose tissue; SFT: sum of the 4 skinfold thickness measurements (biceps + triceps + subscapular + suprailiac). Variables for adjusted analysis: infant sex, pregnancy duration, respective breastfeeding status, maternal pre-pregnancy BMI, AUC $_{Glucose}$ (OGTT) and gestational weight gain.

increased total fat mass and insulin levels in newborns from obese mothers and thereby bringing forward insulin resistance *in utero* without maternal diabetes. However, in the study of Catalano et al. [7], OGTT was performed in the 2nd trimester and a subsequent glucose tolerance challenge in late pregnancy was not performed to exclude GDM in obese women, whereas in our study glucose tolerance was also analyzed in late pregnancy. Our findings on adipose tissue development and distribution within the first year are consistent with data from several studies reporting that GDM offspring overweight at birth diminished within the 1st year *pp* [9,29,30]. Interestingly, these studies found that infant overweight reemerged at the age of 2–3 years. In this context, GDM and reduced maternal insulin sensitivity (IS $_{OGTT}$ index) were reported to be independent predictors for both slower infant weight gain up to month-6 [31] and reduced SFT at year-1 [32]. In contrast, other investigators showed increased body weight and weight/length-ratio in 6-month-old children in relation to pregravid obesity and gestational weight gain or found persistent increased SFT at year-1 in LGA (large for gestational age) offspring born to GDM mothers [33,34].

Apart from maternal variables, cord plasma markers emerged as important indicators for weight and fat mass growth in early childhood; thus, cord insulin levels were inversely related to infant weight gain at year-2 [35]. Moreover, elevated cord blood leptin levels were identified to be related to slower infant weight gain up to month-6 [31], year-2 [36] and year-3 [37]. Altogether, it is tempting to speculate that increased intrauterine and perinatal insulin levels initiated a temporarily prolonged increase in adipose tissues in GDM offspring up to week-6, a postnatal time-period where GDM offspring insulin have returned already to a normal level. Afterwards, during subsequent time up to year-1, weight and adipose tissue growth normalized, because these insulin-mediated effects faded away. However, a long-term impact of maternal and fetal hyperglycemia on later infancy and adolescence obesity risk is still plausible as indicated by epidemiological studies [11,12,38]. In addition, the impact of early postnatal critical periods of programming was highlighted by Péneau et al. [39] showing that high infant BMI at year-1 and early rapid infant weight gain were risk factors for the development and persistence of overweight at the age of 7–9 years.

We found that neonatal PPA at week-1 is an independent predictor for PPA at infant age of 1 year. These data on PPA may mirror intrauterine influences on early adipose tissue development and programming effects with potentially sustained unfavorable effects at later stages in infancy or childhood. This proposed relationship warrants evaluation in future studies with larger cohorts. The importance of investigating specific changes in early adipose tissue distribution as we performed in this study is supported by recent insights into distinct neonatal fat depots assessed by magnetic resonance tomography (MRT) [40,41]. The authors described significantly increased intra-hepatocellular lipids in newborns in relation to pregravid BMI and GDM, but

Table 5 Regression of growth and fat mass parameters at year-1 on respective neonatal assessments

	Respective parameters at year-1					
		Unadjusted analysis		Adjusted analysis		
	N	β	P-value	β	P-value	Adjusted model r^2
Birth weight	41	0.294	0.062	0.179	0.289	0.149; p = 0.085
Birth ponderal index	41	0.248	0.117	0.161	0.342	0.130; p = 0.109
SFT, week-1	41	−0.012	0.939	−0.082	0.666	−0.074; p = 0.746
SCA, week-1	36	0.006	0.863	−0.260	0.227	−0.260; p = 0.277
PPA, week-1	36	0.520	0.002	0.486	0.010	0.275; p = 0.027

β: standardized regression coefficient; PPA: preperitoneal adipose tissue; r^2: coefficient of determination; SCA: subcutaneous adipose tissue; SFT: sum of the 4 skinfold thickness measurements (biceps + triceps + subscapular + suprailiac). Variables for adjusted analysis: infant sex, pregnancy duration, breastfeeding status at month-4, maternal pre-pregnancy BMI, AUC $_{Glucose}$ (OGTT) and gestational weight gain.

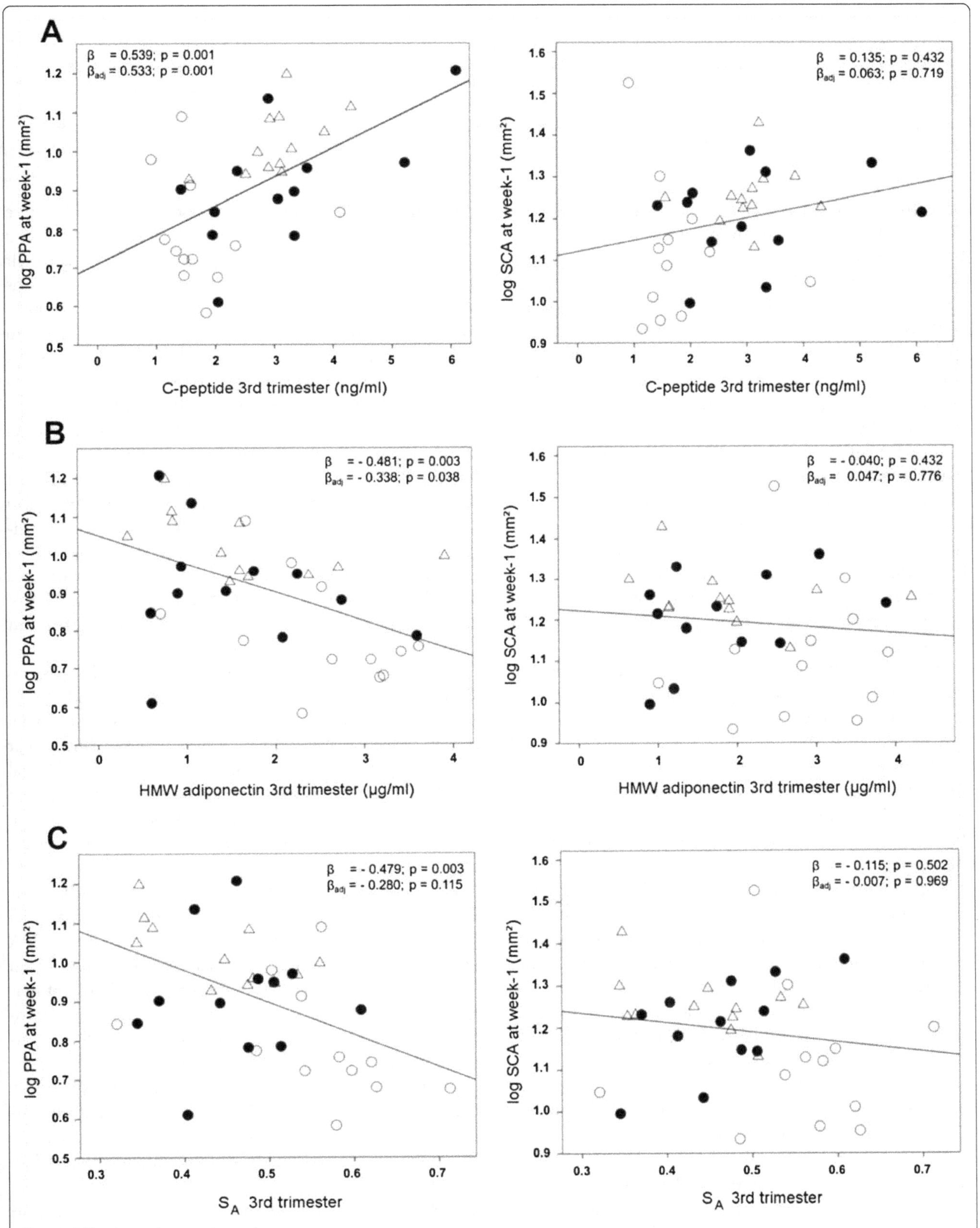

Figure 1 (See legend on next page.)

(See figure on previous page.)

Figure 1 Regression of PPA and SCA at week-1 on maternal plasma C-peptide and adiponectin levels at 3rd trimester. Maternal C-peptide **(A)**, HMW adiponectin **(B)** and S_A **(C)** are presented in relation to neonatal PPA and SCA, respectively. β: unadjusted standardized regression coefficient. $β_{adj}$: standardized regression coefficient adjusted for the variables infant sex, pregnancy duration, maternal pre-pregnancy BMI, AUC $_{Glucose}$ (OGTT) and gestational weight gain. The plotted regression lines indicate the results of the unadjusted analyses. HMW: high molecular weight; Log: logarithmic; PPA: preperitoneal adipose tissue; S_A: HMW-total adiponectin ratio; SCA: subcutaneous adipose tissue; open circles: lean group; black circles: obese group; open triangles: obese GDM group.

conflicting results have been reported regarding the effect of maternal obesity on abdominal fat in neonates [40,41]. Brumbaugh et al. [40] did not find a difference in intra-abdominal fat per body length in infants of obese mothers with GDM, whereas Modi et al. [41] showed the positive relationship between maternal BMI and abdominal fat in newborns, but did not discriminate between subcutaneous and intra-abdominal fat. Apart from that, PPA was demonstrated to be a good approximation for intra-abdominal fat assessed by computer tomography (CT) [19].

More recently, research interest has started to particularly focus on comprehensively analyzing the distribution and accumulation of distinct fat depots in the body, especially the abdominal fat in longitudinal studies and their relation to metabolic biomarkers. Our data indicate that cord plasma insulin was positively related to neonatal SFT and fat mass that is in line with the results reported by Brunner et al. [35]. Importantly, for the first time, we showed that cord insulin levels emerged as independent predictors for PPA and SCA at week-1 after birth. Interestingly, Tamura et al. [42] have shown that insulin levels are strongly related to PPA and SCA in 9-15-year old children. In addition, Cnop et al. [43] reported that insulin sensitivity was inversely correlated with visceral, but not with subcutaneous fat, whereas leptin levels were stronger related to subcutaneous fat amount in adults. Moreover, increased PPA was recently determined as cardiovascular risk factor in obese children [15] and non-obese adults [16,44]. Considering these studies and our data on cord plasma insulin levels with SCA and PPA in neonates, we speculate that increased neonatal PPA and SCA results from insulin-mediated early metabolic malprogramming which may have the potency to contribute to adverse effects later in life. Therefore, increased PPA at birth might be indicative for both later obesity and cardiovascular risk.

With regard to maternal lipid levels during pregnancy and the recurrently described hypertriglyceridemia in GDM [45,46], we found that total and LDL cholesterol levels were significantly lower in obese women than in the lean group, whereas triglyceride levels were similar in all groups at the 3rd trimester. In addition these maternal differences were not reflected in cord plasma where cholesterol and triglyceride levels were rather alike. Our data on both maternal cholesterol and triglyceride levels for all study groups are consistent with several studies [47-52]. According to Meyer et al. [51] and Scifres et al. [52], obese women exhibit higher levels for triglycerides, total and LDL cholesterol at the beginning of pregnancy than their lean counterparts, but these differences decrease towards term reaching similar or even slightly lower levels in obese women. Regarding the relation between maternal and cord LDL and total cholesterol levels, published data are not consistent, and sometimes even opposing levels between newborn and mother have been described [49,53].

In pregnant women, it is known that HMW and total adiponectin are closely related to glycemia, insulin sensitivity and β-cell function [54]. We found that obese mothers, characterized by hyperinsulinemia and increased HOMA-IR-index, had decreased HMW adiponectin and S_A which is in line with recent data from animal and clinical studies reporting that insulin is a negative regulator of adiponectin, preferentially HMW oligomer, secretion [55]. In contrast, in the present study, total and HMW adiponectin levels in cord plasma were not affected by maternal obesity and GDM, as has been described [7,56,57]. Umbilical cord total and HMW adiponectin levels have been associated with neonatal weight, ponderal index and body fat [56,58-60], but similar associations did not emerge in our pilot study (Additional file 3). There was also no significant association between insulin and adiponectin levels in neonates (Additional file 3) indicating that the regulation of fetal adiponectin might be different from adult metabolism [59].

Another important finding of our study was that maternal C-peptide levels were positively and maternal HMW adiponectin levels inversely related to infant PPA at week-1. This strongly suggests that maternal insulin and HMW adiponectin levels are major regulators of maternal metabolism which might impact fetal and newborn PPA growth. Moreover, the observed significant relationships of maternal C-peptide and HMW adiponectin levels with PPA, but not with subcutaneous adipose tissues (SFT and SCA) at week-1 implicate that changes in maternal insulin sensitivity indirectly influences the growth of specific fat compartments during fetal development observed in the neonates.

Although this pilot study was limited by a small participant number and imbalanced offspring sex distribution in the group of obese mothers with GDM as well as the short observational follow-up period, it emphasizes the need to apply ultrasonography as useful method to generate new parameters to characterize longitudinally adipose tissue growth and distribution and their association to blood markers and obesity risk.

Conclusion

This study shows that maternal pregravid obesity combined with GDM but not maternal obesity alone led to offspring neonatal hyperinsulinemia and increased offspring fat mass until week-6. These findings together with the knowledge from published reports on lean pregnant women with GDM corroborate GDM as the pivotal cause of newborn hyperinsulinemia. However, the observed short adverse impact of intrauterine hyperglycemia on neonatal adipose tissue growth seems to vanish within the first year of life. Importantly, the identification of maternal C-peptide and HMW adiponectin levels as novel potential predictors for distinct PPA growth in newborns might be indicative for obesity risk in later life. Recently, increased PPA was determined as cardiovascular risk factor in obese children and non-obese adults. Therefore, increased PPA at birth might be not only indicative for later obesity risk, but also for cardiovascular risk in adulthood. These aspects should be evaluated in relation to the treatment of pregravid obesity and GDM by dietary and lifestyle intervention studies in larger cohorts, since there is an urgent need for the reduction of offspring obesity and the identification of reliable predictors for offspring obesity risk and its relation to cardiovascular risk factors.

Additional files

Additional file 1: Figure S1. Inter-observer agreement for the ultrasonographic measurement of preperitoneal and subcutaneous fat assessed by the Bland-Altman plot. From 120 randomly chosen ultrasonographic images, 180 subcutaneous and preperitoneal adipose tissue areas were independently assessed by a second observer. The mean of the differences (bias) was −0.17 mm^2 and the *Limits of Agreement* were −0.65 mm^2 (mean - 2 SD) and 0.31 mm^2 (mean + 2 SD). SD: standard deviation.

Additional file 2: Table S1. Regression of infant fat distribution parameter at all ages investigated on plasma maternal C-peptide and adiponectin levels at 3rd trimester.

Additional file 3: Table S2. Spearman and partial correlations of cord plasma adiponectin levels with cord plasma insulin and newborn adipose tissue parameters.

Abbreviations

BMI: Body mass index; GDM: Gestational diabetes mellitus; HMW: High molecular weight; HbA1c: Hemoglobin A1c; HDL: High-density lipoprotein; HOMA-IR: Homeostasis model of assessment-insulin resistance; ICC: Interclass coefficient; LDL: Low-density lipoprotein; LGA: Large for gestational age; OGTT: Oral glucose tolerance test; pp: Post partum; PPA: Preperitoneal adipose tissue; S_A: HMW-total adiponectin ratio; SCA: Subcutaneous adipose tissue; SFT: Sum of the 4 skinfold thickness measurements (biceps + triceps + subscapular + suprailiac); SGA: Small for gestational age.

Competing interests

All the authors declare the absence of financial interests that may be relevant to the submitted work.

Authors' contributions

HH and BLB designed research. KTMS gave scientific advice and clinical support. KU was responsible for data collection and trial management, laboratory analysis and performed the statistical analyses. KP performed inter-observer analysis of ultrasonography data. KG supported statistical analysis. KU and BLB wrote the manuscript. All authors read the manuscript and approved the final version.

Acknowledgements

The authors thank all the families who participated in the study. We are grateful to Manuela Hubersberger for her excellent technical assistance in the laboratory. We thank Ulrike Amann-Gassner for study design and protocol development, and Tibor Schuster for statistical advice. We appreciate the support of Ernst Rummeny for giving access to the ultrasonographic system and Verena Schulte for helping the team with ultrasonographic measurements.

Author details

[1]PhD Graduate School 'Nutritional adaptation and epigenetic mechanisms', ZIEL - Research Center for Nutrition and Food Sciences, Technische Universität München, Freising-Weihenstephan, Germany. [2]Clinical Nutritional Medicine Unit, ZIEL - Research Center for Nutrition and Food Sciences, Technische Universität München, Freising-Weihenstephan, Germany. [3]Biochemistry Unit, ZIEL - Research Center for Nutrition and Food Sciences, Technische Universität München, Freising-Weihenstephan, Germany. [4]Else Kröner-Fresenius-Center for Nutritional Medicine, Wissenschaftszentrum Weihenstephan, Klinikum rechts der Isar, Uptown München Campus D, Technische Universität München, Munich, Germany. [5]Abteilung für Geburtshilfe und Perinatalmedizin der Frauenklinik, Technische Universität München, Munich, Germany.

References

1. Ogden CL: **Prevalence of obesity and trends in body mass index among US children and adolescents, 1999–2010.** *JAMA* 2012, **307**:483–490.
2. Blüher S, Meigen C, Gausche R, Keller E, Pfäffle R, Sabin M, Werther G, Odeh R, Kiess W: **Age-specific stabilization in obesity prevalence in German children: A cross-sectional study from 1999 to 2008.** *Int J Pediatr Obes* 2011, **6**:e199–206.
3. Fisher S, Kim S, Sharma A, Rochat R, Morrow B: **Is obesity still increasing among pregnant women? Prepregnancy obesity trends in 20 states, 2003–2009.** *Prev Med* 2013, **56**:372–378.
4. Kurth B: **Erste Ergebnisse aus der "Studie zur Gesundheit Erwachsener in Deutschland" (DEGS).** *Bundesgesundheitsbl* 2012, **55**:980–990.
5. Torloni MR, Betrán AP, Horta BL, Nakamura MU, Atallah AN, Moron AF, Valente O: **Prepregnancy BMI and the risk of gestational diabetes: a systematic review of the literature with meta-analysis.** *Obes Rev* 2009, **10**:194–203.
6. Catalano PM, McIntyre HD, Cruickshank JK, McCance DR, Dyer AR, Metzger BE, Lowe LP, Trimble ER, Coustan DR, Hadden DR, Persson B, Hod M, Oats JJN: **The hyperglycemia and adverse pregnancy outcome study: associations of GDM and obesity with pregnancy outcomes.** *Diabetes Care* 2012, **35**:780–786.
7. Catalano PM, Presley L, Minium J, Hauguel-de Mouzon S: **Fetuses of obese mothers develop insulin resistance in utero.** *Diabetes Care* 2009, **32**:1076–1080.
8. Sewell MF, Huston-Presley L, Super DM, Catalano P: **Increased neonatal fat mass, not lean body mass, is associated with maternal obesity.** *Am J Obstet Gynecol* 2006, **195**:1100–1103.
9. Schaefer-Graf UM, Pawliczak J, Passow D, Hartmann R, Rossi R, Buhrer C, Harder T, Plagemann A, Vetter K, Kordonouri O: **Birth weight and parental BMI predict overweight in children from mothers with gestational diabetes.** *Diabetes Care* 2005, **28**:1745–1750.
10. Catalano PM, Farrell K, Thomas A, Huston-Presley L, Mencin P, Mouzon SH D, Amini SB: **Perinatal risk factors for childhood obesity and metabolic dysregulation.** *Am J Clin Nutr* 2009, **90**:1303–1313.
11. Boerschmann H, Pfluger M, Henneberger L, Ziegler A, Hummel S: **Prevalence and predictors of overweight and insulin resistance in offspring of mothers with gestational diabetes mellitus.** *Diabetes Care* 2010, **33**:1845–1849.

12. Gillman MW, Rifas-Shiman S, Berkey CS, Field AE, Colditz GA: **Maternal gestational diabetes, birth weight, and adolescent obesity.** *Pediatr* 2003, **111**:e221–e226.
13. Clausen TD, Mathiesen ER, Hansen T, Pedersen O, Jensen DM, Lauenborg J, Damm P: **High prevalence of type 2 diabetes and Pre-diabetes in adult offspring of women with gestational diabetes mellitus or type 1 diabetes: the role of intrauterine hyperglycemia.** *Diabetes Care* 2007, **31**:340–346.
14. Clausen TD, Mathiesen ER, Hansen T, Pedersen O, Jensen DM, Lauenborg J, Schmidt L, Damm P: **Overweight and the metabolic syndrome in adult offspring of women with diet-treated gestational diabetes mellitus or type 1 diabetes.** *J Clin Endocrinol Metabol* 2009, **94**:2464–2470.
15. Polat TB, Urganci N, Caliskan KC, Akyildiz B: **Correlation of abdominal fat accumulation and stiffness of the abdominal aorta in obese children.** *J Pediatr Endocrinol Metab* 2008, **21**:1031–1040.
16. Liu KH, Chan YL, Chan WB, Kong WL, Kong MO, Chan JCN: **Sonographic measurement of mesenteric fat thickness is a good correlate with cardiovascular risk factors: comparison with subcutaneous and preperitoneal fat thickness, magnetic resonance imaging and anthropometric indexes.** *Int J Obes Relat Metab Disord* 2003, **27**:1267–1273.
17. Medina-Bravo P, Meza-Santibáñez R, Rosas-Fernández P, Galván-Duarte R, Saucedo-García R, Velázquez-López L, Torres-Tamayo M: **Decrease in serum adiponectin levels associated with visceral Fat accumulation independent of pubertal stage in children and adolescents.** *Arch Med Res* 2011, **42**:115–121.
18. Holzhauer S, Zwijsen RML, Jaddoe VWV, Boehm G, Moll HA, Mulder PG, Kleyburg-Linkers VA, Hofman A, Witteman JCM: **Sonographic assessment of abdominal fat distribution in infancy.** *Eur J Epidemiol* 2009, **24**:521–529.
19. Mook-Kanamori D, Holzhauer S, Hollestein L, Durmus B, Manniesing R, Koek M, Boehm G, van der Beek E, Hofman A, Witteman J, Lequin M, Jaddoe V: **Abdominal fat in children measured by ultrasound and computed tomography.** *Ultrasound Med Biol* 2009, **35**:1938–1946.
20. Coustan DR, Lowe LP, Metzger BE, Dyer AR: **The Hyperglycemia and Adverse Pregnancy Outcome (HAPO) study: paving the way for new diagnostic criteria for gestational diabetes mellitus.** *Am J Obstet Gynecol* 2010, **202**:654. e1–654.e6.
21. Hauner H, Much D, Vollhardt C, Brunner S, Schmid D, Sedlmeier E, Heimberg E, Schuster T, Zimmermann A, Schneider KM, Bader BL, Amann-Gassner U: **Effect of reducing the n-6:n-3 long-chain PUFA ratio during pregnancy and lactation on infant adipose tissue growth within the first year of life: an open-label randomized controlled trial.** *Am J Clin Nutr* 2012, **95**:383–394.
22. Westrate J, Deurenberg P: **Body composition in children: proposal for a method for calculating body fat percentage from total body desity or skinfold-thickness measurements.** *Am J Clin Nutr* 1989, **50**:1104–1115.
23. Weststrate JA, Deurenberg P, van Tinteren H: **Indices of body fat distribution and adiposity in Dutch children from birth to 18 years of age.** *Int J Obes* 1989, **13**:465–477.
24. Bland JM, Altman DG: **Statistical methods for assessing agreement between two methods of clinical measurement.** *Lancet* 1986, **1**:307–310.
25. Pedersen J: *The pregnant diabetic and her newborn: problems and management.* Baltimore: The Williams and Wilkins Company; 1967.
26. Regnault N, Botton J, Heude B, Forhan A, Hankard R, Foliguet B, Hillier TA, Souberbielle J, Dargent-Molina P, Charles M: **Higher cord C-peptide concentrations Are associated with slower growth rate in the 1st year of life in girls but Not in boys.** *Diabetes* 2011, **60**:2152–2159.
27. Colomiere M, Permezel M, Riley C, Desoye G, Lappas M: **Defective insulin signaling in placenta from pregnancies complicated by gestational diabetes mellitus.** *Eur J Endocrinol* 2008, **160**:567–578.
28. Ferraro ZM, Qiu Q, Gruslin A, Adamo KB: **Characterization of the insulin-like growth factor axis in term pregnancies complicated by maternal obesity.** *Hum Reprod* 2012, **27**:2467–2475.
29. Whitaker RC, Pepe MS, Seidel KD, Wright JA, Knopp RH: **Gestational diabetes and the risk of offspring obesity.** *Pediatr* 1998, **101**:e9.
30. Silverman BL, Rizzo T, Green OC, Cho NH, Winter RJ, Ogata ES, Richards GE, Metzger BE: **Long-term prospective evaluation of offspring of diabetic mothers.** *Diabetes* 1991, **40**(Suppl 2):121–125.
31. Parker M, Rifas-Shiman SL, Belfort MB, Taveras EM, Oken E, Mantzoros C, Gillman MW: **Gestational glucose tolerance and cord blood leptin levels predict slower weight gain in early infancy.** *J Pediatr* 2011, **158**:227–233.
32. Hamilton JK, Odrobina E, Yin J, Hanley AJ, Zinman B, Retnakaran R: **Maternal insulin sensitivity during pregnancy predicts infant weight gain and adiposity at 1 year of age.** *Obesity* 2009, **18**:340–346.
33. Deierlein AL, Siega-Riz AM, Adair LS, Herring AH: **Effects of Pre-pregnancy body mass index and gestational weight gain on infant anthropometric outcomes.** *J Pediatr* 2011, **158**:221–226.
34. Vohr BR, McGarvey ST: **Growth patterns of large-for-gestational-age and appropriate-for-gestational-age infants of gestational diabetic mothers and control mothers at age 1 year.** *Diabetes Care* 1997, **20**:1066–1072.
35. Brunner S, Schmid D, Hüttinger K, Much D, Heimberg E, Sedlmeier E, Brüderl M, Kratzsch J, Bader BL, Amann-Gassner U, Hauner H: **Maternal insulin resistance, triglycerides and cord blood insulin in relation to post-natal weight trajectories and body composition in the offspring up to 2 years.** *Diabet Med* 2013, **30**:1500–1507.
36. Brunner S, Schmid D, Hüttinger K, Much D, Brüderl M, Sedlmeier E, Kratzsch J, Amann-Gassner U, Bader BL, Hauner H: **Effect of reducing the n-6/n-3 fatty acid ratio on the maternal and fetal leptin axis in relation to infant body composition.** *Obesity* 2013, **22**:217–224.
37. Boeke CE, Mantzoros CS, Hughes MD,L, Rifas-Shiman S, Villamor E, Zera CA, Gillman MW: **Differential associations of leptin with adiposity across early childhood.** *Obesity* 2013, **21**:1430–1437.
38. Hillier TA, Pedula KL, Schmidt MM, Mullen JA, Charles M, Pettitt DJ: **Childhood obesity and metabolic imprinting: the ongoing effects of maternal hyperglycemia.** *Diabetes Care* 2007, **30**:2287–2292.
39. Péneau S, Rouchaud A, Rolland-Cachera M, Arnault N, Hercberg S, Castetbon K: **Body size and growth from birth to 2 years and risk of overweight at 7–9 years.** *Int J Pediatr Obes* 2011, **6**:e162–169.
40. Brumbaugh DE, Tearse P, Cree-Green M, Fenton LZ, Brown M, Scherzinger A, Reynolds R, Alston M, Hoffman C, Pan Z, Friedman JE, Barbour LA: **Intrahepatic Fat is increased in the neonatal offspring of obese women with gestational diabetes.** *J Pediatr* 2012, **162**:930–936.
41. Modi N, Murgasova D, Ruager-Martin R, Thomas EL, Hyde MJ, Gale C, Santhakumaran S, Dore CJ, Alavi A, Bell JD: **The influence of maternal body mass index on infant adiposity and hepatic lipid content.** *Pediatr Res* 2011, **70**:287–291.
42. Tamura A, Mori T, Hara Y, Komiyama A: **Preperitoneal fat thickness in childhood obesity: association with serum insulin concentration.** *Pediatr Int* 2000, **42**:155–159.
43. Cnop M, Landchild MJ, Vidal J, Havel PJ, Knowles NG, Carr DR, Wang F, Hull RL, Boyko EJ, Retzlaff BM, Walden CE, Knopp RH, Kahn SE: **The concurrent accumulation of intra-abdominal and subcutaneous fat explains the association between insulin resistance and plasma leptin concentrations Distinct metabolic effects of two fat compartments.** *Diabetes* 2002, **51**:1005–1015.
44. Tadokoro N, Murano S, Nishide T, Suzuki R, Watanabe S, Murayama H, Morisaki N, Saito Y: **Preperitoneal fat thickness determined by ultrasonography is correlated with coronary stenosis and lipid disorders in non-obese male subjects.** *Int J Obes Relat Metab Disord* 2000, **24**:502–507.
45. Qiu C, Rudra C, Austin MA, Williams MA: **Association of gestational diabetes mellitus and Low-density lipoprotein (LDL) particle size.** *Physiol Res* 2007, **56**:571–578.
46. Herrera E, Ortega-Senovilla H: **Disturbances in lipid metabolism in diabetic pregnancy – are these the cause of the problem?** *Best Pract Res Clin Endocrinol Metab* 2010, **24**:515–525.
47. Vahratian A, Misra VK, Trudeau S, Misra DP: **Prepregnancy body mass index and gestational age-dependent changes in lipid levels during pregnancy.** *Obstet Gynecol* 2010, **116**:107–113.
48. Dube E, Ethier-Chiasson M, Lafond J: **Modulation of cholesterol transport by insulin-treated gestational diabetes mellitus in human full-term placenta.** *Biol Reprod* 2013, **88**:16.
49. Dube E, Gravel A, Martin C, Desparois G, Moussa I, Ethier-Chiasson M, Forest J, Giguere Y, Masse A, Lafond J: **Modulation of fatty acid transport and metabolism by maternal obesity in the human full-term placenta.** *Biol Reprod* 2012, **87**:14.
50. Schaefer-Graf UM, Meitzner K, Ortega-Senovilla H, Graf K, Vetter K, Abou-Dakn M, Herrera E: **Differences in the implications of maternal lipids on fetal metabolism and growth between gestational diabetes mellitus and control pregnancies.** *Diabet Med* 2011, **28**:1053–1059.

51. Meyer BJ, Stewart FM, Brown EA, Cooney J, Nilsson S, Olivecrona G, Ramsay JE, Griffin BA, Caslake MJ, Freeman DJ: **Maternal obesity is associated with the formation of small dense LDL and hypoadiponectinemia in the third trimester.** *J Clin Endocrinol Metabol* 2013, **98:**643–652.
52. Scifres CM, Catov JM, Simhan HN: **The impact of maternal obesity and gestational weight gain on early and mid-pregnancy lipid profiles.** *Obesity (Silver Spring)* 2014, **22:**932–8.
53. Sivakumar K, Bari MF, Adaikalakoteswari A, Guller S, Weickert MO, Randeva HS, Grammatopoulos DK, Bastie CC, Vatish M: **Elevated fetal adipsin/acylation-stimulating protein (ASP) in obese pregnancy: novel placental secretion via hofbauer cells.** *J Clin Endocrinol Metabol* 2013, **98:**4113–4122.
54. Retnakaran R, Connelly PW, Maguire G, Sermer M, Zinman B, Hanley AJG: **Decreased high-molecular-weight adiponectin in gestational diabetes: implications for the pathophysiology of Type 2 diabetes.** *Diabet Med* 2007, **24:**245–252.
55. Wang Y, Lam KSL, Yau M, Xu A: **Post-translational modifications of adiponectin: mechanisms and functional implications.** *Biochem J* 2008, **409:**623–633.
56. Ballesteros M, Simon I, Vendrell J, Ceperuelo-Mallafre V, Miralles RM, Albaiges G, Tinahones F, Megia A: **Maternal and cord blood adiponectin multimeric forms in gestational diabetes mellitus: a prospective analysis.** *Diabetes Care* 2011, **34:**2418–2423.
57. Luo Z, Nuyt A, Delvin E, Fraser WD, Julien P, Audibert F, Girard I, Shatenstein B, Deal C, Grenier E, Garofalo C, Levy E: **Maternal and fetal leptin, adiponectin levels and associations with fetal insulin sensitivity.** *Obesity* 2013, **21:**210–216.
58. Weyermann M, Beermann C, Brenner H, Rothenbacher D: **Adiponectin and leptin in maternal serum, cord blood, and breast milk.** *Clin Chem* 2006, **52:**2095–2102.
59. Basu S, Laffineuse L, Presley L, Minium J, Catalano PM, Hauguel-de Mouzon S: **In utero gender dimorphism of adiponectin reflects insulin sensitivity and adiposity of the fetus.** *Obesity* 2009, **17:**1144–1149.
60. Inoue M, Itabashi K, Nakano Y, Nakano Y, Tobe T: **High-molecular-weight adiponectin and leptin levels in cord blood Are associated with anthropometric measurements at birth.** *Horm Res* 2008, **70:**268–272.

Maternal obesity and its relation with the cesarean section: A hospital based cross sectional study in Iraq

Waqar Al-Kubaisy[1,3], Mazin Al-Rubaey[2*], Redhwan A Al-Naggar[1,3], Ban Karim[2] and Nor Aini Mohd Noor[1,4]

Abstract

Background: Obesity during pregnancy is reported in approximately one in five pregnant women worldwide. It increases the risk of pregnancy complications many of which necessitate Cesarean section (CS). This study determines the association between obesity and type of delivery.

Methods: A cross-sectional study involving 404 pregnant women was carried out at Al-Yarmouk Teaching Hospital, Baghdad, Iraq. Women with hypertension, diabetes, preterm labor, fetal presentation other than cephalic presentation and multiple gestations were excluded from the study. BMI and past obstetric history were recorded.

Results: The overall rate of CS was 38%. The overall mean body mass index (BMI) was 25.0 ± 4.52 Kg/m^2 and it was significantly higher among women who delivered by cesarean section. Significantly high rate of CS was found in primigravida and multigravida women with high BMI. Moreover, all obese multigravid women with history of previous CS were delivered by CS. The rate of CS was higher in women with primary level education when compared to women with secondary or tertiary education. CS was significantly lower in women with a previous history of abortion.

Conclusion: Obese women with or without a previous history of CS are at a higher risk of having a CS and should therefore be considered as high risk and managed appropriately during pregnancy. Weight management prior to or during pregnancy could help reduce the need for CS.

Keywords: Obesity, Cesarean section, Route of delivery, Iraq

Background

Obesity is most commonly measured as a weight to height ratio and expressed as body mass index (BMI) [1]. It is an internationally accepted method that provides a reliable way to assess obesity related health problems. The prevalence of obesity in adults is increasing worldwide, particularly among women of child bearing age. In Iraq, according to the Ministry of Health report the prevalence of obesity in women in reproductive age was 38.2% in 2006 [2]. Moreover in Baghdad between 1997 and 2007 the prevalence of obesity among women in reproductive age increased from 23.6 to 25% [3,4]. Globally the prevalence of maternal obesity has also increased, rising from 9-10% in the early 1990's to 16 - 19% in the year 2000 [5-7]. In Dublin, 19% of women in their 1st trimester were obese [8]. Similarly in US, obesity among pregnant women ranged from 18.5 -38.3% [9]. Maternal obesity is defined as women who have a BMI ≥30 Kg/m^2 at first antenatal visit [5]. It is calculated by dividing pre-pregnancy weight in kilograms (Kg) by height in meter square (m^2) [6]. It is evident that obesity increases the risk of pregnancy complications. In obese mothers, the perinatal morbidity such as pre-eclampsia and gestational diabetes is high [10-12]. Obesity is associated with increased rates of cesarean section (CS) [12]. Several recent reports document rates of CS 32% in USA [10], 19.1% in Saudi Arabia [11], 9.29% in Jordan [13] and 20.1% in Iraq [14]. Interestingly also the rates of CS in Baghdad city were 17.9, 19 and 28.7% in 2007, 2009 and 2011; respectively [15,16].

* Correspondence: maziniraq2003@gmail.com
[2]Community Medicine Department, Faculty of Medicine, AL-Mustanseryah University, Baghdad, Iraq
Full list of author information is available at the end of the article

Table 1 Characteristic profile of Iraqi pregnant women based on the mode of delivery (n = 404)

Variable	Total		NVD		CS		χ^2	P value
	No	%	No	%	No	%		
Age (years)								
<20	50	12.4	30	60.0	20	40.0	4.661	0.324
20—24	134	33.2	83	61.9	51	38.1		
25—29	100	24.8	67	67.0	33	33.0		
30—34	82	20.3	52	63.4	30	36.6		
≥35	38	9.4	18	47.4	20	52.6		
Husband occupation								
Non-governmental	238	58.2	141	59.2	97	40.8	1.17	0.191
Governmental	166	41.1	109	65.7	57	34.3		
Women's level of education								
Less than Secondary	274	67.8	160	58.4	114	41.6	4.39	0.036
Secondary and higher	130	32.2	90	69.2	40	30.8		
History of Abortion								
No	373	92.3	225	60.3	148	39.7	4.19	0.04
Yes	31	7.7	25	80.6	6	19.4		
Pregnant women classifications								
Primigravida	149	36.9	95	63.8	54	36.2		
Multigravida without CS	149	36.9	111	74.5	38	25.5	28.9	<0.001
Multigravida with CS	106	26.2	44	41.5	62	58.5		

Dietz *et al.* (2005) showed that the rate of cesarean section was 14.3% in lean gravid women and 42.6% in obese women [17]. A linear relationship between BMI and cesarean delivery has been reported [18]. Obese women were 6 times more likely to have cesarean section due to cephalo-pelvic disproportion or failure to progress than non-obese women [19].

Earlier studies in Iraq have not evaluated the association of maternal obesity with other factors like parity and previous cesarean section, which are known risk factors for cesarean section. Therefore, the aim of this study was to determine the association of increased BMI among primigravid, multigravida with and without history of CS with the mode of delivery in the current pregnancy.

Methods

A cross-sectional study was conducted at Obstetrics Department of Al-Yarmouk Teaching Hospital, Baghdad, Iraq from January to May 2012. Ethical approval was obtained from the Ethics Committee at Ministry of Health, Baghdad, Iraq. A convenience sample of 404 pregnant women attending the labor room with induced or spontaneous labor was collected. Informed consent was obtained from each participant. The inclusion criteria were women with normal pregnancy (no pathological conditions) at ≥ 37 weeks of gestation. Primigravida and multigravida with normal pregnancy and live cephalic singleton fetuses were included. Pregnant women with elective cesarean section, hypertension, and diabetes were excluded. In addition,

Table 2 Mean BMI of 404 Iraqi pregnant women in relation to route of delivery

Variable	No	Mean ± SD	Test of significance	p value
All women	404	25.05 ± 4.25		
Primigravidae	149	24.31 ± 4.41		
Multigravidae without CS	149	25.27 ± 4.67	F = 3.562	0.029
Multigravidae with CS	106	25.77 ± 4.34		
Current pregnancy with				
NVD		22.85 ± 2.82	Z = 15.848	<0.001
CS		28.62 ± 4.49		

Table 3 Mode of delivery of Iraqi pregnant women and BMI (n = 404)

Variable	Total		NVD		CS		x^2	P value
	N	%	N	%	N	%		
BMI								
Underweight (<18.5)	15	3.7	13	86.7	2	13.3		
Normal weight (18.5-24.9)	206	51.0	187	90.8	19	9.2		
Overweight (25-29.9)	116	28.7	42	36.2	74	63.8	180.1	<0.001
Obese (≥30)	67	16.6	8	11.9	59	88.1		

multiple gestations, and abnormal lie fetus at time of labor were also excluded. Each participant was interviewed using a well constructed questionnaire. The questionnaire include socio-demographic (age, education and husband's occupation) and obstetrical (parity, history of abortion, type of previous delivery) information. In addition, height and weight were measured and the pre-pregnancy weight was calculated by subtracting 12.5 Kg from the current weight. The average weight gain during pregnancy is estimated as 12.5 Kg [5]. Statistical analysis was done using tests contained in SPSS 20. Descriptive data are presented in frequencies, simple percentages. Chi-square (x^2) test was used to evaluate the associations between categorical variables. ANOVA was used to test the significance of differences between more than two means and Z test was used to test the significance of difference of two means. A p-value of < 0.05 was considered significant.

Results

A total of 404 women were included in this study. More than half of them (58%) were 20-30 years old and more than two thirds (68%) had less than secondary school education. Out of 404 women 154 (38.2%) their current pregnancy were ended by CS. Significant association between mother's education and type of delivery ($p = 0.036$) was present. Women with lower primary education had significantly higher rate of CS (41.6%) than those with secondary school and above education (30.8%) ($p = 0.036$). Women with history of previous abortion showed significantly lower rate of CS compared to women with no history of abortion ($p = 0.04$). However, this study showed that the mode of delivery was neither associated with the age of the women nor with the occupation of the husband ($p = 0.324$, $p = 0.191$; respectively). Regarding the relationship between gravidity of the mother and mode of delivery, multigravidae with previous history of CS had a significantly higher rate of CS (58.5%) in the current pregnancy when compared to other two groups ($p < 0.001$) (Table 1). The overall mean BMI in the study subjects was 25.05 ± 4.25 kg/m^2 (ranging from 16.2 to 39.1) (Table 2). More than half (51%) of the participants were within the normal range of BMI. However, 45.3% were overweight and obese (Table 3). Significant variation in mean BMI was detected among mothers with different gravidity (Table 2). The highest mean BMI was among the multigravidae with a previous history of CS (25.77 ± 4.34 Kg/m^2), while primigravidae had the lowest mean BMI (24.31 ± 4.41; $p = 0.029$) (Table 2). Studying the relationship between mode of delivery in the current pregnancy and BMI level, we gave an evidence that pregnant women whom their pregnancy ended by CS, their BMI was (28.62 ± 4.49) significantly higher ($p < 0.001$) than (22.85 ± 2.82) those whom delivered normally (Table 2). Moreover, with increasing BMI (≥25) above normal, CS was significantly increased steadily ($p < 0.001$) (Table 3). All obese (BMI ≥ 30) multigravidae with a previous history of CS were delivered via CS. CS for the current pregnancy was significantly higher among obese (BMI ≥ 30) primi and multigravida women without previous history of CS (85.7% and 78.3% respectively; $p < 0.001$) compared to non-obese primagravidae and multigravidae (28.1% and 15.9%, respectively) (Table 4).

Discussion

In this study many factors "for example diabetes mellitus, hypertension, fetal presentation other than cephalic and multiple pregnancies" that may relate to CS were excluded. In spite of that, the rate of CS delivery was higher than (22.6%, 33.3%) that reported previously in Iraq [16,20], Saudi Arabia [11], Jordan [13], USA [10] and Pakistan, where it was reported as 32.3% [21]. Moreover, mean BMI of the pregnant women who delivered via

Table 4 Gravidity and mode of delivery based on BMI (n = 404)

Gravidity	BMI < 30		BMI ≥ 30		x^2	p value
	NVD	CS	NVD	CS		
Primi gravid	92 (71.9%)	36 (28.1%)	3 (14.3%)	18 (85.7%)	25.89	<0.001
Multigravida without CS	106 (84.1%)	20 (15.9%)	5 (21.7%)	18 (78.3%)	39.85	<0.001
Multigravida with CS	44 (53%)	39 (47%)	0	23 (100)		

cesarean section was significantly higher than those via vaginal delivery. In addition, there was a significant positive association between BMI and the rate of CS. As BMI increased the rate of CS too increased, suggests that the high rate of CS in our study is mostly due to the high BMI of these women. Our finding is in agreement with Kominarek's *et al.*, (2010) in US [22] who found that cesarean deliveries increased significantly across the different classes of obesity. Similarly, Tosson and Al-hussaini in Egypt, (2005) [23] as well as Perlow *et al.*, (1992) [24] suggested that BMI was significantly related to the mode of delivery. Cnattingham *et al.*, (1998) in reported that obese women due to their large body volume, more time may be taken for oxytocin to reach the optimal tissue level [25]. Also presence of excess intra abdominal adipose tissue itself could mechanically obstruct the progression of labor, this could, overtime, compromise fetoplacental circulation and cause fetal distress and necessitating CS. Although higher rate of CS was found among women aged 35 years and above, this finding was however not significant, which is in contrast to the findings of Perlow *et al.*, (1992) [24].

Our findings are also in agreement with an earlier study [26], where it was reported that women with high BMI and previous history of CS are less likely to have normal vaginal delivery during the next pregnancy. In this study it was noted that none of those obese (BMI ≥ 30) women with a previous history of CS had ended by normal vaginal delivery. Moreover, a significantly high proportion of obese (BMI ≥ 30) primigravida or multi gravidae with no history of CS in this study had their current pregnancy ended by CS. The significantly higher rate of cesarean section among women with lower educational level supports the findings of another study in Baghdad [27]. The possible explanation is that the women with higher education are more likely to take care of their weight and body shape and practice a healthy lifestyle such as regular exercise and healthy diet. Another explanation is that low educational level may lead to poor utilization of health services during pregnancy.

Conclusion

This study showed a significant association between BMI and increased risk of cesarean delivery. Obese women should therefore be considered as high risk and managed appropriately during pregnancy. Weight management should be implemented in the primary care clinics to counsel women to reduce their weight.

Competing interests

The authors declare that they have no competing interests.

Authors' contribution

WA study design and writing the manuscript. MA study design, obtaining ethical approval from Ministry of Health, Iraq, data collection and writing the manuscript, RA statistical data analysis and writing the manuscript. BK data collection. NA agreed to be accountable in all aspects of the work, data interpretation, critical revision of the manuscript, final approval and final editing. All authors read and approved the final manuscript.

Acknowledgements

The authors would like to thank the Obstetrics Department staff at Al-Yarmouk Teaching Hospital for their support. We extend our thanks to all women who participated in this study.

Financial disclosure statement

No funding.

Author details

[1]Population Health and Preventive Medicine Department, Faculty of Medicine, Universiti Teknologi MARA (UiTM), Selangor, Malaysia. [2]Community Medicine Department, Faculty of Medicine, AL-Mustanseryah University, Baghdad, Iraq. [3]Drug Discovery & Health Community of Research, Universiti teknologi MARA (UiTM), 40450 Shah Alam, Selangor, Darul Ehsan, Malaysia. [4]Humanity and Quality of life, Universiti teknologi MARA (UiTM), 40450 Shah Alam, Selangor, Darul Ehsan, Malaysia.

References

1. Gray DS, Fujioka K: **Use of relative weight and body mass index for the determination of adiposity.** *J Clin Epidemiol* 1991, **44**(6):545–550.
2. Ministry of Health, Iraqi: *Chronic Non-Communicable Disease Risk Factors Survey in Iraq*, A STEP Wise Approach .Ministry of Health, Directorate of Public Health, Ministry of Planning and Developmental Cooperation, Central Organization for Statistics &Information Technology; 2006.
3. Al-Twail NG, Abdulla NM, Abdul Ameer AJ: **Prevalence of and factors associated with overweight and obesity among a group of Iraqi women.** *Eastern Mediterranean Health Journal* 2007, **13**(2):14. 50-55.
4. Swidan A: *Nutritional status assessment of female 10-60 years*, Household survey. Baghdad, General Federation of Iraqi women; 1997.
5. Davies GA, Maxwell C, McLeod L, Gagnon R, Basso M, Bos H, Delisle MF, Farine D, Hudon L, Menticoglou S, Mundle W, Murphy-Kaulbeck L, Ouellet A, Pressey T, Roggensack A, Leduc D, Ballerman C, Biringer A, Duperron L, Jones D, Lee LS, Shepherd D, Wilson K: **SOGC clinical practice guidelines: obesity in pregnancy.** *Int J Gyn Obstet* 2010, **110**(2):167–173.
6. WHO: *Obesity: Preventing and managing the global epidemic.* Geneva: World Health Organization; 2000.
7. WHO: **Obesity, Preventing and managing the global epidemic.** In Report of WHO Consultation Obesity. WHO-Technical Report, 2000; N: 894. http://www.who.int/dietphysicalactivity/publications/facts/obesity/en/. Accessed in January 10, 2013.
8. Fattah C, Farah N, Barry S, O'conner N, Stuart B, Turner M: **Maternal weight and body composition in the first trimester of pregnancy.** *Acta Obest and Gynecol Scand* 2010, **89**:952–955.
9. Galtier- Dereure F, Boenger C, Bringer J: **Obesity and pregnancy: Complication and Cost.** *Am J Clin Nutr* 2000, **71**((suppl):1245–1285.
10. Hamilton BE, Martin JA, Ventura SJ: *Births: Preliminary data for 2007. National Vital Statistics reports, U.S. Department of Health and Human services.* Hyattsville, MD: National Center for Health Statistics; 2009. **57** (12).
11. Ba'qeel HS: **King Abdulaziz medical centre: cesarean delivery.** *Ann- Saudi Med* 2009, **29**(3):179–183.
12. Reece EA: **Perspectives on obesity, pregnancy and birth outcomes in the United States: The scope of the problem.** *Am J Obestet Gynecol* 2008, **198:**23–27.
13. Hindawi IM, Meri ZB: **Cesarean Section Rate in Jordan.** *Saudi Med* 2004, **25**(11):1631–1635.
14. Ministry of Health: *Multiple Indicator Cluster Survey Final Report, Iraq 2006 (MICS 3), Central Organization for Statistics & Information Technology, Kurdistan Regional Office.* Iraq: United Nations Children Fund; 2007.
15. Al-dobony SJ: *Rate, Indications and risk factors of cesarean section in maternity hospital in Baghdad city*, hD thesis, Iraqi Board of Medical Specialization, community medicine; 2009.
16. Ministry of Planning: *Women Integrated Social and Health Survey*, Governorate Report (I-WISH 2011), Iraq, Central Statistical Organization-CSO. 2012.

17. Dietz PM, Callaghan WM, Morrow B, Cogswell ME: **Population-based assessment of the risk of primary cesarean delivery due to excess pre-pregnancy weight among nulliparous women delivering term infants.** *Matern Child Health J* 2005, **9**:237–244.
18. Barau G, Robillard PY, Hulsey TC, Dedecker F, Laffite A, Gérardin P, Kauffmann E: **Linear association between maternal body mass index and risk of cesarean section in term deliveries.** *BJOG* 2006, **113**:1173–1177.
19. Young TK, Woodmansee B: **Factors that are associated with cesarean delivery in a large private practice: The importance of pre-pregnancy body mass index and weight gain.** *Am J Obstet Gynecol* 2002, **187**:312–332.
20. Ministry of Health: *Department of Health Vital Statistic.* Iraq: Vital Statistic registry; 2009.
21. Taher SH, Shabab U: **Effect of obesity on Cesarean section rate.** *J Surg Pakistan* 2005, **15**(2):93–96.
22. Kominiarek MA, Vanveldhuisen P, Hibbard J, Landy H, Haberman S, Learman L, Wilkins I, Bailit J, Branch W, Burkman R, Gonzalez-Quintero VH, Gregory K, Hatjis C, Hoffman M, Ramirez M, Reddy UM, Troendle J, Zhang J: **The maternal body mass index: a strong association with delivery route.** *Am J Obestet Gyneco* 2010, **203**(3):264. E1-7.
23. Tosson MM, Alhussaini TK: **The impact of maternal obesity on pregnancy outcome at Assuit University Hospital.** *Ass Univ Bull Env Res* 2005, **8**(2):1–11.
24. Perlow JH, Morgan MA, Montgomery D, Towers CV, Porto M: **Perinatal outcome in pregnancy complicated by massive obesity.** *AJOG* 1992, **167**(4):958–962.
25. Cnattingham R, Cnattingham S, Notzon FC: **Obstacles to reducing cesarean section rates in a low cesarean setting: The effect of maternal age, height and weight.** *Obstet Gynecol* 1998, **92**:205–206.
26. Edward RK, Haresberger S, Johnson IM, Treloar RW, Cruz AC: **Deciding on route of delivery for obese women with prior cesarean delivery.** *Am J Obeset Gynecol* 2003, **189**:385–390.
27. Mohammed BS: ***Risk factors of cesarean section in AL –Yarmouk hospital:*** *PhD thesis, Iraqi Board of Medical Specialization, community medicine*; 2006.

Ethnic variation in stillbirth risk and the role of maternal obesity: analysis of routine data from a London maternity unit

Nicole Penn[1], Eugene Oteng-Ntim[2], Laura L Oakley[3*] and Pat Doyle[3]

Abstract

Background: Approximately 5 in 1,000 deliveries in England and Wales result in stillbirth, with little improvement in figures over the last few decades. The aim of this study was to investigate the association between clinical and socio-demographic factors and stillbirth, with a particular focus on ethnicity and obesity.

Methods: Analysis of routine maternity data on 53,293 singleton births occurring in a large London teaching hospital between 2004 and 2012. Logistic regression was used to investigate risk factors for stillbirth and to explore potential effect modification.

Results: 53,293 deliveries occurred during the time period, of which 329 resulted in a stillbirth (6.2 per 1,000 births). Compared to White women, non-White ethnicity was associated with a doubling of the odds of stillbirth (aOR for Black women 2.15, 95% CI 1.56-2.97; aOR for South Asian women 2.33, 95% CI 1.42-3.83). Obese women had a trend towards higher odds of stillbirth compared to women of recommended BMI (aOR 1.38, 95% CI 0.98-1.96), though this was not significant (p 0.07). Both higher parity (≥2 compared to para 1) and hypertension were associated with a higher odds of stillbirth (parity ≥2 aOR 1.65, 95% CI 1.13-2.39; hypertension aOR 1.84, 95% CI 1.22-2.78) but there was no evidence that area deprivation or maternal age were independently associated with stillbirth in this population. There was some evidence of effect modification between ethnicity and obesity (p value for interaction 0.06), with obesity a particularly strong risk factor for stillbirth in South Asian women (aOR 4.64, 95% CI 1.84-11.70).

Conclusions: There was a high prevalence of stillbirth in this multi-ethnic urban population. The increased risk of stillbirth observed in non-White women remains after adjusting for other factors. Our finding of possible effect modification between ethnicity and obesity suggests that further research should be conducted in order to improve understanding of the interplay between ethnicity, obesity and stillbirth.

Keywords: Stillbirth, Obesity, Ethnicity

Background

In 2012 the prevalence of stillbirth in England and Wales was 4.9 stillbirths per 1,000 total births [1], with an overall decline in prevalence over the preceding decade [2]. However, there is little evidence of improvement in stillbirth rates among singleton pregnancies during this time [3].

Identifying the cause of stillbirth can be challenging due to the plurality of classification systems, many of which result in a high proportion of cases remaining unexplained [4]. Common causes in UK studies are congenital anomaly, antepartum haemorrhage, maternal medical conditions and infection [5,6]. Meta-analysis of studies conducted in high-income countries has identified the following risk factors for stillbirth; overweight and obesity, pre-existing diabetes and pre-existing hypertension, advanced maternal age, primiparity, illicit drug use, low education and low socioeconomic status, no antenatal care, pregnancy-related hypertension, small for gestational age, post-term pregnancy, and previous stillbirth [7]. Many of these associations have been confirmed in UK studies [6,8-10].

* Correspondence: laura.oakley@lshtm.ac.uk
[3]Department of Non-communicable Disease Epidemiology, London School of Hygiene and Tropical Medicine, Keppel Street, London WC1E 7HT, UK
Full list of author information is available at the end of the article

The UK 2009 Perinatal Mortality report found Black women nationally to have twice the odds of stillbirth compared to White women, while Asian women had a smaller but significant increase of 60% in their odds of stillbirth compared to White women [2]. Nationally women of these ethnicities account for only a small proportion of births. However, 2009 estimates suggest that 40.5% of London's population is from a non-White British background [11], with this proportion likely to be higher among the maternal population due to the younger age structure of non-White ethnic groups. Previous studies have reported that among women living in London, Black and Asian women have a higher risk of stillbirth compared to White women [6,12]. In the UK, Black women have higher rates of obesity in pregnancy compared to White women [13]. Little is known about the role of obesity in explaining the higher risk of stillbirth observed in Black and South Asian women in the UK, although there is evidence from other high income countries that the association between obesity and obstetric outcomes varies by ethnicity [14,15]. These studies, predominately conducted in the US, may not be generalizable to the UK due to differences in the composition of ethnic groups between the two countries.

The aim of this study was to investigate the association between clinical and socio-demographic factors and stillbirth in an urban UK population, with a particular focus on the role of ethnicity and obesity. The study population, from south London, is ethnically diverse and has relatively high levels of deprivation and maternal obesity compared to the UK as a whole.

Methods

Data were extracted from a routine database kept on all patients delivering at Guy's and St Thomas's Hospital Foundation Trust (GSTT). The hospitals managed by this Trust are located in south London, UK. Direct patient identifiers were removed from the dataset before analysis and ethical approval was granted by the London School of Hygiene and Tropical Medicine Ethics committee. All 53,293 deliveries between January 2004 and May 2012 which ended in a singleton livebirth or stillbirth were included in this analysis.

Outcome

The primary outcome was stillbirth, defined as 'a baby delivered with no signs of life known to have died after 24 completed weeks of pregnancy' [16]. For the purposes of international comparison, a the number of stillbirths according to the WHO recommended threshold of 28 weeks is presented as an (Additional file 1: Table S1).

Explanatory variables

Ethnicity was classified as White (British, Irish, White Other), Black (Black African, Black Caribbean, Other Black), South Asian (Indian, Pakistani, Bangladeshi, Asian Other), or Other (Chinese, Mixed, Other). Maternal age was grouped as <20 years, 20–24 years, 25–29 years, 30–34 years, 35–39 years and 40+ years for descriptive tables and modelled as a continuous variable for regression modelling.

Deprivation was measured by the English Indices of Multiple Deprivation (IMD); a recognised scoring system for area-based deprivation based on census data covering seven different domains [17]. The IMD (2007) score was calculated using postcode at antenatal care booking, and scores were mapped to national IMD quintiles with quintile 1 as the least deprived and quintile 5 as the most deprived.

Maternal body mass index (BMI) was calculated from the mother's height and weight recorded at booking (weight in kg/(height in m)^2) and categorised as 'underweight' (<18.5), 'recommended' (18.5-24.9), 'overweight' (25–29.9), or 'obese' (30+); implausible values (<13, >70) were coded as missing. We created a second BMI variable for use in sensitivity analyses, applying lower thresholds for South Asian women only (overweight ≥23, obese ≥27.5) as discussed in recent NICE guidance [18].

Women were considered to be a 'hypertension' case when any pre-existing or pregnancy related hypertension was recorded, and a 'diabetes' case when any pre-existing type 1 or 2 or gestational diabetes was recorded. This information was recorded prospectively i.e. before delivery. Parity was categorised into three groups (nulliparous – para 0, para 1, or para 2+), with para 1 as the reference group to reflect the increased risk of stillbirth in primiparous women [7]. Additional explanatory variables were marital status (single vs. in a relationship), and smoking status at booking (yes/no).

Statistical analysis

We calculated the prevalence of stillbirth as the number of singleton stillbirths divided by the total number of births after 24 completed weeks, presented per 1,000 total singleton births. Odds ratios for the association between explanatory factors and stillbirth were calculated using univariate and multivariable logistic regression. Obesity and ethnic group were considered the main explanatory factors and were included in all multivariable models, other variables were included in multivariable modelling where there was evidence that they were independently associated with stillbirth ($p < 0.05$ for at least one parameter using the Wald test after adjustment for other variables). Potential effect modification between ethnicity and BMI, parity and area deprivation was explored using an interaction term in the final logistic regression model. Interaction terms assessed as $p < 0.05$ using the Wald test were considered significant; and p values <0.1 assessed as providing possible evidence of interaction.

To account for the fact that some women contributed more than one birth to the analysis, all confidence intervals were calculated using robust standard errors.

Where data were missing for >10% observations for a variable included in multivariable analysis, a sensitivity analysis was run using the final model fitting a dummy category for missing data to ensure similar results were obtained using the full sample. Additionally, to address the debate surrounding the use of conventional BMI thresholds to assess risk of chronic health conditions in South Asian populations [18], the final multivariable model was repeated using lower BMI thresholds for South Asian women. The results of this model were compared to the main analysis.

All statistical analysis was conducted using Stata version 13.

Results

Prevalence of stillbirth

Of the 53,293 singleton births in this analysis, 329 resulted in stillbirth: an overall rate of 6.2 stillbirths per 1,000 births (95% CI 5.5-6.9) (Table 1). There was slight variation in the stillbirth rate by year of delivery, with the highest rate mid-period in 2008/09. The prevalence of stillbirth was higher in all non-White groups compared to White women: 9.1 per 1,000 for both South Asian and Black women, 6.9 for other ethnic groups, and 3.8 for White women (Additional file 2: Table S2).

For the 202 stillbirths where results of the initial exam were reported, nearly two-thirds (64%, n = 129) were known to be antepartum deaths due to a reported macerated appearance. A further 36% (n = 73) of stillbirths were reported as fresh intrauterine deaths however it cannot be known how many of those were the consequence of an antepartum rather than intrapartum cause. The majority (62.0% n = 204) of stillbirths occurred before 37 weeks gestation and only 10% were delivered after 40 weeks gestation.

Characteristics of the sample

Table 2 describes the characteristics of the mothers in the sample. In summary, 59% of mothers were aged 30 and over at the time of delivery, the majority of mothers were either White (49.5%) or Black (32.5%), and nearly four-fifths (79%) lived in the two most deprived IMD quintiles nationally. More than 30% of mothers were overweight or obese and 58% were nulliparous. One quarter (26.6%) of all women were single. Key characteristics stratified by ethnicity are presented as an (Additional file 1: Table S1).

For both smoking status and BMI there were considerable levels of missing data (11% and 20% respectively); for all other variables less than 2% of records were missing data.

Univariate analysis

The results of univariate logistic regression are presented in Table 2. Maternal age (modelled as a continuous variable) was significantly associated with stillbirth (OR 1.02 per unit increase in age, 95% CI 1.00-1.04, p 0.039), with the highest odds of stillbirth occurring in women ≥40 years. Area deprivation, as measured by IMD, did not appear to be associated with stillbirth in this crude analysis, nor did single status or smoking status. Women with two or more previous children had a higher odds of stillbirth compared to women with only one previous child and women of all ethnicities had higher odds of stillbirth than White women. Both overweight women and obese women had a higher odds of stillbirth compared to women of recommended BMI (OR for overweight women: 1.36, 95% CI 1.00-1.86, p = 0.046; obese women: OR 1.97, 95% CI 1.44-2.68, P < 0.001).

Multivariable analysis

Ethnicity remained strongly associated with stillbirth in multivariable analysis (Table 3). Using White women as the comparison group, Black women had twice the odds of stillbirth (aOR 2.15, 95% CI 1.56-2.97, p < 0.001) and South Asian women 2.3 times the odds (aOR 2.33, 95% CI 1.42-3.83, p < 0.001).

The dose response association between maternal BMI and stillbirth observed in univariate analysis was somewhat attenuated after adjustment, with no evidence of increased odds of stillbirth among overweight women (aOR 1.03, 95% CI 0.75-1.42, p 0.85), and the OR for obese women just over the p 0.05 significance level (aOR 1.38, 95% CI 0.98-1.96, p 0.07).

Table 1 Crude stillbirth rate by year of delivery (n = 53,293)

		Total births		Stillbirths		Stillbirth rate (per 1,000 total births)	Crude OR (95% CI)	p value
		n	(%)	n	(%)			
All births		53,293		329		6.2		
Year of delivery	2004/05	11,361	(21.3)	70	(21.3)	6.2	ref	
	2006/07	12,347	(23.2)	79	(24.0)	6.4	1.04 (0.75-1.43)	0.82
	2008/09	13,241	(24.8)	96	(29.2)	7.3	1.18 (0.86-1.61)	0.30
	2010/11/12[1]	16,344	(30.7)	84	(25.5)	5.1	0.83 (0.60-1.15)	0.26

[1] 6 months of data for 2012 combined with 2010/11.

Table 2 Univariable analysis of clinical and socio-demographic factors associated with stillbirth (n = 53,293)

		Total births		Stillbirths		Crude OR (95% CI)	p value
		n = 53293	(%)	n = 329	(%)		
Ethnicity	White	26,390	(49.5)	99	(30.1)	ref	
	Black	17,337	(32.5)	157	(47.7)	2.43 (1.88-3.13)	<0.001
	Asian	2,957	(5.5)	27	(8.2)	2.45 (1.60-3.75)	<0.001
	Other	5,790	(10.9)	40	(12.2)	1.85 (1.27-2.69)	0.001
	Missing	*813*	*(1.5)*	6	*(1.8)*		
Deprivation (IMD)	Quintile 1 (least deprived)	1,636	(3.1)	7	(2.1)	0.64 (0.30-1.37)	0.25
	Quintile 2	3,056	(5.7)	16	(4.9)	0.78 (0.46-1.32)	0.36
	Quintile 3	6,072	(11.4)	31	(9.4)	0.76 (0.51-1.14)	0.19
	Quintile 4	23,997	(45.0)	151	(45.9)	0.94 (0.74-1.20)	0.64
	Quintile 5 (most deprived)	18,147	(34.1)	121	(36.8)	ref	
	Missing	*385*	*(0.7)*	3	*(0.9)*		
Maternal age	<20 yrs	2,041	(3.8)	11	(3.3)	0.84 (0.44-1.58)	0.58
	20-24 yrs	7,217	(13.5)	39	(11.9)	0.84 (0.56-1.24)	0.38
	25-29 yrs	12,125	(22.8)	78	(23.7)	ref	
	30-34 yrs	17,473	(32.8)	100	(30.4)	0.89 (0.65-1.20)	0.45
	35-39 yrs	11,441	(21.5)	74	(22.5)	1.00 (0.73-1.39)	0.97
	40+ yrs	2,996	(5.6)	27	(8.2)	1.40 (0.90-2.18)	0.13
	Per year increase in age					*1.02 (1.00-1.04)*	*0.039*
BMI	Underweight	1,413	(2.7)	7	(2.1)	1.01 (0.47-2.16)	0.98
	Recommended	24,423	(45.8)	120	(36.5)	ref	
	Overweight	10,503	(19.7)	70	(21.3)	1.36 (1.00-1.84)	0.046
	Obese	6,339	(11.9)	61	(18.5)	1.97 (1.44-2.68)	<0.001
	Missing	*10,615*	*(19.9)*	*71*	*(21.6)*	*1.36 (1.02-1.83)*	*0.04*
Parity	Nulliparous	30,856	(57.9)	168	(51.1)	1.03 (0.76-1.36)	0.85
	Para 1	13,196	(24.8)	70	(21.3)	ref	
	Para 2+	9,170	(17.2)		(27.7)	1.88 (1.37-2.57)	<0.001
	Missing	*71*	*(0.1)*	*0*	*(0.0)*		
Single status	Married or living with partner	38,987	(73.2)	240	(72.9)	ref	
	Single	14,167	(26.6)	88	(26.7)	1.01 (0.79-1.29)	0.94
	Missing	*139*	*(0.3)*	1	*(0.3)*		
Smoking	Non-smoker at booking	44,205		278	(84.5)	ref	
	Smoker at booking	3,327		26	(7.9)	1.01 (0.79-1.29)	0.29
	Missing	*5,761*	*(10.8)*	*25*	*(7.6)*		
Hypertensive disorders	No hypertension	50,721	(95.2)	295	(89.7)	ref	
	Hypertension	2,572	(4.8)	34	(10.3)	2.29 (1.61-3.26)	<0.001
Diabetes	No diabetes	52,064	(97.7)	317	(96.4)	ref	
	Diabetes	1,229	(2.3)	12	(3.6)	1.61 (0.90-2.87)	0.11

After adjustment, women with two or more previous births had a higher odds of stillbirth (aOR 1.65, 95% CI 1.13-2.39, p 0.009) compared to women with only one previous birth. Hypertension was associated with a near doubling of the odds of stillbirth (aOR 1.84, 95% CI 1.22-2.78, p 0.004).

The final logistic regression model was run on an expanded sample including observations with missing data on BMI, fitting a dummy category for 'BMI – missing'. The results of this analysis were not notably different from the analysis using the restricted sample (Additional file 3: Table S3).

Table 3 Multivariable analysis of clinical and socio-demographic factors associated with stillbirth (n = 42,043)

		Adjusted OR[1] (95% CI)	p value
Ethnicity	White	ref	
	Black	2.15 (1.56-2.97)	<0.001
	Asian	2.33 (1.42-3.83)	0.001
	Other	1.99 (1.32-3.01)	0.001
Maternal age	*per year increase in age*	1.03 (1.01-1.06)	0.012
BMI	Underweight	1.04 (0.49-2.23)	0.911
	Recommended	ref	
	Overweight	1.03 (0.75-1.42)	0.847
	Overweight	1.38 (0.98-1.96)	0.068
Parity	Nulliparous	1.28 (0.92-1.79)	0.137
	Para 1	ref	
	Para 2+	1.65 (1.13-2.39)	0.009
Hypertensive disorders	No hypertension	ref	
	Hypertension	1.84 (1.22-2.78)	0.004

[1]Odds ratios adjusted for all other variables in table.

Effect modification

There was no evidence of interaction between ethnicity and either parity or deprivation in either stratified univariable analysis or multivariable analysis. However, stratified analysis suggested potential effect modification between ethnicity and maternal BMI. Among White and Black women, there was a consistent dose response relationship between increasing BMI from the recommended weight category onwards (recommended, overweight, and obese) and stillbirth rate. However, the relationship between BMI and stillbirth risk was exceptional among South Asian women with a disproportionately high stillbirth rate observed among obese women (Figure 1). To further investigate the possibility of effect modification an interaction term was included in the adjusted regression model with maternal BMI modelled as a binary variable (obese vs. not obese, underweight women included in the reference category) in order to maximise power. The Wald statistic for the interaction term provided some evidence ($p = 0.05$) of effect modification. Stratified adjusted odds ratios (Table 4) demonstrate that obesity is a strong independent risk factor for stillbirth among South Asian women, though there was little evidence that obesity was associated with stillbirth in other ethnic groups.

South Asian specific BMI thresholds

Applying lower thresholds for overweight and obesity in South Asian women resulted in a higher proportion of South Asian women being classified as overweight or obese (52.4% vs. 34.1% using conventional thresholds). In multivariable analysis (Additional file 4: Table S4a) the odds ratio for the association between South Asian ethnicity and stillbirth was very slightly attenuated by using lower BMI thresholds to define overweight and obesity (aOR for South Asian women using alternative BMI thresholds 2.26, 95% 1.37-3.72; aOR using conventional thresholds 2.33, 95% 1.42-3.83). In stratified analysis (Additional file 4: Table S4b), the OR for the association between obesity and stillbirth in South Asian women was considerably lower using alternative BMI

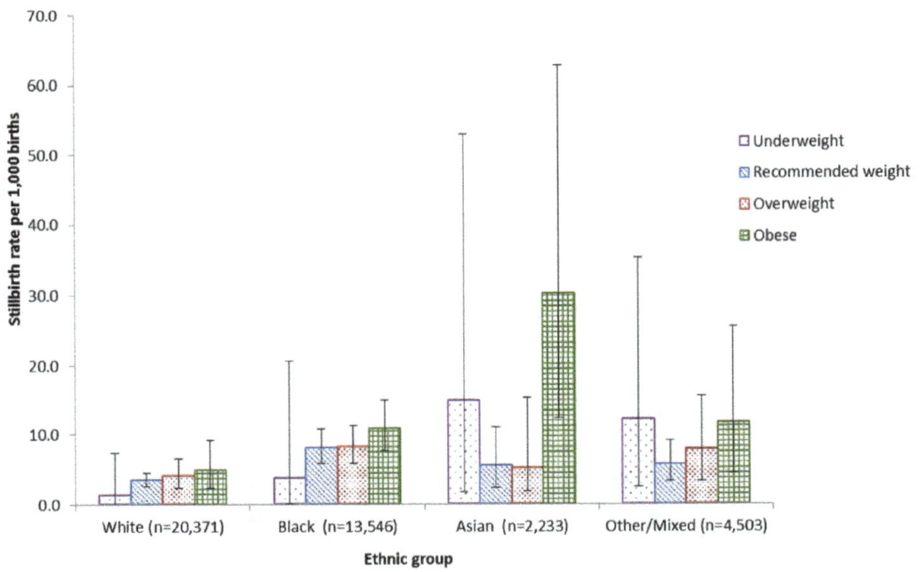

Figure 1 Stillbirth rate by maternal BMI category and ethnic group.

Table 4 Adjusted odds ratios for the association between obesity and stillbirth, stratified by ethnic group

		Births	Stillbirths	Stillbirth rate (per 1,000 total births)	Adjusted OR[1] (95% CI)	p value
		n	n			
White	Not obese	19116	68	3.6	ref	
	Obese	2032	10	4.9	1.32 (0.68-2.57)	0.41
Black	Not obese	10326	83	8.0	ref	
	Obese	3503	38	10.8	1.14 (0.76-1.71)	0.52
Asian	Not obese	2137	13	6.1	ref	
	Obese	232	7	30.2	4.64 (1.84-11.70)	0.001
Other	Not obese	4240	28	6.6	ref	
	Obese	513	6	11.7	1.60 (0.68-3.78)	0.28

[1]Adjusted for maternal age, hypertension and parity.

thresholds (aOR 2.83, 95% CI 1.17-6.85 vs. aOR 4.64, 95% CI 1.84-11.70).

Discussion

Main findings

In this study conducted using a diverse urban population, a number of maternal clinical and socio-demographic factors were independently associated with stillbirth. In particular, non-White ethnicity was significantly associated with stillbirth after adjustment for factors, and there was evidence to suggest that the association between obesity and stillbirth varied by ethnic group. A notable observation was the high risk of stillbirth in obese South Asian women.

Strengths and limitations

This study was conducted using a unique maternal population: urban, multi-ethnic and with a high degree of deprivation. A large number of variables were available for analysis, although the information was not available (or incomplete) for some variables of interest, for example likely timing of fetal death (antepartum or intrapartum), classification of stillbirth type (underlying cause and associated factors), previous complications, fetal growth restriction, and congenital anomalies. In particular, fetal growth restriction and congenital anomalies have been hypothesised as variables key in explaining the increased risk of stillbirth in non-White women. For most included variables there was a low level of missing data. However, for BMI, approximately 1 in 5 mothers had missing data and these women were not included in final adjusted models. This is a significant limitation of the analysis. Although there was little evidence that women with missing BMI differed with respect to any key characteristics, the group with missing BMI tended to be slightly older, less deprived, less likely to have diabetes, and more likely to be nulliparous (data not shown). All these characteristics are associated with a lower prevalence of obesity, suggesting that women with missing BMI may be more likely to be non-obese (i.e. data are "missing not at random"). This is clinically plausible, as BMI may be more likely to be measured by clinicians where women are visibly overweight. Sensitivity analysis including a dummy category for 'BMI – missing' showed that the estimates were highly similar when the women with missing BMI were included in the models. The fact that women with missing BMI status appear to have an increased odds of stillbirth in univariate analysis suggests that these women may have other risk indicators which were unmeasured in our analysis.

The relative rarity of stillbirth in this population means estimates in sub-group analysis have in some cases been calculated from a small number of events, resulting in wide confidence intervals. The analysis was likely underpowered to examine interaction, with only 27 stillbirths in one of the key groups of interest (South Asian women) group. In addition, under-reporting of hypertensive and diabetic conditions may have led to residual confounding by these factors in the adjusted analysis. Information on whether diabetes was pre-existing or gestational was not available for all diabetes cases, so we chose to combine these two conditions. This may have had the effect of underestimating the stillbirth risk associated with pre-existing diabetes as there is little evidence that gestational diabetes is associated with stillbirth [8].

Ethnicity was self-reported by mothers and recorded by the midwife at booking. For the analysis reported here, ethnicity was combined into four categories (White, South Asian, Black and Other). Although in many cases, more detailed description of ethnicity was available (for example, 'Black-African'), this was not well reported and general categories such as 'Black British' were frequently used. Although collapsing ethnicity into four groups helped to maximise statistical power, it is acknowledged that the inability to look at risk factors among individual ethnic groups is a limitation of this study. In addition, we were unable to look at association between country of birth and stillbirth: at least one previous study reported that the risk of stillbirth for different ethnic groups varied by country of birth (UK vs. non-UK) [8].

Although we had information on smoking, this was only recorded at booking. For those women who are smoking at the start of pregnancy, there is evidence that smoking behaviour tends to fluctuate throughout pregnancy as women attempt to cut down and/or cease smoking [19] and therefore smoking at booking can only be regarded as a proxy for smoking behaviour throughout pregnancy.

Interpretation

The prevalence of stillbirth in this urban population was 6.2 per 1000 total births. This figure is considerably higher than reported national figures between 2004 and 2012, despite the fact that multiple births were excluded from our study population. It is however, encouraging to note that stillbirth appears to be declining in this population when compared to reported rates of 7.3-8.5 per 1,000 between 2000 and 2010 [20]. The higher prevalence of stillbirth is likely to be in part attributable to the ethnic diversity of this population, and the fact that GSTT is a tertiary referral centre providing specialist care to pregnant women with complex medical conditions.

In this study Black and South Asian ethnicity, obesity, parity and hypertension were all found to be independent risk factors for stillbirth. Although the odds ratios for the association between stillbirth and deprivation, maternal age and diabetes showed trends in line with previous studies (i.e. for advanced maternal age and diabetes the ORs were higher, ORs for lower deprivation were lower), p values were not statistically significant. This may be because the analysis was underpowered to look at these exposures given the rarity of stillbirth. Additionally, most women in this population were considered relatively deprived on a national IMD scale, making it difficult to assess the relationship between deprivation and stillbirth.

In this population, multivariable analysis found that Black and South Asian women had twice the odds of stillbirth compared to White women. This finding is consistent with the results of previous studies reporting a higher risk of stillbirth among non-White women [8]. It has been hypothesised that the increased risk of stillbirth among Black and South Asian women is in part attributable to higher rates of obesity, diabetes, pre-eclampsia and hypertension, high parity and greater deprivation. However, diabetes and deprivation did not have a confounding effect on this relationship in our analysis, and higher odds of stillbirth for all non-White groups remained after parity and hypertension were adjusted for.

Our finding that obesity and ethnicity interact in relation to stillbirth is a novel finding. Specifically, our results suggest that obese South Asian women have a significantly higher risk of stillbirth compared to obese White women. Interestingly, an earlier study conducted using the same population found the effect of obesity on diabetes was significantly stronger in South Asian women compared to White women [21]. Our findings in relation to stillbirth may reflect differences in metabolic susceptibility. They should be considered alongside an increasing body of evidence concluding that the association between obesity and chronic disease (e.g. diabetes) varies by ethnicity. It has been recommended that lower BMI cut-offs should be used to indicate South Asians at higher risk of ill health [22], with a recent suggestion that a similar approach could be extended to Black African and African-Caribbean groups. By using the same BMI obesity threshold for all ethnic groups in our main analysis, it may be that we captured a more 'extreme' obese group of South Asian women. To address this concern we ran a sensitivity analysis, the results of which suggest that although the odds of stillbirth associated with obesity are slightly lower for South Asian women when using lower BMI cut-offs, the findings remain significant.

The general increase in stillbirth risk observed in Black women and women from 'other' non-White backgrounds may be attributable to 'social' or 'biological' factors not measured in this study. In terms of social factors, proximal factors such as education, support or knowledge, differences in antenatal screening practice and attitudes to accessing care may be key to explaining the increased risk of stillbirth. In a biological model of causation the intermediaries may be factors such as differences in natural length of gestation [12] and birthweight [23], or higher rates of congenital anomaly due to increased prevalence of diabetes, obesity and consanguinity [24,25].

Conclusion

This study, conducted in a diverse population with a higher than average stillbirth rate, confirms that ethnicity is an important risk factor for stillbirth. The findings of this study also provide some evidence that the association between obesity and stillbirth differs by ethnic group, with obesity a key risk factor for stillbirth among South Asian women, but less so women from other ethnic backgrounds. This finding is important when clinically assessing high risk pregnancies. Further research is needed into the mechanism by which ethnicity acts to raise the risk of stillbirth in women, particularly in terms of the role of obesity in this relationship.

Ethical approval

Ethical approval was granted by the London School of Hygiene and Tropical Medicine Ethics committee (ref. 012–326, approved 03 June 2013).

Additional files

Additional file 1: Table S1. Clinical and socio-demographic factors by stillbirth (≥28 weeks). This table presents the number of births and stillbirths by clinical and socio-demographic factors, limited to births ≥28 weeks. This repeats some of the information in Table 2 using the WHO definition of stillbirth as deaths occurring at ≥28 weeks gestational age.

Additional file 2: Table S2. Clinical and socio-demographic factors by ethnic group. This table presents clinical and socio-demographic factors by ethic group, presenting the number of births and stillbirths by ethnic group for all the clinical and socio-demographic factors included in Table 2.

Additional file 3: Table S3. Multivariable analysis of clinical and socio-demographic factors associated with stillbirth, using a dummy category for BMI missing (n = 52,403). This table presents the results from a model equivalent to Table 3, including a dummy category for BMI missing.

Additional file 4: Table S4a. Multivariable analysis of the association between ethnic group and stillbirth, and obesity and stillbirth, using lower BMI thresholds for South Asian women. This table shows the adjusted odds ratios for the association between ethnic group and stillbirth, and obesity and stillbirth, using ethnicity-specific thresholds for BMI. These results can be compared to those in Table 3. **Table S4b.** Adjusted odds ratios for the association between obesity and stillbirth using lower BMI thresholds for South Asian women, stratified by ethnic group. This table shows odds ratios stratified by ethnic group for the association between obesity and stillbirth using ethnicity-specific thresholds for BMI. These results can be compared to those in Table 4.

Competing interests

The authors declare that they have no competing interests.

Authors' contributions

EO, NP and PD conceived the study and all authors contributed to the design of the study. NP, PD and LO designed and conducted the analysis. All authors were involved in the interpretation of the data. All authors wrote the initial draft of the manuscript and contributed to revising consecutive drafts. All authors read and approved the final version of the manuscript.

Author details
[1]King's College London School of Medicine, Capital House, King's College, London SE1 3QD, UK. [2]Guy's and St Thomas' NHS Foundation Trust, Westminster Bridge Road, London SE1 7EH, UK. [3]Department of Non-communicable Disease Epidemiology, London School of Hygiene and Tropical Medicine, Keppel Street, London WC1E 7HT, UK.

References

1. Office for National Statistics (ONS): *Births in England and Wales 2012.* London: ONS; 2013.
2. Centre for Maternal and Child Enquiries (CMACE): *Perinatal Mortality 2009.* London: CMACE; 2011.
3. Seaton SE, Field DJ, Draper ES, Manktelow BN, Smith GC, Springett A, Smith LK: **Socioeconomic inequalities in the rate of stillbirths by cause: a population-based study.** *BMJ Open* 2012, **2**(3).
4. Flenady V, Froen JF, Pinar H, Torabi R, Saastad E, Guyon G, Russell L, Charles A, Harrison C, Chauke L, Pattinson R, Koshy R, Bahrin S, Gardener G, Day K, Petersson K, Gordon A, Gilshenan K: **An evaluation of classification systems for stillbirth.** *BMC Pregnancy Childbirth* 2009, **9**(1):24.
5. Shankar M, Navti O, Amu O, Konje J: **Assessment of stillbirth risk and associated risk factors in a tertiary hospital.** *J Obstet Gynecol* 2002, **22**(1):34–38.
6. Smeeton NC, Rona RJ, Dobson P, Cochrane R, Wolfe C: **Assessing the determinants of stillbirths and early neonatal deaths using routinely collected data in an inner city area.** *BMC Med* 2004, **2**(1):27.
7. Flenady V, Koopmans L, Middleton P, Frøen JF, Smith GC, Gibbons K, Coory M, Gordon A, Ellwood D, McIntyre HD: **Major risk factors for stillbirth in high-income countries: a systematic review and meta-analysis.** *Lancet* 2011, **377**(9774):1331–1340.
8. Gardosi J, Madurasinghe V, Williams M, Malik A, Francis A: **Maternal and fetal risk factors for stillbirth: population based study.** *BMJ* 2013, **346:**f108.
9. Kenny LC, Lavender T, McNamee R, O'Neill SM, Mills T, Khashan AS: **Advanced maternal age and adverse pregnancy outcome: evidence from a large contemporary cohort.** *PLoS One* 2013, **8**(2):e56583.
10. Tennant PWG, Rankin J, Bell R: **Maternal body mass index and the risk of fetal and infant death: a cohort study from the North of England.** *Hum Reprod* 2011, **26**(6):1501–1511.
11. Office of National Statistics: *Population Estimates for Ethnic Group (experimental) Mid-2009.* London: ONS; 2011.
12. Balchin I, Whittaker JC, Patel RR, Lamont RF, Steer PJ: **Racial variation in the association between gestational age and perinatal mortality: prospective study.** *BMJ* 2007, **334**(7598):833.
13. Heslehurst N, Rankin J, Wilkinson JR, Summerbell CD: **A nationally representative study of maternal obesity in England, UK: trends in incidence and demographic inequalities in 619[thinsp]323 births, 1989–2007.** *Int J Obes (Lond)* 2010, **34**(3):420–428.
14. Steinfeld JD, Valentine S, Lerer T, Ingardia CJ, Wax JR, Curry SL: **Obesity-related complications of pregnancy vary by race.** *J Matern Fetal Med* 2000, **9**(4):238–241.
15. Ramos GA, Caughey AB: **The interrelationship between ethnicity and obesity on obstetric outcomes.** *Am J Obstet Gynecol* 2005, **193**(3, Supplement):1089–1093.
16. Royal College of Obstetricians and Gynaecologists (RCOG): *Late Intrauterine Fetal Death and Stillbirth.* London: RCOG; 2010.
17. Department of Communities and Local Government: *Index of Multiple Deprivation. The English Indices of Deprivation.* London: Department of Communities and Local Government; 2007.
18. National Institute for Health and Care Excellence: *Assessing Body Mass Index and Waist Circumference Thresholds For Intervening To Prevent Ill Health and Premature Death Among Adults from Black, Asian and Other Minority Ethnic Groups in The UK (Nice Guidelines Ph46).* Manchester: NICE; 2013.
19. Pickett KE, Rathouz PJ, Kasza K, Wakschlag LS, Wright R: **Self-reported smoking, cotinine levels, and patterns of smoking in pregnancy.** *Paediatr Perinat Epidemiol* 2005, **19**(5):368–376.
20. Tezcan B, Khazaezadeh N, Ash A, Oteng-Ntim E: **Social disparity and intrauterine death: from politics to policies.** *J Obstet Gynaecol* 2011, **31**(6):507–508.
21. Oteng-Ntim E, Kopeika J, Seed P, Wandiembe S, Doyle P: **Impact of obesity on pregnancy outcome in different ethnic groups: calculating population attributable fractions.** *PLoS One* 2013, **8**(1):e53749.
22. WHO EC: **Appropriate body-mass index for Asian populations and its implications for policy and intervention strategies.** *Lancet* 2004, **363**(9403):157.
23. Kelly Y, Panico L, Bartley M, Marmot M, Nazroo J, Sacker A: **Why does birthweight vary among ethnic groups in the UK? Findings from the Millennium Cohort Study.** *J Public Health* 2009, **31**(1):131–137.
24. Dornhorst A, Paterson CM, Nicholls JSD, Wadsworth J, Chiu DC, Elkeles RS, Johnston DG, Beard RW: **High prevalence of gestational diabetes in women from ethnic minority groups.** *Diabet Med* 1992, **9**(9):820–825.
25. Bundey S, Alam H, Kaur A, Mir S, Lancashire R: **Why do UK-born Pakistani babies have high perinatal and neonatal mortality rates?** *Paediatr Perinat Epidemiol* 1991, **5**(1):101–114.

Permissions

All chapters in this book were first published in P&C, by BioMed Central; hereby published with permission under the Creative Commons Attribution License or equivalent. Every chapter published in this book has been scrutinized by our experts. Their significance has been extensively debated. The topics covered herein carry significant findings which will fuel the growth of the discipline. They may even be implemented as practical applications or may be referred to as a beginning point for another development.

The contributors of this book come from diverse backgrounds, making this book a truly international effort. This book will bring forth new frontiers with its revolutionizing research information and detailed analysis of the nascent developments around the world.

We would like to thank all the contributing authors for lending their expertise to make the book truly unique. They have played a crucial role in the development of this book. Without their invaluable contributions this book wouldn't have been possible. They have made vital efforts to compile up to date information on the varied aspects of this subject to make this book a valuable addition to the collection of many professionals and students.

This book was conceptualized with the vision of imparting up-to-date information and advanced data in this field. To ensure the same, a matchless editorial board was set up. Every individual on the board went through rigorous rounds of assessment to prove their worth. After which they invested a large part of their time researching and compiling the most relevant data for our readers.

The editorial board has been involved in producing this book since its inception. They have spent rigorous hours researching and exploring the diverse topics which have resulted in the successful publishing of this book. They have passed on their knowledge of decades through this book. To expedite this challenging task, the publisher supported the team at every step. A small team of assistant editors was also appointed to further simplify the editing procedure and attain best results for the readers.

Apart from the editorial board, the designing team has also invested a significant amount of their time in understanding the subject and creating the most relevant covers. They scrutinized every image to scout for the most suitable representation of the subject and create an appropriate cover for the book.

The publishing team has been an ardent support to the editorial, designing and production team. Their endless efforts to recruit the best for this project, has resulted in the accomplishment of this book. They are a veteran in the field of academics and their pool of knowledge is as vast as their experience in printing. Their expertise and guidance has proved useful at every step. Their uncompromising quality standards have made this book an exceptional effort. Their encouragement from time to time has been an inspiration for everyone.

The publisher and the editorial board hope that this book will prove to be a valuable piece of knowledge for researchers, students, practitioners and scholars across the globe.

List of Contributors

Valerie Mueller
Department of Obstetrics & Gynecology, McMaster University, 1280 Main St. West, Hamilton, ON L8S 4L8, Canada

Sarah D McDonald
Department of Obstetrics & Gynecology, McMaster University, 1280 Main St. West, Hamilton, ON L8S 4L8, Canada
Department of Radiology, McMaster University, 1280 Main St. West, Hamilton, ON L8S 4L8, Canada
Department of Clinical Epidemiology & Biostatistics, McMaster University, 1280 Main St. West, Hamilton, ON L8S 4L8, Canada

Christina K Park, Joseph Beyene and Binod Neupane
Department of Clinical Epidemiology & Biostatistics, McMaster University, 1280 Main St. West, Hamilton, ON L8S 4L8, Canada

Eleanor Pullenayegum
Child Health Evaluative Sciences Program, Hospital for Sick Children, 555 University Avenue, Toronto, ON M5G1X8, Canada

Keyna Bracken
Department of Family Medicine, McMaster University, 1280Main St. West, Hamilton, ON L8S 4L8, Canada

Wendy Sword
Department of Clinical Epidemiology & Biostatistics, McMaster University, 1280 Main St. West, Hamilton, ON L8S 4L8, Canada
School of Nursing, McMasterUniversity, Hamilton, ON L8S 4L8, Canada

Helen McDonald
Midwifery Education Program, McMaster University, 1280 Main St. West, Hamilton, ON L8S 4L8, Canada

Valerie H Taylor
Department of Psychiatry, Women's College Hospital, 76 Grenville St,Toronto, ON M5S 1B1, Canada

Melissa Brouwers
Department of Clinical Epidemiology & Biostatistics, McMaster University, 1280 Main St. West, Hamilton, ON L8S 4L8, Canada
Department of Oncology, McMaster University, 1280 Main St. West, Hamilton, ON L8S 4L8, Canada

Lyn Ebert
Faculty of Health & Medicine School of Medicine & Public Health, University of Newcastle, Callaghan, NSW, Australia

Shanna M. Fealy
School of Nursing & Midwifery University of Newcastle, Port Macquarie Campus, Port Macquarie 2444, NSW, Australia
Faculty of Health & Medicine School of Medicine & Public Health, University of Newcastle, Callaghan, NSW, Australia
Maternity Care Services, The Port Macquarie Base Hospital, Port Macquarie, NSW, Australia

Rachael M. Taylor
Faculty of Health & Medicine School of Medicine & Public Health, University of Newcastle, Callaghan, NSW, Australia
Mothers and Babies Research Centre, University of Newcastle, University Drive, Callaghan 2308, NSW, Australia
Hunter Medical Research Institute, Newcastle, NSW, Australia

Maralyn Foureur
School of Nursing & Midwifery University of Newcastle, Port Macquarie Campus, Port Macquarie 2444, NSW, Australia
Centre for Midwifery, Child and Family Health, Faculty of Health, University of Technology Sydney, Broadway, Ultimo, NSW 2007, Australia

John Attia
Hunter Medical Research Institute, Newcastle, NSW, Australia
Centre for Clinical Epidemiology and Biostatistics, School of Medicine & Public Health, University of Newcastle, Callaghan, NSW, Australia
Division of Medicine, John Hunter Hospital, Newcastle, NSW, Australia

Alessandra Bisquera
Hunter Medical Research Institute, Newcastle, NSW, Australia
Centre for Clinical Epidemiology and Biostatistics, School of Medicine & Public Health, University of Newcastle, Callaghan, NSW, Australia

Alexis J. Hure
Faculty of Health & Medicine School of Medicine & Public Health, University of Newcastle, Callaghan, NSW, Australia
Hunter Medical Research Institute, Newcastle, NSW, Australia

Judith G. M. Jelsma
Department of Public and Occupational Health and, Amsterdam Public Health research institute, VU University Medical Centre, Van der Boechorststraat 7, 1081BT Amsterdam, Amsterdam, The Netherlands

David Simmons
Institute of Metabolic Science, Addenbrookes Hospital, Cambridge, England, UK
Macarthur Clinical School, University of Western Sydney, Campbelltown, NSW, Australia

Nina Gobat and Stephen Rollnick
School of Medicine, Cardiff University, Cardiff, Wales, UK

Kinga Blumska, Ewa Wender-Ożegowska and Agnieszka Zawiejska
Medical Faculty I, Poznan University of Medical Sciences, Poznan, Poland

Goele Jans
KU Leuven Department of Development and Regeneration: Pregnancy, Fetus and Neonate Gynaecology and Obstetrics, University Hospitals Leuven, Leuven, Belgium

Elisabeth R. Mathiesen
Center for Pregnant Women with Diabetes, Departments of Endocrinology and Obstetrics, Rigshospitalet, Faculty of Health Sciences, University of Copenhagen, Copenhagen, Denmark

Annunziata Lapolla and Maria G. Dalfrà
Universita Degli Studi di Padova, Padova, Italy

Dorte M. Jensen and Liselotte Andersen
Odense University Hospital, Odense, Denmark

Frank J. Snoek
Department of Medical Psychology, Amsterdam Public Health research institute, VU University Medical Centre, Amsterdam, The Netherlands
Department of Medical Psychology, Academic Medical Centre, Amsterdam, The Netherlands

Mireille N. M. van Poppel
Department of Public and Occupational Health and, Amsterdam Public Health research institute, VU University Medical Centre, Van der Boechorststraat 7, 1081BT Amsterdam, Amsterdam, The Netherlands
Institute of Sport Science, University of Graz, Graz, Austria

K. Cheney and K. Black
Women's and Babies, Royal Prince Alfred Hospital, Missenden Road, Camperdown, Sydney, NSW 2050, Australia
Discipline of Obstetrics, Gynaecology and Neonatology, The University of Sydney, Sydney, NSW 2006, Australia

S. Berkemeier
Division of Obstetrics and Gynaecology, Campbelltown Hospital, Sydney, NSW 2560, Australia

K. A. Sim
The Boden Institute, Charles Perkins Centre, The University of Sydney, Sydney, NSW 2006, Australia

A. Gordon
Discipline of Obstetrics, Gynaecology and Neonatology, The University of Sydney, Sydney, NSW 2006, Australia
Charles Perkins Centre, The University of Sydney, Sydney, NSW 2006, Australia

Sara Holton and Jane Fisher
Jean Hailes Research Unit, Monash University, Level 4/553 St Kilda Road, Melbourne, Victoria 3004, Australia

Christine East
Maternity Services, Monash Health and Monash University, Monash Medical Centre, 246 Clayton Rd, Clayton, Victoria 3168, Australia

Yawen Shao, Jie Qiu, Baohong Mao, Wei Dai, Xiaochun He, Hongmei Cui, Xiaojuan Lin, Ling Lv, Zhongfeng Tang, Sijuan Xu, Min Zhou, Xiaoying Xu, Weitao Qiu and Qing Liu
Gansu Provincial Maternity and Child Care Hospital, 143 North Road, Qilihe District, Lanzhou, Gansu Province 730050, China

Huang Huang, Dennis Wang and Nan Zhao
Yale University School of Public Health, 60 College Street, New Haven, CT 06520, USA

Yawei Zhang
Yale University School of Public Health, 60 College Street, New Haven, CT 06520, USA
Yale School of Medicine, New Haven, CT, USA

Cassandra Vieten
California Pacific Medical Center Research Institute, 475 Brannan Street, San Francisco, CA 94120, USA
Institute of Noetic Sciences, 625 Second Street, # 200, Petaluma, CA 94952, USA

Helané Wahbeh
Institute of Noetic Sciences, 625 Second Street, # 200, Petaluma, CA 94952, USA

Kimberly Coleman-Phox and Elissa Epel
Center for Health and Community, University of California, San Francisco, 3333 California St., Suite 465, San Francisco, CA 94143-0844, USA

Barbara A. Laraia
Center for Health and Community, University of California, San Francisco, 3333 California St., Suite 465, San Francisco, CA 94143-0844, USA
School of Public Health, University of California, Berkeley, 207-B University Hall, Berkeley, CA 94720-7360, USA

Jean Kristeller
Department of Psychology, Indiana State University, Terre Haute, Indiana 47809, USA

Nancy Adler
Center for Health and Community, University of California, San Francisco, 3333 California St., Suite 465, San Francisco, CA 94143-0844, USA
Department of Psychology, Indiana State University, Terre Haute, Indiana 47809, USA

Nicole R. Bush
Center for Health and Community, University of California, San Francisco, 3333 California St., Suite 465, San Francisco, CA 94143-0844, USA
Department of Pediatrics, University of California, San Francisco, 550 16th Street, San Francisco, CA 94158, USA

Larissa G. Duncan
School of Human Ecology, University of Wisconsin-Madison, 1300 Linden Drive, Madison, WI 53706, USA

Christine M. Olson
Division of Nutritional Sciences, 406 Savage Hall, Cornell University, Ithaca, NY 14853, USA

Susan W. Groth
School of Nursing, University of Rochester, Elmwood Ave., Rochester, NY 14642, USA

Meredith L. Graham and Myla S. Strawderman
Division of Nutritional Sciences, 352 MVR Hall, Cornell University, Ithaca, NY 14853, USA

Jennifer E. Reschke and Isabel Diana Fernandez
Department of Public Health Sciences, University of Rochester School of Medicine and Dentistry, 265 Crittenden Blvd, CU420644, Rochester, NY 14642, USA

Z. Sui, C. Cramp and A. R. Deussen
The Robinson Research Institute, Discipline of Obstetrics and Gynaecology, School of Paediatrics and Reproductive Health, The University of Adelaide, Adelaide, VIC 3168, Australia

L. J. Moran
The Robinson Research Institute, Discipline of Obstetrics and Gynaecology, School of Paediatrics and Reproductive Health, The University of Adelaide, Adelaide, VIC 3168, Australia
Monash Centre for Health Research Implementation, School of Public Health and Preventive Medicine, Monash University, Clayton, Australia

S. A. McNaughton
Institute for Physical Activity and Nutrition (IPAN), Deakin University, Geelong, VIC, Australia

R. M. Grivell and J. M. Dodd
The Robinson Research Institute, Discipline of Obstetrics and Gynaecology, School of Paediatrics and Reproductive Health, The University of Adelaide, Adelaide, VIC 3168, Australia
Department of Perinatal Medicine, Women's & Babies Division, Women's and Children's Hospital, North Adelaide, Adelaide, Australia

Amy C. O'Higgins, Anne Doolan, Thomas McCartan, Laura Mullaney, Clare O'Connor and Michael J. Turner
UCD Centre for Human Reproduction, Coombe Women and Infants University Hospital, Dublin 8, Ireland

Emma Molyneaux and Louise M. Howard
Section of Women's Mental Health, Institute of Psychiatry, Psychology & Neuroscience at King's College London, London, England

Shahina Begum, Annette L. Briley, Paul T. Seed and Lucilla Poston
Department of Women and Children's Health, King's College, London, England

Hongying Wu and Jiayi Yue
Department of Gynaecology and Obstetrics, Liaocheng People's Hospital, Liaocheng 252000, Shandong Province, People's Republic of China

Shaniece Criss
Department of Health Sciences, Furman University, 3300 Poinsett Hwy, Greenville, SC 29613, USA

Emily Oken, Lauren Guthrie and Marie-France Hivert
Obesity Prevention Program, Department of Population Medicine, Harvard Medical School and Harvard Pilgrim Health Care Institute, 401 Park Drive Suite 401E, Boston, MA, USA02215

Anke Diemert, Mirja Pagenkemper, Gudula Hansen, Alina Drozdowska, Kurt Hecher and Petra Arck
Department of Obstetrics and Fetal Medicine, University Medical Center Hamburg-Eppendorf, Martinistrasse 52, Hamburg 20246, Germany

Susanne Lezius
Institute for Medical Biometry and Epidemiology, University Medical Center Hamburg-Eppendorf, Hamburg 20246, Germany

Birgit C. Zyriax
Preventive Medicine, University Heart Center, University Medical Center Hamburg-Eppendorf, Hamburg, Hamburg

Jayne R. Rice, Miguel Angel Luque Fernandez, Yasmin V. Barrios, Bizu Gelaye and Michelle A. Williams
Department of Epidemiology, Harvard T.H. Chan School of Public Health, 677 Huntington Ave, K501, Boston, MA, 02115 USA

Vicky Motta
Instituto Nacional Materno Perinatal de Lima, Lima, Peru

Gloria T. Larrabure-Torrealva
Instituto Nacional Materno Perinatal de Lima, Lima, Peru
Departamentos de Medicina y Ginecología y Obstetricia Universidad Nacional Universidad Nacional Mayor de San Marcos, Lima, Peru

Mirtha Grande
Asociación Civil de Proyectos en Salud, AC.PROESA, Lima, Peru

Sixto Sanchez
Universidad de Ciencias Aplicadas, Lima, Peru
Asociación Civil de Proyectos en Salud, AC.PROESA, Lima, Peru

Linda de Wit and Judith G. M. Jelsma
Department of Public and Occupational Health, EMGO+ Institute for Health and Care Research, VU University Medical Centre, Van der Boechorststraat 7, 1081BT Amsterdam, The Netherlands

Mireille N. M. van Poppel
Department of Public and Occupational Health, EMGO+ Institute for Health and Care Research, VU University Medical Centre, Van der Boechorststraat 7, 1081BT Amsterdam, The Netherlands
Institute for Sport Science, University of Graz, Graz, Austria

Annick Bogaerts
Department of Healthcare Research, PHL University College, Limburg Catholic University College, Hasselt, Belgium

Ewa Wender-Ozegowska and Agnieszka Zawiejska
Akademia Medyczna im Karola Marcinkowskiego, Poznan, Poland

Pablo Rebollo
BAP Health Outcomes Research SL, Oviedo, Spain

Annunziata Lapolla and Maria G. Dalfrà
Universita Degli Studi di Padova, Padova, Italy

Alessandra Bertolotto
Università di Pisa, Pisa, Italy

Fidelma Dunne
National University of Ireland, Galway, Ireland

Dorte M. Jensen and Liselotte Andersen
Odense University Hospital, Odense, Denmark.

Frank J. Snoek
Department of Medical Psychology, EMGO+ Institute for Health and Care Research, VU University Medical Centre, Amsterdam, The Netherlands
Department of Medical Psychology, Academic Medical Centre, Amsterdam, The Netherlands

Mufiza Zia Kapadia
Department of Obstetrics and Gynecology, McMaster University, Hamilton, Canada

Anca Gaston
School of Kinesiology, University of Western Ontario, London, Ontario, Canada

Sherry Van Blyderveen
New Leaf Psychology, Milton, Canada

Louis Schmidt
Department of Psychology, Neuroscience & Behavior, McMaster University, Hamilton, Canada

Joseph Beyene
Department Clinical Epidemiology and Biostatistics, McMaster University, Hamilton, Canada

Helen McDonald
Midwifery Education Program, Department of Family Medicine, McMaster University, Hamilton, Canada

Sarah D McDonald
Division of Maternal-Fetal Medicine, Departments of Obstetrics & Gynecology, Radiology, and Clinical Epidemiology & Biostatistics, McMaster University, 1280 Main Street West, room 3N52B, Hamilton, Ontario L8S 4K1, Canada

Mariana Santos Felisbino-Mendes, Fernanda Penido Matozinhos and Gustavo Velasquez-Melendez
Department of Maternal and Child Nursing and Public Health, Escola de Enfermagem, Universidade Federal de Minas Gerais (UFMG), Av. Alfredo Balena, 190 - Bairro Santa Efigênia, 30130-100, Belo Horizonte, MG, Brasil

J Jaime Miranda
CRONICAS Center of Excellence in Chronic Diseases, and Department of Medicine, School of Medicine, Universidad Peruana Cayetano Heredia, Lima, Peru

Eduardo Villamor
Department of Epidemiology, School of Public Health, University of Michigan, Ann Arbor, MI, USA

Kirsten Uebel
PhD Graduate School 'Nutritional adaptation and epigenetic mechanisms', ZIEL - Research Center for Nutrition and Food Sciences, Technische Universität München, Freising-Weihenstephan, Germany
Clinical Nutritional Medicine Unit, ZIEL - Research Center for Nutrition and Food Sciences, Technische Universität München, Freising-Weihenstephan, Germany

Kurt Gedrich
Biochemistry Unit, ZIEL - Research Center for Nutrition and Food Sciences, Technische Universität München, Freising-Weihenstephan, Germany

Karina Pusch
Else Kröner-Fresenius-Center for Nutritional Medicine, Wissenschaftszentrum Weihenstephan, Klinikum rechts der Isar, Uptown München Campus D, Technische Universität München, Munich, Germany

Hans Hauner
Clinical Nutritional Medicine Unit, ZIEL - Research Center for Nutrition and Food Sciences, Technische Universität München, Freising-Weihenstephan, Germany
Else Kröner-Fresenius-Center for Nutritional Medicine, Wissenschaftszentrum Weihenstephan, Klinikum rechts der Isar, Uptown München Campus D, Technische Universität München, Munich, Germany

Bernhard L Bader
PhD Graduate School 'Nutritional adaptation and epigenetic mechanisms', ZIEL - Research Center for Nutrition and Food Sciences, Technische Universität München, Freising-Weihenstephan, Germany
Clinical Nutritional Medicine Unit, ZIEL - Research Center for Nutrition and Food Sciences, Technische Universität München, Freising-Weihenstephan, Germany
Else Kröner-Fresenius-Center for Nutritional Medicine, Wissenschaftszentrum Weihenstephan, Klinikum rechts der Isar, Uptown München Campus D, Technische Universität München, Munich, Germany

Karl-Theo M Schneider
Abteilung für Geburtshilfe und Perinatalmedizin der Frauenklinik, Technische Universität München, Munich, Germany

Mazin Al-Rubaey and Ban Karim
Community Medicine Department, Faculty of Medicine, AL-Mustanseryah University, Baghdad, Iraq

Waqar Al-Kubaisy and Redhwan A Al-Naggar
Population Health and Preventive Medicine Department, Faculty of Medicine, Universiti Teknologi MARA (UiTM), Selangor, Malaysia
Drug Discovery & Health Community of Research, Universiti teknologi MARA (UiTM), 40450 Shah Alam, Selangor, Darul Ehsan, Malaysia

Nor Aini Mohd Noor
Population Health and Preventive Medicine Department, Faculty of Medicine, Universiti Teknologi MARA (UiTM), Selangor, Malaysia
Humanity and Quality of life, Universiti teknologi MARA (UiTM), 40450 Shah Alam, Selangor, Darul Ehsan, Malaysia

Nicole Penn
King's College London School of Medicine, Capital House, King's College, London SE1 3QD, UK

Eugene Oteng-Ntim
Guy's and St Thomas' NHS Foundation Trust, Westminster Bridge Road, London SE1 7EH, UK

Laura L Oakley and Pat Doyle
Department of Non-communicable Disease Epidemiology, London School of Hygiene and Tropical Medicine, Keppel Street, London WC1E 7HT, UK

Index

www.ingramcontent.com/pod-product-compliance
Lightning Source LLC
LaVergne TN
LVHW080733210926
848485LV00003B/547
9781639271573